NUTRITION MANUAL FOR AT-RISK INFANTS AND TODDLERS

Janice Hovasi Cox, MS, RD, Editor

Precept Press, Chicago
Division of Bonus Books, Inc.

01 00 99 98 97 5 4 3 2 1

Library of Congress Cataloging-in-Publication Data

Nutrition manual for at-risk infants and toddlers / Janice Hovasi Cox, editor.
p. cm.
Includes bibliographical references and index.
ISBN 0-944496-47-4 (hc)
1. Developmentally disabled children—Nutrition. 2. Diet therapy for children. 3. Diet therapy for infants. 4. Children—Diseases—Nutritional aspects. I. Cox, Janice Hovasi.
RJ233.N886 1997
615.8'54'083—dc21 96-49613

International Standard Book Number: 0-944496-47-4

Precept Press
Division of Bonus Books, Inc.
160 East Illinois Street
Chicago, Illinois 60611

Composition by Point West, Inc., Carol Stream, IL

Printed in the United States of America

The material contained in this volume was submitted as previously unpublished material, except in the instances in which some of the illustrative material was derived.

Great care has been taken to maintain the accuracy of the information contained in the volume. However, neither Precept Press nor the editors can be held responsible for errors or for any consequences arising from the use of the information contained herein.

This book is dedicated to infants and toddlers throughout the world who by reason of disease, disability, or deprivation, do not have enough to eat, and the Spirit that enlightens and impels us to find ways to nourish them.

CONTENTS

PREFACE

The impetus for compiling this book grew from my involvement with health care professionals who provide services to "at-risk" infants and children throughout Michigan in home health agencies, maternal and infant support services, public health departments, WIC programs, Head Start programs, and schools for children who are physically or mentally challenged. Having been involved with the nutrition of infants in the neonatal intensive care unit or in follow-up clinics for infants and children with diseases and disabilities ranging from bronchopulmonary dysplasia and cystic fibrosis to renal disease and multihandicapping conditions for nearly 20 years, I am witness to the growing need for and dependence upon nutrition experts within the community.

The methods and means of providing health care in the United States are undergoing a period of tremendous upheaval. Ethical standards demand that the outcome of services provided continue to eliminate or minimize disease and disability. Cost containment and quality of life issues demand that the processes by which these goals are attained be reviewed, reevaluated, and streamlined to eliminate those that are ineffective, unnecessary, or redundant within systems. Redesigning health care services for children has required that (1) effective screening for health and developmental problems be available and accessible, (2) children with special needs be referred promptly to services that will effect a desired outcome, and (3) families and the communities in which they reside assume ever-increasing responsibilities for identifying and meeting their children's needs.

Recent federal legislation prescribes that infants and children at risk for developmental disability—for any reason, be it physical, emotional, social or psychological—are entitled to nutrition assessment and treatment by recognized experts within the context of family-centered care and using services that already exist. Education and health care leaders in each state must devise their own plans to coordinate and integrate services already in existence and develop education programs to ensure the expertise of the service providers available.[1] Educational programs that lead to certification or registration in the health care professions often do not include training for delivery of services to at-risk infants and children.[2,3] Even within the field of nutrition, programs that prepare participants to become registered dietitians often do not include specific training for this population. Many nutrition service providers are "entry level" professionals who may have limited experience working with this population. Nutrition resources for those who provide services to the at-risk pediatric population need to be concise and "user friendly," recognizing that preservice training or experience in this area of nutrition may be limited.

Many excellent textbooks and manuals address infant and pediatric nutrition for the professional,[4-8] and other volumes contain compilations of nutrition education materials for the parent/caregiver.[9,10] It is not the purpose of this volume to recreate a comprehensive nutrition text, but to provide a convenient reference that specifically addresses the nutritional screening and guidelines for care in the home of at-risk infants and toddlers through 2 years of age in the context of "family-centered care." The two chapters in section 1 provide background information regarding program and staff development. The four chapters in section 2 provide guidelines for nutrition assessment: dietary intake, feeding, growth, and clinical evaluation. A separate section for laboratory assessment has not been included because many community settings do not have access to laboratory facilities. Laboratory assessment is covered in depth in many of the pediatric nutrition references.[4-8] Section 3 deals with specific nutrition issues by diagnoses. These chapters include a brief introduction, a list of important nutritional considerations, examples or case studies used to illustrate important points when necessary, and a list of current and "hallmark" references that provide more detailed or comprehensive information about the topic. It is hoped that these are presented in a concise, user-friendly format. Bulleted lists, tables, charts, or diagrams are employed whenever possible to facilitate each section's use as a reference in the busy clinic or school setting.

As changes within the health care field require professionals and programs to work together to achieve our purpose, many who contribute to the nutritional care of at-risk infants and children will not claim nutrition as their primary discipline or training. It is hoped that physicians, nurses, occupational therapists, physical therapists, social workers, speech pathologists, and teachers as well as dietitians will all find useful information in this volume. If the best possible nutritional outcome is measured by the full achievement of growth and health potential, we must all work together as a cohesive functional family, strengthened by our individual expertise and our common goal.

JANICE HOVASI COX

References

1. The Education of the Handicapped Act Amendments of 1986 (Public Law 99-457) Part H. Department of Education. Early intervention program for infants and toddlers with handicaps; Final regulations. Federal Register 54 (119):26306–26348, June 22, 1989.
2. Michigan's Comprehensive System of Personnel Development, Interdisciplinary Personnel Preparation Committee Final Report. (Presented to the State Interagency Coordinating Council for the Infant and Toddler Early Intervention Program Part H or the Individuals with Disabilities Education Act) Lansing, Mich., December 10, 1993.
3. Accreditation/approval manual for dietetic education programs. Chicago: American Dietetic Association, 1987.
4. Fomon SJ. Nutrition of normal infants. St. Louis: Mosby, 1993.
5. Groh-Wargo S, Thompson M, Cox J, eds. Nutrition for high-risk newborns. rev. ed. Chicago: Precept Press, 1994.
6. Hendricks KM, Walker WA. Manual of pediatric nutrition, 2d ed. Philadelphia: Decker, 1990.
7. Queen PM, Lang CE, eds. Pediatric nutrition handbook. Rockville, Md.: Aspen, 1992.
8. Suskind RM, Lewinter-Suskind L, eds. Textbook of pediatric nutrition, 2d ed. New York: Raven Press, 1993.
9. Aspen Reference Group. Caregiver education guide for children with developmental disabilities. Rockville, Md.: Aspen, 1994.
10. Klein MD, Delaney TA. Feeding and nutrition for the child with special needs: Handouts for parents. Medvescek CR, ed. Tucson: Therapy Skill Builders, 1994.

ACKNOWLEDGMENTS

The editor wishes to give special thanks to the contributing authors for their patience and perseverance throughout the process of writing, editing, and revising this book. The staff at Precept Press, particularly Aaron Cohodes, Debbie Flapan, and Mike McClain, and manuscript editor Rex Olsen must be commended for their enthusiasm, trust, and unlimited patience.

A special thanks also is due Wendy Finsterwald-Watts, RNC, who planted in me the idea for this book in the first place. Peg McConnell, Gwen Armstrong, and Barb Free at the Michigan Department of Public Health nurtured the idea, giving me many wonderful opportunities to work with nutritionists throughout the state. Each experience has been enriching and rewarding.

Though perhaps unknowingly, each family and each child who have entered my life through my work contributed to this book. Many have allowed me to watch and record their growth. Some have taught me compassion, understanding, and the value of perseverance, especially David Matthew, Skylar, and Allison. Others have shown me the "real life" importance of each nutrient, from ascorbic acid to zinc, especially Jennifer, Julian, and Joshua.

The greatest measure of gratitute is extended to my family and friends. Each of us begins in a family, and from whatever strengths its members possess, we draw our initial nurturance that helps us achieve what we set out to do throughout our lives. From mine, it is my mother's resourcefulness, my father's unconditional love, and my sister Geri's loyal encouragement. My husband Steve is my steadfast source of love and emotional support in addition to great backup cook and launderer! Our children, Emily and Daniel, are a boundless source of inspiration, entertainment, enthusiasm for life, and the living of each day with joy—their patience with me throughout this project has been greatly appreciated. And last, but certainly not least, I wish to acknowledge my source of professional encouragement and personal balance, my friend Joyce Ross. A heartfelt thank-you.

CONTRIBUTORS

Sally Bonnema, MA, RD, Pediatric Nutritionist, Food and Nutrition Services, The Children's Hospital at Bronson, Kalamazoo, Michigan

Janice Hovasi Cox, MS, RD, Neonatal and Pediatric Nutritionist, Food and Nutrition Services, The Children's Hospital at Bronson, Kalamazoo, Michigan

Barbara B. Free, MS, RD, Nutrition Consultant, Michigan Department of Public Health, Lansing, Michigan

Dena Goldberg, PhD, RD, Pediatric Nutritionist, Alaska State Health Department, Nutrition Unit, Section of Maternal, Child, and Family Health, Anchorage, Alaska

Karen Gray, OTR, Occupational Therapist, Allegan County Intermediate School District, Allegan, Michigan

Sharon Groh-Wargo, MS, RD, LD, Neonatal Nutritionist, Department of Pediatrics, MetroHealth Medical Center, Cleveland, Ohio

Molly Holland, MPH, RD, CD, Nutritionist, Vermont Department of Health, Children with Special Health Needs, Burlington, Vermont

Ruth Kavalhuna, MA, Child Developmentalist, Calhoun County Intermediate School District, Marshall, Michigan

Wendy King, PT, Pediatric and Neonatal Physical Therapist/Developmental Specialist, Rehabilitation Services, Children's Hospital at Bronson, Kalamazoo, Michigan

Ingrida Mara Melbardis, RD, Pediatric Nutritionist, Food and Nutrition Services, The Children's Hospital at Bronson, Kalamazoo, Michigan

Nancy Nevin-Folino, MEd, RD, CS, LD, Neonatal and Pediatric Nutritionist, Children's Medical Center, Dayton, Ohio

Gloria Pina, RN, CPNP, Pediatric Nurse Practioner, Children's Medical Center, Dayton, Ohio

Peggy Rasche, MS, RD, LD, Pediatric Nutritionist, formerly at Clinical Nutrition Services, Children's Hospital, Columbus, Ohio

Melody Thompson RD, LD, Pediatric Nutritionist, Clinical Nutrition Services, Children's Hospital, Columbus, Ohio

Lori Yelton, MS, RD, Pediatric Nutritionist, Kalamazoo Center for Medical Studies/Michigan State University, Kalamazoo, Michigan

INTRODUCTION

Ruth Kavalhuna, MA

Marcia watched the young mother cradle her 5-month-old baby in her arms and speak softly as the restless infant slowly calmed enough to drift into a light sleep. She remembered the hostile looks of suspicion with which this same young mother had greeted her on their first meeting. She would never forget the infant's howls that had terrorized the entire household for many hours each day. They had been down a difficult path together in the months since that shaky beginning. Now the baby was developing well, and her mother was taking pride in her young child's accomplishments. Marcia wondered what she had said or done that had contributed to the happy success that this mother-and-child pair were enjoying. What could she take from this experience that would be helpful to other families with little children?

Service providers who work with families and their infants and young children have experienced the satisfaction that comes when everything goes well and the family thrives. Unfortunately, many have also experienced the frustration of interaction with families for whom nothing seems to go well. Individuals who select this line of work usually do so with a desire to be supportive to families and a commitment to help infants and young children experience healthy growth and development. With such good intentions, why do so many experience frustration and feelings of futility? Why do service providers, be they nurses, occupational therapists, physical therapists, nutritionists, teachers, or others who have devoted their careers to helping families find themselves facing failure?

An easy answer is to place blame with the family. "They are noncompliant." "They just don't care." "Their problems are so overwhelming that there are no solutions." "They will not follow through." "We have done everything we can, but the family doesn't take advantage of the opportunities we offer them." It takes courage to ask the ensuing questions: "Why could this family not accept the sincere and essential assistance that was offered?" "What could we do to make our assistance and services more acceptable to such families?"

Service providers come from their educational and training experiences with an abundance of knowledge, a wealth of skills, and a driving desire to apply what they have learned. Those who have been in the field for some time have learned so much about infants, toddlers, mothers, and—sometimes—even fathers. They believe that they have seen just about everything at least once and are anxious to save families the difficulties of learning the "hard way."

It is so easy to move quickly into an interaction with a family, gathering essential data, assessing existing needs, writing a service plan (care plan, therapy plan, nutrition plan, etc.), and implementing the program with service delivery. Indeed, agency and program forms and time lines often encourage this quick, efficient approach to the initiation of early intervention with families.

We are learning that it is at this early stage of the process that the seeds of failure are often sown. A "one size fits all" process does not seem to be appropriate for all, or even most, families. Service providers begin the process with a desire to identify problems and needs, then determine how their expertise can be helpful. Families approach the interaction from a variety of positions. Nearly all families are initially more attentive to the manner in which service providers present themselves than to any other aspect of the interaction. As the often-heard saying goes, "People don't care how much you know until they know how much you care."

When service providers engage in interactions with a family, they are stepping into a world that has its own history, culture, set of values, operational rules, and a multitude of personal experiences and feelings. Service providers bring their own beliefs, history, culture, values, and personal experiences to each interaction. These viewpoints are sometimes very different from those of the family. Because of the unspoken yet powerful differences in perspectives, service providers are wise to focus initial time and attention on learning about the family's way of experiencing their lives.

Ruth Humphry believes that "teamwork of parents and professionals is needed in all aspects of early intervention, particularly in feeding."[1] Because feeding is basic to the relationship between the parent and the infant or child, it is extremely important to gather information in a supportive, nonthreatening manner. Working with families regarding feeding and nutritional issues requires acknowledgment of the influences of cultural practices, family traditions, societal or family pressures, and even commercial advertising. When feedings are not successful, parents may have feelings of failure or loss in self-confidence or control. The individual strengths and needs of both the parents and the infant or child must be objectively and respectfully considered. Building a strong, positive rapport with the parents engenders trust and develops a cooperative spirit and willingness to accept and implement changes in feeding when changes are truly needed.[2]

Communication Failures

Communication failures often happen between individuals when each assigns different meanings or values to words, events, or persons. When Caroline, a clinic nurse, discovered that three of Maria's children were underweight, she encouraged the young mother to apply for food stamps. Caroline talked about the expense of purchasing food for the five children, about the importance of good nutrition in growth and development, and about how food stamps could stretch the family's food dollars. When Maria responded that she would talk to her husband and uncle about this, Caroline felt frustrated and remarked that Maria's uncle was never helpful in raising the children and didn't even live in the same city. Maria looked ashamed and said no more. Caroline did not know that in Maria's family, Uncle Theo was the patriarch. If Maria and her husband could obtain his support, the whole family would approve and agree with their decision to accept financial help. Without the support of her uncle, Maria would have to suffer heavy criticism and be seen as an inadequate mother by her family and community. If Caroline had understood that Maria's uncle could be the best ally to the plan, she might have suggested ways to present the issue to him. Because Caroline had a different history and cultural reference to the role of an uncle, she became a barrier to the very help she desired to bring to Maria and her family.

Discovering the individual perspective of families is best accomplished by the temporary suspension of the service provider's own attitudes and values. Putting thoughts and values "on the shelf" for a time allows the service provider to focus observation and listening skills objectively and respectfully on the family's point of view. This does not mean forsaking personal values; rather, it is a means for initiating a relationship with the family where they are. From this mutual starting point, the process of assessing strengths and needs and the development of a service plan can begin with the commitment of both service providers and family members. Families are more willing to communicate and interact with service providers who listen and take the time to comprehend their perspectives. They feel valued, supported, and hopeful regarding the difficulties with which they are struggling.

Jerod was five months old when Sondra began following him as an outpatient for failure to thrive. His mother, Carla, reported that he frequently vomited, so she fed him only small amounts of formula at each feeding. After a period of observation and a medical workup for gastroesophageal reflux, Sondra was confused. They revealed no abnormalities, not even occasional spitting up. When Sondra watched Carla feeding Jerod, she noted that Carla terminated the feeding before Jerod had given any sign of being ready to stop. When he protested, Carla offered the pacifier instead of giving him more to eat. Sondra was tempted to feel angry with Carla for withholding food from her hungry baby and for being so insensitive to Jarod's cues. She decided, instead, to discover how Carla viewed this dilemma.

When Sondra asked Carla what would happen if they tried giving Jarod larger amounts of formula at each feeding, the anxious mother replied that she was sure he would vomit. This seemed very frightening to her. Sondra gently probed further, "If Jarod vomited, what would happen?" Carla began to cry and told the story of her first baby, who had died in the night of sudden infant death syndrome (SIDS). She explained that she thought she was responsible for the baby's death because she had overfed him and he had choked to death on his vomit. It became clear to Sondra that Carla was trying to make sure that she would never put Jarod's life in jeopardy by overfeeding him, as she believed she had done with her first baby. When Sondra understood Carla's reason for feeding Jarod such small amounts of formula, she began to help Carla understand what had happened in the past. They worked together as Carla developed the courage to allow her baby to take larger amounts of formula so that he would obtain the nourishment he needed to grow and develop.

Careful attention to the living arrangement gives service providers a wealth of information for understanding what life is like for a particular family. The availability of the necessities of life, the presence of kitchen appliances and facilities, the arrangement of furniture, the presence of toys and books, the availability of help from others, the location in the community, and many other observable characteristics provide insight into the values, expectations, strengths, and needs of a family. Careful observation of interactions among individuals, including nonverbal forms of communication, provides valuable information to sensitive service providers.

Justine observed that the proud parents of twin boys had established a workable schedule for sharing the care responsibilities for their babies. One twin was experiencing some minor feeding problems, and Justine was visiting the home every few days to support the family and monitor the baby's weight gain. When she observed some discomfort on the father's part and guessed that he had a problem with so much extra attention being given to the one twin, she began to hold and interact with the other twin at each visit. The father smiled his approval. Justine made the remark that she could see that these parents were being very careful to let both babies know that they were important as individuals. The father explained that his twin cousins had grown up believing that one was the "good twin" and the other was the "bad twin," and he didn't want this to happen to his sons.

Asking Questions

Learning to ask questions that enable family members to express their ideas and feelings can assist service providers. "How do the people in your family feel about breast-feeding and bottle-feeding?" "It sounds like your grandma believes that it will spoil your 2-year-old if you let him eat whenever he wants, is that right?" "In your opinion, it's not good to let children learn to waste food, is it?" "Tell me about a typical day with your baby." Questions like these are concrete and focus on specific, significant family beliefs and practices. Service providers gain insight and convey the message that the family's perspective is important. Such questions present opportunities for the family to share information and feelings with service providers who can then become their partners in finding solutions to their difficulties.

Toward increasing cultural awareness, service providers may engage in formal or informal research about particular cultural groups with which they know they will be interacting. Such research provides valuable basic information, but should always be used solely as an introduction to a particular cultural group. Within all communities, there is wide variation that cannot be reduced to a single, standardized description. For this reason, it is helpful to be honest with a family that has cultural perspectives and practices with which service providers are not familiar. Service providers may explain their wish to honor the family's customs and declare their need for guidance from the family to learn what is acceptable. Some cultures do not engage in open criticism of others, and family members would be uncomfortable in correcting service providers' errors. For some, it would be more acceptable for the service provider to ask, "What is the proper way to do (this or that)?" Requesting direction from families as to the manner in which they prefer to have things done nearly always strengthens their working relationship with the service providers, whether or not cultural differences are present.

The 'Cultural Consultant'

It may be impossible for a service provider to be culturally competent in all of their interactions with families. The assistance of a language interpreter or "cultural consultant" may be helpful in facilitating engagement and interactions with a family from a cultural group that is new to the service provider. A cultural consultant is an individual who is of the same culture as the family and who has lived in the United States long enough to have gained a basic understanding of the English language, mainstream attitudes, and cultural practices. This person may pose the service provider's questions to the family in a manner consistent with their customs and communication styles. Such a consultant can give service providers on-the-spot advice to aid in understanding the family's strengths and viewpoints.

Sonia asked a cultural consultant to accompany her when she made a home call on a family that had just immigrated. When they arrived, the mother and the consultant engaged in excited conversation, and Sonia could see that the family was delighted to meet someone from their home country. The visit went well, and Sonia remarked on what beautiful children this family had. Sonia helped complete the necessary forms so that the family could obtain financial aid to purchase food for the children. When she and the interpreter were on the way back to the office, Sonia asked if there was anything that she needed to know for future visits with this family. The consultant explained that parents in this family's culture do not consider it proper to praise chilren for their physical beauty or good behavior. It is believed that this will cause the children to become prideful and selfish, and that they will grow up without the ability to put the welfare of the family above their own personal desires. Sonia realized that she had presented a dilemma to the family when she only intended to offer a compliment. She also acknowledged that without the aid of her consultant, she might have repeated this behavior many times.

All of the children described in these stories have individual nutritional needs. All of the families of these children have their own unique way of experiencing their lives. The chapters that follow provide a wealth of information to accomplish the identification and treatment of nutrition and feeding problems—the science of nutritional care. But it is the art of nutritional care—the entering into families' lives with compassion, understanding, flexibility, and a sense of humor—that actually allows the science of nutritional care to work.

Service providers enter relationships with families with the goal of helping to alleviate the pressures and problems that interfere with parents' ablilities to support the healthy growth and development of their babies and toddlers. Although success rewards both families and service providers in many of these relationships, there are always interactions that frustrate everyone involved. Service providers might ask themselves what transpired in successful interactions that did not occur in interactions that seemed to fail. Reviewing successful experiences is sure to reveal a spirit of cooperation between family members and service providers.

Individuals wish to be approached by others who demonstrate a genuine interest in their thoughts, feelings, and ideas. This is as true of the alliance between service provider and family as it is of all other relationships. Service providers who listen and observe, ask questions about beliefs and customs, and demonstrate a desire to understand the strengths, priorities, and needs of the family promote the growth of relationships built upon trust and mutual respect. The rewards of strong family–service provider teams are thriving, healthy children; empowered, satisfied families; and effective, energized service providers.

References

1. Humphrey R. Impact of feeding problems on the parent-infant relationship. Infants Young Child 3(3):30–38, 1991.
2. Wolf LS, Glass RP. Feeding and swallowing disorders in infancy: Assessment and management. Tucson: Therapy Skill Builders, 1992.

SECTION I

PROVIDING NUTRITION SERVICES

Nutrition Manual for At-Risk Infants and Toddlers
Janice Hovasi Cox, editor

1

EARLY INTERVENTION

Molly Holland, MPH, RD, CD

By definition, children with "special health needs" require more than the usual pediatric care to reach their full potential for growth and development. The term *early intervention* applies to infants and children from birth to 5 years who have special health needs that increase their risk for delayed cognitive, physical, communication, adaptive skill, social, or emotional development.[1-3] Factors that contribute to these delays in growth and development include congenital or acquired conditions, chronic illness, and adverse psychosocial environment. Early intervention implies changing outcomes by timely identification and treatment or management of factors that contribute to delayed development. The purpose of this chapter is to provide background information about early intervention and the population served, the importance of nutrition in early intervention, and the purpose, scope and content of nutrition services included in a community-based setting.

Background

Earlier diagnosis of rare or life-threatening conditions and sophisticated technology delivering prompt and innovative medical and/or surgical treatment have increased the life expectancy for prematurely born and medically fragile infants. Other conditions such as human immunodeficiency virus (HIV) infection and increased prenatal drug and/or alcohol abuse have expanded the population of children with special health needs. It has been estimated that 10–15% of children in the United States have special health needs.[4]

Outcome research reveals that early intervention and treatment of medical and developmental conditions has these effects:

The author wishes to thank Beverly MacCarty, Vermont Part H coordinator, for her valuable comments and suggestions. This chapter was funded in part by the Vermont University Affiliated Program. U.S. Department of Health and Human Services, Bureau of Maternal and Child Health Training Grant no. MCJ509412.

- Decreases utilization of special education services in later years[5]
- Ultimately reduces costs and increases educational attainment[6]
- Improves developmental outcome for infants with biological conditions such as Down syndrome and cerebral palsy[7]
- Improves developmental outcome for very low birth weight infants[8]
- Allows families to better cope with the stresses associated with their child's medical or developmental problems.

Although early intervention services for infants and toddlers have existed to one degree or another for many years, the past 10 to 20 years have brought dramatic changes in how and where these services are provided. In the past, many infants and children with chronic illness or disabling conditions remained hospitalized or lived in long-term care facilities. The philosophical shift toward "deinstitutionalization" in recent decades now places most of these infants and children within their families and communities.[9] Cost containment has also driven the delivery of health care to a more community-based model. Managed care systems prefer primary services that are provided within the community and home environment over hospital and long-term care facility services.

Provision of services for infants and children with special health needs in family-centered, community-based care programs empowers families but brings them new responsibilities. The elements of family centered care given in table 1-1 have served to create new partnerships on many levels toward empowerment of families and helping them manage the responsibilities of caring for their infant or child at home.[10, 11] Professionals from tertiary care hospitals and community-based health, education, mental health, and social service programs across a wide range of disciplines must all work together with parents toward achieving common goals.

During the past 10 years, legislation has become a driving force accompanying these technological, research, cost-containment, and philosophical trends toward family-centered, community-based, comprehensive care for infants and young children with special needs. This force began in 1975 with U.S. Public Law 94-142, the Education of All Handicapped Children Act, which mandated free and appropriate education in the least restrictive environment to all children and young adults ages 5 through 22. The Individuals with Disabilities Act of 1986 (P. L. 99-457, part H) amended the law to include preschool children. The Surgeon General's Report in 1987 pledged national support to children with special health care needs and their families and provided the impetus for the creation, expansion, and improvement of community-based early intervention services on a national level.[12, 13] Subsequent legislation has extended the law to

- Include early intervention for eligible infants and toddlers[3]
- Create a "family-driven" collaborative process between families and professionals[14]
- Provide early intervention services using existing programs, agencies and funding streams[15]
- Design, develop, and implement state-wide interagency coordination of comprehensive and multidisciplinary services.[3]

Table 1-1. Elements of Family-Centered Care

1. Recognition that the family is the constant in the child's life while the service systems and personnel within those systems fluctuate
2. Facilitation of parent/professional collaboration at all levels of health care: care of an individual child; program development, implementation, and evaluation; and policy formation
3. Sharing of unbiased and complete information with parents about their child's care on an ongoing basis in an appropriate and supportive manner
4. Implementation of appropriate policies and programs that are comprehensive and provide emotional and financial support to meet the needs of families
5. Recognition of family strengths and individuality and respect for different methods of coping
6. Understanding and incorporating the developmental needs of infants, children, and adolescents and their families into health care delivery systems
7. Encouragement and facilitation of parent-to-parent support
8. Assurance that the design of health care delivery systems is flexible, accessible, and responsive to families

Shelton TL, Jeppson ES, Johnson BH, Family-centered care for children with special health care needs. Washington, D.C.: Association for the Care of Children's Health, 1987. Reprinted with permission.

Table 1-2. Elements of an Individual Family Service Plan (IFSP)

IFSP elements include statements on the following:
- The child's present levels of development
- Family resources, priorities, and concerns
- How to enhance development of infants and toddlers with disabilities
- Major outcomes expected, including criteria, procedures, and timeliness to achieve specific goals
- Specific early intervention services that will help the child and family
- Projected dates for initiating services and their duration
- Name of the service coordinator responsible for helping the family implement and coordinate the plan
- Steps to help the child and family with the transition to preschool services at age 3.

Solomon, R. Pediatricians and early intervention: everything you need to know but are too busy to ask. Inf Young Children. 7(3) 1995; 46. Reprinted with permission. © 1995, Aspen Publishers.

Although the early intervention legislation is specific in many ways, eligibility varies from state to state. Each program in every state provides services in a multitude of ways and settings. Provision of services depends on the needs of the child and family and how the local agencies and programs are best able to meet these needs. Services may be provided in the home or at clinics, hospital outpatient departments, or community health centers. Services may be provided as one-on-one therapy, or group therapy (such as play groups or parent support groups), or several professionals may provide services jointly.

The goal of early intervention programs is to meet the individual needs of every eligible child and family in achieving their potential for growth, development, and independence. An individualized family service plan (IFSP), as outlined in table 1-2, is developed for each child by an interdisciplinary team. This team includes the family and recognized experts from various disciplines, including but not limited to those listed in table 1-3. Once a plan has been established and implemented, it is the responsibility of the team, either as individuals or as a group, to evaluate progress toward identified goals and revise the IFSP if needed.[16]

Importance of Nutrition in Early Intervention

When an infant or child is enrolled in an early intervention program, myriad services and opportunities become available. Services offered to each child and family are determined by evaluations, discussions, and decisions made during the process of developing an IFSP. Often, the need for nutrition services is overlooked when other more imminent or acute issues are raised by the family or other providers. However, reports indicate that 40–90% of infants and children with special health needs have at least one nutrition-related problem.[17, 18] Careful consideration of each infant's or child's nutritional needs are essential for the following reasons:

Table 1-3. Early Intervention Services

May include but are not limited to the following:

Vision services	Service coordination (birth to 3 yr)
Family training	Screening/assessment
Counseling	Home visits
Social work services	Occupational therapy
Psychological services	Special instruction
Medical services	Assistive technology
Nutrition services	Physical therapy
Medical services for diagnostic or evaluation purposes	Health services necessary to enable child to benefit from other services

Reference: U.S. Department of Education.[3]

- The time period of birth to age 3 is critical in terms of growth and maturation of all body systems (e.g., brain growth, organ and tissue development).
- All children, whether or not they have special health needs, require good nutrition to achieve their genetic potential for growth and development.[19]
- Behaviorally, undernourished infants and children become apathetic, and interactions with the environment decrease. Also, attention span and exploratory behaviors decline, possibly exacerbating the effects of malnutrition on mental development.[20]
- When children have special health needs, they are at increased risk for developing nutrition problems that can further affect growth and development as listed in table 1-4.[21]
- Feeding problems, if they cause a decline in nutritional status, may lead to other problems, such as reduced immunity and increased illness, decreased activity or strength, and problems with elimination, skin integrity, and oral health. Each of these problems may in turn impair feeding, thus creating a self-perpetuating cycle.[22]

Table 1-4. Chronic Condtions with Associated Nutrition-Related Problems

	Problems and factors contributing to high nutritional risk													
	Child-related										Caregiver-related			
DISORDER	Altered nutrient needs	Altered energy needs/intake	Problems with oral cavity	Nutrient deficiencies	Constipation/diarrhea	Poor appetite	Delayed feeding skills	Malabsorption	Nutrient-drug interactions	Maladaptive behaviors	Lack of knowledge	Difficulty understanding diet	Does not limit intake	Inappropriate feeding practices
Asthma (moderate to severe)		●		●		●			●					
Visual impairment							●			●				
Mental retardation		●	●		●		●			●				●
Congenital heart disease	●	●		●		●		●	●		●			
Seizure disorder	●								●		●			
Cerebral palsy		●	●	●	●	●	●		●		●		●	●
Arthritis	●	●									●			
Paralysis		●			●		●			●	●		●	
Diabetes mellitis											●	●	●	
Cleft lip/palate		●	●				●				●			●
Down syndrome		●	●		●		●			●	●		●	●
Sickle cell disease	●			●		●								
Neural tube defect		●			●				●				●	
Autism						●			●	●				●
Cystic fibrosis	●	●		●	●	●		●	●		●	●	●	●
Leukemia/cancer	●	●		●	●	●			●					
Phenylketonuria/inborn errors of metabolism	●			●							●	●	●	
Chronic renal failure	●	●		●	●	●			●		●	●		
Bronchopulmonary dysplasia	●	●		●			●		●					
HIV/AIDS	●	●	●	●	●	●	●	●	●		●			
Gastrointestinal disorders	●			●	●	●		●						

Adapted with permission from Dwyer JT, Freedland J.[21]

- Feeding is central to the development of a relationship between infant or child and parent, forming the foundation for trust and social interaction. When feeding is not successful, families may feel a strong sense of failure, worry, and distress.[23]
- A well-nourished infant or child can be more responsive to the many other therapies required toward achieving goals set forth in the IFSP.[24]

Team members must learn how to identify nutrition problems and how nutrition specialists can contribute to positive outcomes in families of children with special health needs. Nutritionists with training and skills in caring for infants and young children with special health needs and in family-centered care must be available.

Components of Nutritional Care in Early Intervention

To successfully meet the nutritional needs of infants and children who require early intervention, several components of nutrition services delivery must be identified and developed. These components fall into four general areas: direct delivery of nutrition care, program development, personnel preparation, and coordination of nutrition services with other community resources (see figure 1-1). In some ways, these components are very similar to the delivery of nutrition services to any population. The framework described here uses the philosophy and terminology of early intervention programs so that unique aspects can be easily identified in a familiar model.

Nutrition care Nutrition evaluation Development of nutrition care plan Monitoring Cultural competence Family-centered care	**Programmatic/systems** Nutrition screening Referral criteria Data collection Reimbursement Quality assurance Advocacy Job description/staffing pattern
Care coordination With other community nutrition resources Team's approach to monitoring Parent/professional collaboration Coordination with other RDs	**Personnel preparation** Nutrition Early intervention Family-centered care

Figure 1-1. Components of delivery of nutrition services in early intervention.

Nutrition Care Components of Nutrition Services

The primary role of the nutritionist in early intervention is to provide nutrition assessment, develop care plans, monitor progress, and make referrals to other resources to accomplish nutrition goals. This role has been further defined by early intervention legislation as given in table 1-5.

Table 1-5. Definition of Nutrition Services in Early Intervention

- Conducting individual assessments in:
  - Nutrition history and dietary intake
  - Anthropometric, biochemical, and clinical variables
  - Feeding skills and feeding problems
  - Food habits and food preferences
- Developing and monitoring appropriate plans to meet nutritional needs based on the findings of the nutritional assessment
- Making referrals to appropriate community resources to carry out nutrition goals

Reference: U.S. Department of Education. Early intervention program for infants and toddlers with handicaps; final regulations. Federal Register 54(119): 34 CFR Part 303.12, (d) (7), p 26,312, 1989.

Nutrition evaluation. Not every infant or child who requires early interntion services requires a full nutrition assessment. Screening each infant or child for the presence of nutrition problems or increased risk of nutrition problems is discussed later, but should identify those who may benefit from a more in-depth nutrition assessment and treatment plan. When completing a nutrition evaluation, several factors must be considered in order to maintain a family-centered approach:

- The emphasis and focus should be on identifying the family's concerns, perceptions, and priorities. These should each be included in the plan of care.
- The language used in verbal communication with the family and in the written report should avoid jargon, abbreviations, or terms that may be unfamiliar to the parents. This report is given to the family and is used to develop the comprehensive individual family service plan.
- The positive *outcome*, rather than the *problem* should be the focus of the nutrition care plan. For example, "Lisa (mother) would like Ben to *eat more foods by mouth* and *be less dependent on his gastrostomy feeding tube*" identifies the positive outcome, rather than the problem, which is that Ben requires most of his feedings by gastrostomy tube, making him more dependent on his family and less mobile throughout the day.
- The family's strengths should be identified, including available resources, family supports, knowledge, skills, and understanding that will help them successfully implement the plan.

Nutrition care plan. Including each of the following components in the nutrition care plan enhances its incorporation into the overall IFSP. A nutrition care plan based on the assessment should include:

- *Long-term nutrition goals or outcomes.* These goals encompass broad areas the family has identified to meet the child's needs. Goals may relate to growth, nutritional status, feeding skills or abilities, tolerance of food textures, mealtime behaviors, the family's nutrition knowledge, access to food or nutrition programs, or learning how to integrate the child's special dietary needs into the family's eating habits. Table 1-6 provides examples of nutrition-related outcomes.
- *Objectives, activities, or strategies.* Sometimes goals may seem overwhelming or unattainable. Breaking long-term goals down into smaller steps makes progress more obvious. Individual objectives, activities, or strategies should be observable or measurable and developed specifically to meet identified goals. Table 1-7 illustrates how objectives may be written to reflect desired outcomes.
- *Timetable for evaluation.* A timetable of anticipated progress toward meeting goals allows parents and other members of the early intervention team to develop reasonable expectations and a means to measure progress.
- *Identification of who will monitor or provide follow-up.* Parents should be given adequate information so that they can actively participate in the evaluation process and tell when their child is progressing well and when not. Assigning responsibility for follow-up helps to assure that the family will reach identified goals, revising the means of reaching those goals if needed.

Monitoring. Although in most cases the nutritionist monitors the progress toward reaching the goals and accomplishing the objectives set forth in the nutrition care plan, other providers may be involved in this function. Other providers who may monitor portions of the nutrition care plan might include:

Table 1-6. Examples of Nutrition-Related Outcomes

Develop or refine self-feeding skills
Improve oral-motor function
Improve mealtime behavior
Identify and communicate nutrition needs
Improve food preparation skills
Improve growth rates
Maintain lab data (i.e., serum glucose, phenylalanine levels, etc.) within normal limits

Horsley J. Nutrition issues facing children with special health care needs. Nutr Focus 9(3):1–5, 1994. Nutrition Section, CHDD, University of Washington, Seattle.

Table 1-7. Examples of Nutrition Outcomes and Objectives for a Child with Spina Bifida

Nutrition outcome no. 1:	Susan would like Kyle to maintain his weight and continue to grow linearly to achieve a weight/height within normal limits on the pediatric growth chart
Nutrition objection no. 1:	Kyle will limit his daily intake of infant formula to 32 oz, which will be decreased as baby foods are introduced into his diet
Nutrition objective no. 2:	Kyle will be weighed and measured monthly and his growth will be plotted on a pediatric growth chart
Nutrition objective no. 3:	Kyle's parents will demonstrate an understanding of Kyle's calorie and nutrient needs relative to his growth, activity level, and bowel program
Nutrition outcome no. 2:	Susan would like Kyle to accept an increased variety of foods and textures in his diet
Nutrition objective no. 1:	Kyle will try at least one new baby food each week at home beginning with infant cereal and advancing to infant fruits and vegetables
Nutrition objective no. 2:	Kyle will advance to junior foods and other textures and cup drinking within six months

Note: Each objective also has strategies and a specific starting date and an endpoint at which it would be evaluated. A so each objective was assigned to a person who supervised the activity and monitored the process.

Horsley J. Nutrition issues facing children with special health care needs. Nutr Focus 9(3):1–5, 1994. Nutrition Section, CHDD, University at Washington, Seattle. Reprinted with permission.

- Registered nurses may monitor growth, biochemical changes, and bowel patterns.
- Feeding therapists (often occupational therapists or speech and language pathologists) may monitor introduction of new food types/textures or caregiver feeding practices.
- Special educators or social workers may monitor success at changing mealtime behaviors.
- Service coordinators may monitor successful enrollment in food supplemental programs or procurement of special food supplements.

Coordination and communication between the nutritionist and other providers involved in monitoring portions of the nutrition care plan are critical to success. This "transdisciplinary" model of care becomes easier once relationships between providers are established.

Cultural competence. Recognizing cultural differences, especially as they relate to feeding, is a critical but often overlooked aspect of nutritional care. Cultural competence is defined as knowledge and interpersonal skills that allow individuals to increase their understanding and appreciation of cultural differences and similarities within, among, and between groups.[25] The development of cultural competence moves through stages, providing nutritionists with understanding and skills to more effectively transmit nutrition information to families with cultures different from their own.[25] On occasion, traditional food habits or beliefs may conflict with the child's nutritional or developmental needs. Because professionals working with families have tremendous power in early feeding relationships, they need to be able to understand how culture affects the family's actions, attitudes, and beliefs.[26] Observation, discussion, a neutral and understanding attitude, and being prepared for conflict when different cultural beliefs or attitudes emerge are strategies for becoming more culturally competent.[26]

Family-centered care. Being family centered requires building partnerships with families and working together to meet the needs of the child. This represents a major shift from the traditional professional-centered model in which the health care professional is considered the expert who makes most of the decisions, with or without family input. The first step toward becoming family centered is to identify family characteristics, such as those listed in table 1-8, that must be incorporated into the development of a nutrition care plan. Becoming family-centered in the true sense of the word may mean that professionals need to reevaluate their interactions with families, recognizing that when partnerships develop, everyone succeeds.[27] A self-assessment of attitudes and practices toward family-centered care is given in figure 1-2. Assessments of nutrition services by families and other providers can also be used.

Program/System Components of Nutrition Services

In order to provide successful nutrition service for families and providers in early intervention programs, several program or system components need to be recognized and addressed. These include:

Table 1-8. Checklist for Identifying Family Characteristics

Siblings and ages, the amount of time they require from parents—does feeding decrease available time?
Number of adults significantly involved with the child and their roles
Perspectives of family relatives about feeding difficulties
Family work schedules
Information about the primary caregiver's typical day
How does the family want you to work with them?
How many suggestions can the family realistically handle at one time?

Meilhan K. Promoting partnerships between health care providers and parents of children with special health care needs. Nutr Focus 8(3) 1–5, 1993. Nutrition Section, CHDD, University of Washington, Seattle. Reprinted with permission.

Nutrition screening. Screening is the process of identifying infants or children who exhibit nutrition problems or are at increased risk for developing these problems. Screening should be conducted on *each* infant and child in a program. It should be simple enough to complete/administer that it can be completed by others. Also, it should be valid and reliable in identifying those with nutrition problems or at increased risk for developing such problems.

Although some nutrition problems are obvious to parents and other providers, many may be subtle at first. Infants and children who are at risk for developing nutrition-related problems may not be identified unless standardized screening methods are used.[28] Using standardized screening tools such as those given in appendixes A and B, the CHEWS, [29], PEACH,[30], or NFIT[31] helps to reliably identify infants and children with nutritional problems or at increased risk of developing these problems.

Ideally, the nutrition screening should be completed as part of the initial intake process; however, it may be more realistically incorporated in a later phase of the evaluation time frame if the program has a complex intake process.[28] The development of a nutrition screening process is as important as the screening tool itself. Administrative and program staff support must be obtained to ensure long-term success.[31] Training each person who will be involved in the screening and referral process and the periodic evaluation of the process is essential.[32]

Referral criteria. Criteria based on the screening tool used are developed to guide referral of infants and children who would benefit from nutrition intervention. Examples are given in appendixes A and B.

Data collection. It is important that program providers, planners, and administrators receive information/data about the nutrition services being provided. This information is useful in evaluating services, planning future program development, and in holding discussions with site staff, regional planning groups (e.g., interagency coordinating councils), administrators, policymakers, and sources of funding. It is also useful for advocacy efforts to assure access to nutrition services.[28]

Data may include objective information such as demographics, sources of referral, enrollment numbers, nutritional risk factors, and outcomes. Subjective information may include parent and other provider evaluations of services, program accomplishments, and the like. Individual program data may be combined with the data from other nutrition programs such as the Food Supplemental Program for Women, Infants, and Children (WIC) to establish a state-wide data bank. These may be integrated with other nutritional surveillance data systems such as the state maternal and child (Title V) data system.[28]

Reimbursement. There are many issues related to reimbursement of nutrition services in early intervention programs. Public and/or private payment for screening, assessment and follow-up services, and for special nutritional products is not available in all states.[2] In a survey to determine funding sources for early intervention nutrition services in all 50 states, sources were shown to include Title V grants, WIC, Medicaid, Early and Periodic Screening, Diagnosis and Treatment (EPSDT) programs, Department of Education, private health insurance companies, and state and local sources. Federal legislation in various amendments to P.L. 99-457 (Part H) allocates limited funds to be used "as a last resort," but other avenues of funding are necessary. Health insurance reimbursement through third-party billing is a growing source of reimbursement.[6] Some states have legislation concerning third-party billing that can help finance nutrition services.

Quality assurance. Maintaining high standards of practice is a critical component of any service delivery system. The American Dietetic Association has published quality assurance guidelines and standards of practice for nutrition service delivery to children with special health care needs.[33] Another publication, although not specific to nutrition services, was written by a group of parents, health care providers, and policymakers.[34] It identifies standards or indicators for individual services, team characteristics, agency responsibilities, and state guidelines for support.

Family-Centered Nutrition Services Rating Scale

Nutritionists' Scale

For each statement, please circle the number that best describes your feelings and opinions

	Rarely		Sometimes		Always	
1. The Early Intervention program helps families get nutrition services from other agencies	1	2	3	4	5	N/A
2. I help families get services from other agencies	1	2	3	4	5	N/A
3. Nutrition services are planned with a family's transportation and scheduling needs in mind	1	2	3	4	5	N/A
4. The IEP (Individualized Education Plan), or IFSP (Individualized Family Service Plan), or Nutrition Care Plan is used as a tentative "plan of action" that responds to changes with the child or family	1	2	3	4	5	N/A
5. I offer information in a variety of ways that is complete and clear	1	2	3	4	5	N/A
6. I communicate with other professionals and agencies that a family uses	1	2	3	4	5	N/A
7. I understand that a family balances their child's dietary needs with the other needs of their family	1	2	3	4	5	N/A
8. I provide information to help families explain their child's dietary or other needs to brothers, sisters, friends, and other family members	1	2	3	4	5	N/A
9. I respect and create ways for families to be involved in making decisions about nutrition	1	2	3	4	5	N/A
10. I help families feel they can make a positive difference in their child's life, particularly with feeding and nutrition	1	2	3	4	5	N/A
11. I explain the findings of the nutrition assessment to the family at the time of the assessment	1	2	3	4	5	N/A
12. I ask families about the information they have received from doctors and others	1	2	3	4	5	N/A
13. I offer to visit families in their homes	1	2	3	4	5	N/A
14. Families are treated as the true experts on their child with planning and providing nutrition services	1	2	3	4	5	N/A
15. I respect differences among children, families, and families' ways of life	1	2	3	4	5	N/A
16. I ask families' opinions and include them in the process of evaluating their child	1	2	3	4	5	N/A
17. I create an open climate for families to ask questions	1	2	3	4	5	N/A
18. I help families use problem-solving skills for making decisions about themselves and their child's nutrition and feeding	1	2	3	4	5	N/A
19. The Early Intervention program and/or I make it easier for families to meet and discuss feeding and nutrition concerns with others as needed	1	2	3	4	5	N/A
20. Families receive complete copies of all nutrition reports about their child and family	1	2	3	4	5	N/A

Figure 1-2. Instrument for self-assessment of attitudes and practices toward family-centered care. (Source: Julia Allen, MS, RD, Rhode Island Department of Health. Adapted with permission from Summers JA, Turnbull AP, Murphy DL, et al. Beach Center on Families and Disabilities, University of Kansas.)

This manual can be used by a wide audience not only for evaluation, but education, training, and advocacy.[4] Components of Part H legislation also address quality assurance of service delivery, and the assessment of nutrition services should be included.

Job descriptions and staffing patterns. In early intervention programs, a core staff usually coordinates the program and provides services. Consultants and part-time staff may be hired or contracted with to provide additional services as needed. Through interagency agreements, many services (including nutrition) are provided on a consulting basis. Many programs do not have a nutritionist as a member of the core staff unless that person is acting in additional capacities.

Staffing patterns and job descriptions vary, depending on the size of the program, the availability of qualified nutrition personnel, and the program goals or model of service delivery[28] (an example is given in table 1-9). As programs change or grow, data collection, quality assurance, and advocacy efforts may be used to support increased availability and expanded function of nutrition services.

Advocacy. Many do not fully appreciate the importance of or recognize the efforts to advocate nutrition services. Advocacy takes many forms, including increasing the awareness of the needs and issues of others, promoting services or programs, influencing public policy and legislation, and identifying gaps in current systems.[4] Advocacy for individual families can, in the long run, help support programs on the local level. Parents and nutritionists should advocate that the program include nutrition screening as part of the initial intake process so that parental concerns, nutritional problems, or nutritional risk factors can be identified and treated in a timely manner.

On a higher level, advocacy through coalition building is a recognized and useful technique. Establishing a state or regional planning group to ensure the provision of nutrition services can serve many functions, including advocacy for nutrition services. Becoming involved at the policymaking level and acquiring membership on state or local interagency coordinating councils provides nutritionists with opportunities to influence decisions about personnel preparation, role definitions, and scope of services. Other disciplines represented on these committees have the

Table 1-9. Staffing Patterns for Nutritionists Working in Early Intervention Programs

Full time (4–5 days/wk)
- Conducts nutrition screening and assessments
- Participates in care conferences and IFSP meetings
- Coordinates implementation of nutrition care plan, including making outside referrals, monitoring plan
- Provides follow-up as needed and coordinates with other providers
- Acts as service coordinator for nutrition-intensive cases
- Participates in child/parent groups and other staff activities
- Provides education and training to staff, parents, and other community providers
- Other staff duties dependent on site's model

Part time (one site 2–3 days/wk)
- Conducts assessments on children referred for nutritional evaluations
- Coordinates implementation of nutrition care plan, including making outside referrals
- Provides follow-up as needed or coordinates with other providers
- Limited team conferences
- Provides consultation to service coordinators
- Acts as service coordinator for nutrition-intensive cases (as time permits)
- Participates in child/parent groups and other staff activities (as time permits)
- Provides education and training to staff and parents (as time permits)

Consultant (covers several sites or one site; time varies with program)
- Conducts assessments on children referred for nutritional evaluations
- Coordinates implementation of nutrition care plan, including making outside referrals
- Provides limited follow-up as needed or coordinates follow-up with other providers
- Provides consultation to service coordinators
- Provides education and training to staff and parents (as time permits)
- Provides limited service coordination (as time permits)

Adapted from Bayerl C, Ries JD, et al. Early start: Nutrition services in early intervention. Office of Nutrition, Bureau of Family and Community Health, Massachusetts Department of Public Health, 1994.

opportunity to learn more about what a nutritionist does and how nutritionists can be effective interventionists and advocates for families.[35]

Personnel Preparation

The preparation and training of nutritionists is imperative in providing high-quality services to families and other providers. Nutritionists must be competent in pediatric nutrition, providing recommendations for infants and children with complex feeding problems, anticipatory guidance, and general nutrition advice. Additional training is often needed in how early intervention programs work, developing individual family service plans, referral processes, interdisciplinary teamwork, service coordination, and family-centered care.[2, 23] (Chapter 2 provides a closer look at nutrition service provider competencies and educational resources to achieve these competencies.)

Care Coordination

Legislation relative to early intervention was not meant to set up a separate system of services, but to coordinate services that already existed.[3] To accomplish family-centered, comprehensive, and coordinated care, nutritionists must incorporate several factors into each assessment and care plan.

Coordination of nutrition services with other services or programs. Once the nutrition assessment is completed, a plan of care is developed with the family and other team members, using available services. Referral to other agencies or programs is expected. These may include other nutritionists, food supplemental programs, and/or nutrition education programs. Potential resources for assistance with nutrition services are listed in table 1-10. Referral to physicians, nursing agencies, feeding therapists, mental health, or social service agencies may also be needed as nutrition impacts and is impacted by many aspects of health and development.

Coordination with other nutritionists. Infants and children with special health care needs are often involved with tertiary care hospitals during the initial stages or acute episodes of illness as inpatients or by participation in outpatient pediatric subspecialty clinics. If nutritional care is needed, a pediatric nutrition specialist may be consulted. Barriers to receiving care and consistent follow-up at tertiary care centers include lack of transportation, long-distance travel, ability for parents to take time off from work, and poverty.[36]

Parents may be confused or stressed when different providers do not give complete or consistent information or recommendations. Parents have often requested that they be connected to a local program before they leave a tertiary institution.[37] When follow-up care is being planned in connection with hospital discharge, nutrition services that are local and convenient for families should be considered. Communication among nutritionists in tertiary care facilities, WIC programs or other public health agencies, and early intervention programs is necessary to ensure adequate follow-up, provide consistency of care, and coordinate services. Early intervention visits may be able to function as high-risk follow-up nutrition visits for the WIC program. Table 1-11 gives examples of how care can be coordinated between the tertiary care facility and early intervention providers.

Parent/professional collaboration. The goals and strengths of the family must be considered when deciding a course of action to treat or manage a nutritional problem. Parents should be respected as equals because they contribute valuable information and often have excellent suggestions for problem solving if given adequate information and share equally in the decision-making process. Health care providers may initially feel uncomfortable as they experiment with this new type of partnership.[38] If providers focus on the goal—to assist families in meeting their needs and priorities—then collaboration makes sense.

Summary

As nutrition experts, dietitians must be responsive to changes within the health care delivery system and the changing needs of their clients. The redesigning of health care services for infants and children has required that (1) effective screening for health and developmental problems be available and accessible, (2) infants and children with special needs be referred promptly to services that will effect a desired outcome, and (3) families and the communities in which they reside assume ever-increasing responsibilities for identifying and meeting their infants' and children's needs. The early intervention arena provides many opportunities and challenges for dietitians to provide a valuable service.

Table 1-10. Potential Resources for Assistance with Nutrition Services

	Assistance available						
Resources	To assist staff with nutrition program planning, development, and evaluation and with inservice education and training	To provide direct nutrition services to children, e.g., nutrition assessment, development of care plans, counseling, clinical management, and follow-up	To provide specialized therapeutic nutrition management for children	To provide food assistance to children	To provide instruction to families regarding food planning, purchasing, and preparation	Local contact	Phone number
Expert nutrition consultation							
Director or administrator of public health nutrition program in the state health agency	X						
Public health nutrition consultants in state and local health agencies	X						
Nutritionists in special programs serving children with chronic conditions, e.g., pediatric pulmonary centers, genetics treatment centers, university-affiliated programs, and diagnostic evaluation centers	X	X	X				
Educators of public health nutrition professionals in universities, particularly schools of public health	X						
Nutritionists or dieticians working in local child health programs in health departments, hospitals, WIC, EPSDT, Head Start, VNA, etc., and in private practice		X					
Pediatric dietitians in major hospitals affiliated with a medical school			X				
Food assistance resources							
WIC and CSFP				X			
Food stamp program				X			
School feeding and child nutrition programs				X			
Emergency food assistance through churches and community programs				X			
Instruction on food management							
County extension home economists					X		
EFNEP aides					X		
Home economists in community programs, secondary schools, public utilities					X		
Nutrition or dietetic technicians and community aides					X		

WIC—Women, Infants, and Children program; EPSDT—Early and Periodic Screening, Diagnosis, and Treatment program; VNA—Visiting Nurse Association; CSFP—Commodities Supplemental Food Program; EFNEP—Early Food and Nutrition Education Program.

Adapted with permission from: Baer MT, ed. Nutrition services for children with handicaps: A manual for state Title V programs. Los Angeles: University Affiliated Training Program; Center for Child Development and Developmental Disorders, Children's Hospital of Los Angeles, Dec. 1982.

Table 1-11. Examples of Partnership between Community and Tertiary Care Nutrition Providers to Coordinate Services for Children with Pediatric HIV

Nutritional issue	Coordination of community care	Coordination of tertiary care
Child with HIV infection	*Tertiary care nutritionist:* Completes nutritional assessment, identifies present and potential problems, develops care plan, makes appropriate referrals	*Community nutritionist:* Monitors growth and nutritional status, ensures food availability (food stamps, WIC), provides anticipatory guidance, monitors for HIV-related nutritional problems
Child requiring enteral feeding	*Tertiary care nutritionist:* Prescribes product and method and rate of administration, educates caregiver on maintenance of enteral feeds, makes changes as necessary, identifies local nutritionist to coordinate with, sends recipe and plan to local nutritionist	*Community nutritionist:* Monitors growth, documents oral and enteral intakes and checks tolerance, ensures availability of formula, communicates any problems with tertiary care nutritionist
Child with failure to thrive	*Tertiary care nutritionist:* Rules out organic and oral-motor nutritional related reasons for FTT, develops nutrition care plan, makes appropriate referrals, acts in liaison with community nutritionist for coordination	*Community care nutritionist:* Monitors growth, revises plan and recommendations as needed, coordinates efforts with community services (day care, etc.), ensures food availability (WIC, food stamps, etc.)

Adapted with permission from Mugriditchian L, Arent-Fine J, Dwyer J, Holland M, Polhamus B. The nutrition of the HIV infected child. Part II: Care management. Topic Clin Nutr. 7(2): 11-20, 1992. © 1992, Aspen Publishers.

References

1. Ireys HT, Nelson RP. New federal policy for children with special health care needs: Implications for pediatricians. Pediatrics 90:321–27, 1992.
2. Kozlowski BW, Powell JA. Position of the American Dietetic Association: Nutrition services for children with special health needs. J Am Diet Assoc 95:809–12, 1995.
3. U.S. Department of Education. Early intervention programs for infants and toddlers with disabilities: Proposed rule making. Federal Register 57(85):18,994, 1992.
4. Baer MT, Farnan S, Mauer AM. Children with special health care needs. In: Sharbaugh CO, ed. Call to action: better nutrition for mothers, children, and families. Washington, D.C.: National Center for Education in Maternal and Child Health, 1991; 191–208.
5. Chamberlin RW. Developmental assessment and early intervention programs for young children: Lessons learned from longitudinal research. Pediatr Rev 8:237–339, 1987.
6. Environmental Health Law Project. Early intervention advocacy network notebook: New guide to Part H laws and regulations. Washington, D.C., July, 1992.
7. Sholkoff J, Hauser-Cram P. Early intervention for disabled infants and their families: A quantitative analysis. Pediatrics 80:650–58, 1987.
8. Solomon R. Pediatricians and early intervention: Everything you need to know but are too busy to ask. Inf Young Child 7:38–51, 1995.
9. Lucas B. Serving infants and children with special health care needs in the 1990's—are we ready? J Am Diet Assoc 89:1559–1601, 1989.
10. Shelton TL, Jeppson ES, Johnson BH. Family-centered care for children with special health care needs. Washington, D.C.: Association for the Care of Children's Health, 1987.
11. Schuman A, Benham R. Early childhood intervention: A nationwide resource. Semin Pediatr Gastroenterol Nutr 4:8–11, 1993.

12. Surgeon General's Report: Children with special health care needs, Campaign 1987. Commitment to: Family-centered, community-based, coordinated care. Washington, D.C.: U.S. Department of Health and Human Services, Public Health Service, 1987. DHHS (PHS) pub. no. (HRS) D/MC 87–2.
13. Gittler J. Community-based service systems for children with special health care needs and their families. Iowa City: National Maternal and Child Health Resource Center, 1988.
14. Nash J. Public Law 99–457: Facilitating family participation on the multidisciplinary team. J Early Interven 14:318–26, 1990.
15. Walker DK. Building a family-centered early intervention system. In: Gallager and Fullagar, eds. The coordination of health and other services for infants and toddlers with disabilities: The conundrum of parallel systems. Carolina Policy Studies Program, 1992.
16. Horsley J. Nutrition issues facing children with special health care needs. Nutr Focus 9(3):1–5, 1994.
17. Lichtenwalter L, Freeman R, Lee M, et al. Providing nutrition services to children with special needs in a community setting. Top Clin Nutr 8:75–78, 1993.
18. Bayerl CT, Ries JD, Bettencourt MF, et al. Nutrition issues of children in early intervention programs: Primary care team approach. Semin Pediatr Gastroenterol Nutr 4:11–15, 1993.
19. Brizee L, Sophos C, McLaughlin J. Nutrition issues in developmental disabilities. Inf Young Child 2:10–21, 1990.
20. Baer M, Blyer E, Cloud H, et al. Providing early nutrition intervention services: Preparation of dietitians, nutritionists and other team members. Inf Young Child 3:56–66, 1991.
21. Dwyer JT, Freedland J. Nutrition services. In: Wallace HM, Ryan Jr G, Oglesby A, eds. Maternal and child health practices, 3d ed. Oakland, Calif.: Third Party Publishing Co., 1988.
22. Coyner AB. Meeting health needs of handicapped infants. In: Zelle R, Coyner AB, eds. Developmentally disabled infants and toddlers: Assessment and intervention. Philadelphia: Davis, 1983; 1–59.
23. Satter E. Childhood feeding problems. Feelings and their medical significance. Newsletter. Ross Laboratories, Columbus, Ohio, 1990.
24. Kaufman M. Are dietitians prepared to work with handicapped infants? PL 99–457 offers new opportunities. J Am Diet Assoc 89:1602–05, 1989.
25. Bronner Y. Cultural sensitivity and nutrition counseling. Top Clin Nutr 9:13–19, 1994.
26. Phillips C, Cooper R. Cultural dimensions of feeding relationships. Zero to three 12:10–13, 1992.
27. Bishop KK, Woll J, Arango P. Family/professional collaboration for children with special health needs and their families. Burlington, Vt.: Department of Social Work, University of Vermont, 1993.
28. Bayerl C, Ries J. Early start: Nutrition services in early intervention. Boston, Mass.: Office of Nutrition, Bureau of Family and Community Health, Mass. Dept. of Public Health/Eunice Kennedy Shriver Center, University Affiliated Program, 1994.
29. Bujold C, Sadegian K. Nutrition screening questionnaire. Santa Fe, N.M.: New Mexico Health and Environmental Department, CHEWS Nutrition Project, 1988.
30. Campbell MK, Kelsey KS. The PEACH survey: A nutrition screening tool for use in early intervention programs. J Am Diet Assoc 94:1156–58, 1994.
31. Baroni M, Sondel S. A collaborative model for identifying feeding and nutrition needs in early intervention. Inf Young Child 8:15–25, 1995.
32. Admundson J. System development for nutrition services in early intervention. Dietetics in Development and Psychiatric Disorders. Newsletter, Winter 1996; 7–9.
33. American Dietetic Association, Dietitians in Pediatric Practice, Quality Assurance Committee. Quality assurance criteria sets for pediatric nutrition conditions: A model. Chicago: The Association, 1988.
34. New England SERVE. Enhancing quality: Standards and indicators of quality care for children with special health care needs. Boston: New England SERVE, 1989.
35. Hine RJ, Cloud H, Carithers T, et al. Early nutrition intervention services for children with special health care needs. J Amer Diet Assoc 89:1636–39, 1989.
36. McGarr B, Dwyer J, Holland M. Delivering nutrition services in early intervention in rural areas. Inf Young Child 7:52–62, 1995.
37. Washington State Department of Health. Focus groups on nutrition services with parents of children with special health care needs in Washington State. Olympia, Wash. October 1994.
38. Meilahn K. Promoting partnerships between health care providers and parents of children with special health care needs. Nutr Focus 8(3):1–5, 1993.

Nutrition Manual for At-Risk Infants and Toddlers
Janice Hovasi Cox, editor

2

NUTRITION SERVICE PROVIDER COMPETENCIES

Janice Hovasi Cox, MS, RD, and Barbara B. Free, MS, RD

In 1992, a Michigan task force was established in compliance with requirements of the Individuals with Disabilities Education Act (IDEA), Public Law 99-457, part H (now P.L. 102-119) to define competencies, assess training needs, and develop training guidelines for professionals who provide special "early intervention" health care or educational services to infants and children under 3 years of age.[1] The Merrill-Palmer Institute of Wayne State University contracted with the state to develop and coordinate the efforts of this task force, known as the Interdisciplinary Personnel Preparation Committee (IPPC). The IPPC included academic faculty and service provider representatives from each of the following disciplines: medicine, nursing, nutrition, occupational therapy, physical therapy, speech pathology, audiology, psychology, social work, special education, and preprimary education. Parents of infants and children with special needs were also included on this task force to provide guidance and suggestions from the family perspective.

Disciplinary Resource Groups

While the IPPC identified global or interdisciplinary competencies,[2] each of the IPPC representatives separately engaged a group of peer professionals, known as a Disciplinary Resource Group (DRG), to identify competencies and training needs specific to their individual discipline. Qualifications for personnel providing early

Acknowledgments
The authors wish to thank the members of the Michigan Nutrition Disciplinary Resource Group for thoughtful insight and expert contributions toward the identification of competencies and training guidelines for nutrition professionals who provide early intervention services to infants and children with special health care needs. In addition to the authors, who served as cochairs, members of the Nutrition DRG were: Gwen Armstrong, MS, RD; Jenny Bond, PhD, RD; Nancy Fassinger, RD; Juanita McHale, MA, RD; Hope O'Leary, MS, RD; Sally Poux, MPH, RD; Anita Sandretto, PhD, RD; June Ventimiglia, RD; and Audrey Wittrup, MSW.

intervention services are identified in part H of P.L. 99-457 as "entry level requirements that are based on the highest requirements in the State applicable to the profession or discipline."[2] In Michigan, this is interpreted to mean the registered dietitian (RD) as provider of nutrition assessment, treatment, and education.

The Nutrition DRG included experienced RDs from the following programs and institutions: Michigan Department of Public Health; Children's Special Health Care Services; Women, Infants, and Children (WIC) Supplemental Food Program; Head Start (Wayne County); Michigan State University (East Lansing); Oakland County Health Division; Children's Hospital of Michigan (Detroit); University of Michigan School of Public Health (Ann Arbor); University of Michigan Medical Center—Mott's Children's Hospital (Ann Arbor); Edward Sparrow Hospital (Lansing); and Bronson Methodist Hospital (Kalamazoo). These RDs were able to provide diverse perspectives from their experience in professional training programs and in public health, preprimary school, hospital, and clinic settings. A parent and a part H coordinator were also included in this working group to provide guidance and suggestions from the family and the overall program perspectives.

Background information was collected, including (1) the rules and regulations pertaining to nutrition services and training of personnel within the P. L. 99-457, part H,[1] (2) the position of the American Dietetic Association (ADA) regarding the role and training of "early intervention" nutrition service providers,[3] (3) basic training requirements for entry level dietitians established by the ADA,[4] (4) a review of the literature,[5–11] and (5) a review of competencies established in other states.[12, 13]

The Nutrition DRG submitted a list of competencies for dietitians working with at-risk infants and toddlers as presented in table 2-1. Many of these competencies are required in a general way to obtain RD credentials,[14] although prepractice training, which specifically addresses at-risk infants and toddlers, may be limited due to lack of curriculum flexibility or lack of faculty expertise.[5] Competencies that are often acquired beyond entry into the profession, and for which additional training is needed when working with infants and toddlers, were also identified by the Nutrition DRG and are listed in table 2-2. The Merrill-Palmer Institute staff developed a format for assessing training needs of early intervention providers to achieve cross-disciplinary and discipline-specific competencies. Results of this needs assessment in Michigan are given in table 2-3.[15]

Table 2-1. Competencies of Nutrition Service Provider

1. Demonstrates knowledge of the methods used to prevent, reduce severity, or delay the onset of nutrition-related disease and disability in infants and toddlers who are at risk for or who have chronic illness or handicapping conditions
2. Obtains, evaluates, and interprets the following components of the nutrition assessment:
   - Anthropometric/growth measurements
   - Dietary intake
   - Normal, immature, dysfunctional (physical), and behavioral aspects of feeding skills
   - Biochemical and laboratory tests
   - Clinical signs and symptoms of nutritional deficiency, inadequacy, excess or toxicity
3. Identifies and interprets physical, psychosocial and economic environment of the family as it relates to nutritional status. This includes the feeding relationship between the parents/caregivers and the child and the ability of the parents/caregivers to feed the child
4. Identifies energy and nutrient requirements
5. Identifies actual or potential drug and food/nutrient delivery interactions
6. Identifies, develops, implements, and monitors effectiveness, and modifies or revises nutrition interventions for typical and atypical 0 to 2-year-olds, including children with established conditions (chronic disease or handicapping conditions) within the framework of the overall care plan through
   - Feeding recommendations to circumvent dysfunction and promote/enhance normal oral and feeding development
   - Dietary modifications used in the *treatment* of established conditions (chronic diseases or handicapping conditions)
   - Appropriate foods and/or feedings (including foods of normal or modified consistency, infant formulas, tube feedings, nutrient supplements, parenteral nutrient solutions, feeding equipment, etc.)
7. Provides diet instruction, nutrition education, and nutrition counseling to meet the individual medical, physical, and psychosocial needs of the child and family within the framework of the family's learning styles, abilities, and functional level of literacy and understanding
8. Identifies and directs parents/caregivers to resources (including sources of payment), providers, and channels of access to nutrition services and other services available to this population, both public and private
9. Defines scope, content, and delivery of quality nutrition intervention services and evaluates these services to assure/improve quality of care and cost effectiveness.

Reference: Michigan's comprehensive system of personnel development.[2]

Table 2-2. Nutrition Competencies in which More Training is Needed

1. Knowledge of the methods used to prevent, reduce severity, or delay the onset of nutrition-related disease and disability in infants and toddlers who are at risk for or who have chronic illness or handicapping conditions
2. Evaluation and interpretation of growth
3. Evaluation and interpretation of normal, immature, dysfunctional (physical), and behavioral aspects of feeding skills
4. Evaluation of the feeding relationship between child and parent/caregiver as it relates to nutritional status and well-being
5. Identification of energy and nutrient needs for infants and children with chronic disease or handicapping conditions
6. Identification, development, and implementation of nutrition interventions for infants and children with chronic disease or handicapping conditions, including:
   - Feeding recommendations to circumvent dysfunction and promote/enhance normal oral and feeding development
   - Dietary modifications used in the *treatment* of established conditions (chronic diseases or handicapping conditions)
   - Appropriate foods and/or feedings (including foods of normal or modified consistency, infant formulas, tube feedings, nutrient supplements, parenteral nutrient solutions, feeding equipment, etc.)
7. Definition and evaluation of program scope, content, and delivery of nutrition services (both process and outcome components) to assure and improve quality of care and cost effectiveness

Reference: Michigan's comprehensive system of personnel development.[2]

Table 2-3. Education and Training Needs Assessment Survey, State of Michigan*

Cross-discipline competencies
1. Process of coping and adapting to the birth of a child with disabilities or delays
2. Developmental theories and intervention models
3. Current local, state, and federal laws regarding early intervention services
4. Integrating identified goals into daily routines
5. Family-centered interviewing and observational methods
6. Understanding of the various roles and unique contributions of families, paraprofessionals, and professionals involved in early intervention services
7. Identify unique child/family strengths/resources/needs

Nutrition competencies
1. Knowledge of methods used to prevent, reduce severity, or delay the onset of nutrition-related disease and disability in infants and toddlers who are at risk for or who have chronic illness or handicapping conditions
2. Evaluation and interpretation of growth
3. Assessment instruments
4. Identifying and interpreting the physical, psychosocial, and economic environment of the family as it relates to the child's nutritional status
5. Identifying, developing, and implementing nutrition interventions for infants and children with chronic disease or handicapping conditions, including:
   - Feeding recommendations to circumvent dysfunction and promote/enhance normal oral and feeding development
   - Dietary modifications used in the *treatment* of established conditions (chronic diseases or handicapping conditions)
   - Appropriate foods and/or feedings (including foods of normal or modified consistency, infant formulas, tube feedings, nutrient supplements, parenteral nutrient solutions, feeding equipment, etc.)
6. Diet instruction, nutrition education, and nutrition counseling to meet the individual medical, physical, and psychosocial needs of the child and family within the framework of the family's learning styles, abilities, and functional level of literacy and understanding
7. Monitoring the effectiveness of nutrition education and intervention to meet the needs of the child within the framework of the comprehensive care plan

*Sample size: 117 nutrition service providers. Each of the items listed were identified by at least 75% of the respondents as areas in which they needed more education or training.

Reference: Rita Benn.[15]

Continuing Education

Continuing education for dietitians is available in a variety of settings and formats. Workshops offering nutrition training are available through the University of Iowa, the University of Alabama at Birmingham, the University-affiliated programs at the University of Southern California (Los Angeles) and Cincinnati Center for Developmental Disorders, and through other institutions.[16] An individualized competency-based training initiative, "Training for the Care of the Handicapped Child," is available at Riley Hospital for Children, Indianapolis. Other nutrition education opportunities include professional conferences sponsored by the ADA and public health and WIC programs. Publications such as those by Horsley[17] and Bujold,[18] along with medical and nutrition journals, also provide updated information, announcements of educational opportunities, and contacts for developing a network of early-intervention nutrition service providers.

The final report of the IPPC identifies competencies for each of the professional disciplines.[2] Cross-disciplinary competencies such as the theoretical and ethical foundations, interpersonal skills, and advocacy skills included in the report are listed in table 2-4.[2] Whereas this document provides a formidable description of the expert service provider, it is understood that entry level practitioners are not proficient in all areas. The IPPC recommends that training needs of professionals be periodically assessed statewide so that relevant educational programs can be implemented to improve the competency level of service providers.

Table 2-4. Cross-Discipline Competencies

Theoretical foundations
1. Demonstrates understanding of the elements of family-centered care
2.* Uses developmental theories, intervention models, and current research for intervention with infants and toddlers exhibiting established conditions, developmental delay, or risk for developmental delay
3.* Demonstrates understanding of typical and atypical growth and development within the context of each family, including the interdependence of developmental areas and caregiver-child interaction
4. Understands family dynamics and systems, including the contribution of cultural, social, and environmental factors on the family
5.* Demonstrates understanding of the ongoing process of coping and adapting to the birth or identification of a child with disabilities or delays, including anxiety, grief, and loss for both family members and professionals

Legal/ethical foundations
1. Demonstrates ethical practice in working with families, including privacy and confidentiality
2.* Demonstrates knowledge of current local, state, and federal laws regarding early intervention services

Interpersonal/team skills
1. Understands the effect of one's family history, culture, and experiences on developing relationships
2. Demonstrates interpersonal skills that foster trust and successful working relationships
3. Demonstrates sensitive, useful, and clear communication skills (listening, speaking, and writing) with families and other professionals
4.* Utilizes skills as a service coordinator and as a team member for developing, implementing, and evaluating an overall care plan for an individual client
5. Integrates assessments from one's area of expertise with those of other disciplines in developing overall care plan for an individual client
6. Uses group process skills to enhance team functioning
7.* Demonstrates understanding of the various roles and unique contributions of families, paraprofessionals, and professionals involved in early intervention services.

Advocacy skills
1. Supports the family as primary decision-makers and promotes their acquisition of knowledge, skills, and confidence in identifying and carrying out their goals for their child
2. Increases collaboration among families and professionals in policy and program decisions
3. Uses methods of advocacy for families of children with established conditions, developmental delay, or risk for developmental delay

*Didactic and experiential components of the education of entry-level dietitians include many of these cross-disciplinary competencies. Those cross-disciplinary competencies marked with an asterisk are identified as those for which additional training may be needed.

Reference: Michigan's comprehensive system of personnel development.[2]

References

1. The Education of the Handicapped Act Amendments of 1986 (Public Law 99-457) part H. Department of Education. Early intervention program for infants and toddlers with handicaps; Final regulations. Fed Regis 54 (119):26306–348, June 22, 1989.
2. Michigan's comprehensive system of personnel development. Interdisciplinary personnel preparation committee final report. (presented to the State Interagency Coordinating Council for the Infant and Toddler Early Intervention Program Part H or the Individuals with Disabilities Education Act) Lansing, Mich., Dec. 10, 1993.
3. Blyler E, and Lucas B. Position of the American Dietetic Association: Nutrition in comprehensive program planning for persons with developmental disabilities. J Am Diet Assoc 87:1068–74, 1987.
4. Accreditation/approval manual for dietetic education programs. Chicago: American Dietetic Association, 1987.
5. Kaufman M. Are dietitians prepared to work with handicapped infants? PL 99-457 offers new opportunities. J Am Diet Assoc 89:1602–-05, 1989.
6. Hine RJ, Cloud HH, Carithers T, et al. Early nutrition interventions services for children with special health care needs. J Am Diet Assoc 89:1636–39, 1989.
7. Lucas BL. Serving infants and children with special health care needs in the 1990's—are we ready? J Am Diet Assoc 89:1599–1601, 1989.
8. McCollum JA, Bailey DB. Developing comprehensive personnel systems: Issues and Alternatives. J Early Intervent 15:57–65, 1991.
9. Bailey DB, Simeonsson RJ, Yoder DE, et al. Preparing professionals to serve infants and toddlers with handicaps and their families: An integrative analysis across eight disciplines. Except Child 56:26–35, 1990.
10. Bailey DB. Issues and directions in preparing professionals to work with young handicapped children and their families. In: Gallagher J, Trohanis P, Clifford R, eds. Policy implementation and PL 99-457: Planning for young children with special needs. Baltimore: Paul H. Brookes, 1989; 97–132.
11. Bayerl CT, Ries JD. Early start: Nutrition services in early intervention in Massachusetts. Zero to Three 12:29–31, 1992.
12. Zervigon-Hakes A. Competencies for professions serving at-risk and disabled infants, toddlers and their families. Research study submitted to: The Bureau of Education for Exceptional Students, Division of Public Schools, Florida Department of Education and the Florida Interagency Coordinating Council for Infants and Toddlers. Florida Consortium of Newborn Intervention Programs, 1991.
13. Wisconsin Interagency Coordinating Council. Competencies for early intervention personnel. In: Recommendations of the program committee regarding screening and evaluation/assessment, attachment 4. Madison, Wis.: Department of Health and Social Sciences, 1990.
14. Accreditation/approval manual for dietetic education programs. Chicago: American Dietetic Association, 1987.
15. Rita Benn, PhD, Merrill-Palmer Institute, Wayne State University, Detroit, personal communication.
16. National Center for Education in Maternal and Child Health. Nutrition services for children with special health needs: Abstracts of active and completed projects FY 1985–1991. Washington D.C.: National Center for Education in Maternal and Child Health, 1991.
17. Horsley JW. Nutrition issues facing children with special health care needs in early intervention programs and at school. Nutr Focus 9:1–8, 1994.
18. Bujold CR. Public Law 99-457—a review. Building Block for Life 15:1–2, 1992.

Section II

Nutrition Assessment

Nutrition Manual for At-Risk Infants and Toddlers
Janice Hovasi Cox, editor

3

NUTRITION SCREENING AND DIET HISTORY

Janice Hovasi Cox, MS, RD

Maintaining optimal health, growth, and development at any age depends upon many things: access to good medical care, adequate housing, love and a nurturing environment, and good nutritional status. This is particularly true for infants and young children who are in the midst of rapid growth and development and who are particularly vulnerable to infectious disease due to the relative immaturity of their immune systems. Identifying infants and children who are at risk for having poor nutritional status is important if we wish to promote optimal health, growth, and development.

Although evaluation of growth provides a general measure of nutritional outcome, the diet history identifies whether or not the nutrition process is appropriate and adequate. In-depth nutrition assessment of every infant and child is neither practical nor essential. Most infants and children are successfully and adequately nourished, and they grow and develop within expected norms. Nutrition screening is designed to identify which infants or toddlers have—or are at increased risk for having—nutrition-related problems. This chapter provides suggestions for nutrition screening and obtaining diet histories that render accurate information about food intake and feeding practices, particularly those that may place the infant/child at nutritional risk and those that may indicate the need for referral to a registered dietitian experienced in the evaluation and treatment of infants and children with nutrition problems.

Nutrition Screening

A variety of nutrition screening tools are available in local health departments, food supplemental programs, and the literature.[1,2] When developing a screening tool, it is important to consider who will be conducting the screen, their training, and the population being screened. Simple "yes" and "no" questions require fewer skills and less training for those conducting the screen and require less time to complete, but these may be less specific and too selective, identifying more false positives and false negatives. Screening tools that include multiple-choice questions or questions requiring a more general response from the parents may call for more training for those conducting the screen and more time to complete, but these may provide more accurate or useful information.

Policy regarding completion of the nutrition screening tool should be carefully considered. The first contact with a service provider or agency often begins with a "screening" tool. This first interaction establishes a relationship and foundation for other interactions. Feeding practices are affected by culture, family traditions, societal pressures, professional advice, commercial advertising, and the individual nature and perceptions of both the infant/child and the parents. Historical information should be obtained from the parent or other caregiver who feeds the infant/child most frequently. The history they provide not only about specific food intake but their perceptions of the feeding process are invaluable. Because feeding is basic to the relationship between the infant/child and parent, gathering information in a supportive, nonthreatening manner is extremely important. Building a strong positive rapport with the parent engenders trust and develops a cooperative spirit and willingness to accept and implement changes in feeding when changes are truly needed. When feedings are not successful, parents may have feelings of failure or loss in self-confidence or control.[3] These feelings must be acknowledged and respected. General suggestions for obtaining food intake and feeding practice information are given in table 3-1.

Sample nutrition screening tools are given in appendixes A and B. Specific guidelines for nutrition screening are given in the following sections.

Growth Parameters

The focus of the feeding assessment is determined by the adequacy of growth. If growth parameters are within the normal range, the feeding assessment should be focused on the quality of the diet and general information about feeding practices. If growth parameters are above or below the normal range, the feeding assessment must provide more detailed information about the quality and quantity of food consumed, feeding behaviors, and any possible losses of nutrients due to vomiting or diarrhea. If weight for age or weight for length fall below the 5th (or 10th)

Table 3-1. General Suggestions for Obtaining Dietary Intake Information

- Set aside personal attitudes and values so that listening and observation skills can be focused objectively and respectfully on the family's point of view. "People don't care how much you know, until they know how much you care."
- Avoid asking questions that insinuate "blame," particularly if growth is not within normal limits or feeding problems are present. Examples: "How often does your baby usually eat?" is better than "How often do you feed your baby?" or "How much does your baby take at one feeding?" instead of "How much do you feed your baby?"
- If specific information is needed, avoid asking the question so that it can be answered by a simple "yes" or "no." For example, "What kind of formula does your baby drink?" allows the parent to identify a specific feeding, while "Does your baby drink Similac?" does not require the parent to identify specific information. "How do you prepare your baby's formula?" requires a more specific answer than "Do you follow the directions on the can to prepare your baby's formula?"
- Ask the caregiver to describe formula preparation. Have cans, cups, scoops, and bottles available to aid in their description. If the caregiver cannot describe or demonstrate formula preparation, he or she may not be giving infant formula or preparing it accurately. "Do you ever prepare the formula differently?" Overdilution of formula may provide inadequate nutrition. Sometimes families add extra water because they think the baby needs the extra water or they may be trying to make the formula last longer—so they won't run out before they can get more. Overconcentrated formula may be given to help satiate fussy babies, but this may provide inadequate water and/or excessive nutrient intake.
- The amount of breast milk, formula, or food given is often the most difficult to assess. Parents who rely on hunger and satiety cues (as they well should!) rather than the clock and the amount of formula in the bottle may have the most difficulty reporting amounts taken. Questions regarding frequency of formula or food preparation and purchase, amount purchased above food supplemental program allotments, amounts discarded, recorded intake of formula or foods consumed, number of bottles or meals consumed on a daily basis, duration of feedings, sleep schedules, and description of hunger and satiety cues can all help identify amounts taken.
- Ask the caregiver to describe the baby's usual behavior during a feeding. This will help to identify parents' perceptions of hunger and satiety cues, attitudes about feeding, and infant/child feeding behaviors. If they are at a loss for words, you can help by giving them several adjectives or descriptions from which to choose.
- Avoid giving advice while obtaining history information. Making judgments about or changes in child care during the interview may alter the parents' responses to subsequent questions or distract them from providing full and accurate information.
- Asking "Do you have any concerns about your baby's/child's nutrition?" may provide a shortcut to a problem for which parents are seeking help. Addressing this problem first may allow parents to move on to other questions or issues. This may also open the relationship between service provider and parent for teamwork in solving this and other problems in the future.

percentiles or above the 95th (or 90th) percentiles, prompt referral to a registered dietitian may be beneficial in obtaining further nutrition information, identifying the cause of growth deviation, and developing a course of action when one is needed.

Women, Infants, and Children Food Supplemental Program (WIC)

This government-sponsored program provides infant formula, milk, cheese (or sometimes other dairy products), juice, cereal, and eggs in specified quantities to families with limited financial resources and increased medical or nutritional risk. Guidelines for eligibility and food package content are determined by designated state agencies. Knowing the individual state's guidelines facilitates referral when needed and helps to identify the quantity and quality of formula, milk, and/or food intake.

Formula/Milk

Feeding guidelines for infants and children are given in tables 3-2 and 3-3. Use of highly specialized formulas such as Alimentum, Nutramigen, Pregestimil, or Pediasure may indicate that the infant/child has unusual nutritional needs and may need guidance when other foods are added to the diet as development progresses. Use of whole cow's milk during the first year may provide inadequate intake of iron, vitamins C and B_6, and essential fatty acid.

Table 3-2. Feeding Recommendations for Infants

Developmental stage	Age (mo)	Food and amounts* consumed daily
Sucks and swallows liquids; tongue protrusion reflex is predominant; head bobbing	0–3	Breast milk or iron-fortified infant formula only
Sits with minimal support; head is erect and steady; can transfer food from front of tongue to back of mouth and swallows pureed food	4–6	Breast milk or iron-fortified infant formula Dry infant cereal, strained fruits or vegetables in amounts limited so as not to significantly reduce breast milk or formula intake. If breast-fed, may give strained meat to supplement protein and iron intake Juice (2–4 oz)
Sits unsupported, balances head well and has body control; able to mash food with jaw and swallow food of different consistencies; begins self-feeding	7–9	Breast milk or iron-fortified infant formula Dry infant cereal (8–12 tbsp/day) Strained or mashed fruits and vegetables (6–8 tbsp/day) Juice (2–4 oz) Strained or finely ground meats (2–4 tbsp/day) Toast or teething biscuit
Continues increasing skill in biting, chewing and swallowing food; holds cup, uses spoon, and likes self-feeding	10–12	Breast milk or iron-fortified infant formula.† Dry infant cereal (8–12 tbsp/day) Fork-mashed or soft fruits and cooked vegetables (6–8 tbsp/day) Juice (2–4 oz) Ground or chopped meat or meat substitutes (1–2 oz/day) Potato and whole grain or enriched grain products; toast or teething biscuits

*Amounts of formula vary based on energy and growth needs. Recommend according to infant's corrected age/developmental readiness. Amounts for breast milk are not easily identified as supply is usually based on demand.

†Vitamin D-fortified whole milk is not recommended under 1 yr of age. Low-fat or reduced fat milk is not recommended under 2 yr of age.

Note: Fluoride supplements are not recommended until tooth eruption occurs, and are not needed if water supplies contain at least 0.3 ppm (0.3 mg/L); if water supplies contain < 0.3 ppm, a supplement of 0.25 mg may be given.

Reference: Anderson JV, Van Nierop MR, eds. Basic nutrition facts: A nutrition reference. Lansing, Mich.: Michigan Department of Public Health, Center for Health Promotion and Cooperative Extension Service, Michigan State University, 1989.

Table 3-3. Feeding Recommendations for Toddlers (Ages 1–3)

Food groups	Minimum number and portion sizes of servings (for children 1–3 yr)
Vegetables and fruits Include one good source of vitamin A every other day and one good source of vitamin C every day; include one good source of folic acid every day for children over 7 yr of age	6 servings 1 serving = cooked: 2 tbsp canned: 2 tbsp raw: 1/2 small juice: 1/4 cup
Breads and cereals Choose a variety from this group that are enriched, fortified, or whole grain	7 servings 1 serving = 1/2 slice bread 1/4 cup hot cereal 1/2 cup cold cereal 1/4 cup pasta 1/4 cup rice 2-2" crackers
Milk and cheese Choose foods fortified with vitamin D and get adequate exposure to sunlight	5 servings 1 serving = 1/2 cup milk 1" cheese cube 1 slice processed cheese 1/2 slice cheese 1/2 cup cottage cheese 1/2 cup yogurt
Meat, poultry, fish	3 servings 1 serving = 1 oz lean meat, poultry, fish 1 egg 1/2 cup cooked dry beans, peas or lentils 3-1/2 oz tofu 2 tbsp peanut butter
Fat Fat is essential for young children and may be supplied by margarine or vegetable oils	1 tsp
Calories Total average calories supplied from minimum recommended servings	1300 calories
Recommended Daily Allowances Energy intake and ranges which allow for different body sizes and levels of activity	1300 calories (900–1800 calories)

This guide is aimed at meeting the Recommended Daily Dietary Allowances. A variety of foods from each group should be eaten daily.

Note: Fluoride supplements are not recommended if water supplies contain > 0.6 ppm (6 mg/L) for any age group or for children under 3 yr of age if water supplies contain 0.3 to 0.6 ppm. Children up to 3 yr of age may be given 0.25 mg fluoride/day if water supplies contain < 0.3 ppm.[9]

Reference: Anderson JV, Van Nierop MR, eds. Basic nutrition facts: A nutrition reference. Lansing, Mich.: Michigan Department of Public Health, Center for Health Promotion and Cooperative Extension Service, Michigan State University, 1989.

If the cow's milk is low-fat or skim, this may also provide inadequate calorie and excessive protein intake. If goat's milk provides a significant portion of the nutritional intake, overall intake of iron, vitamins C and D, folacin and essential fatty acid may be inadequate. Omission of breast milk, infant or pediatric formulas, and cow's milk from the diet or use of other imitation milks or milk substitutes may render a diet deficient in many nutrients.[4]

The parents may be able to identify the daily volume of intake easily. If not, or if an unusual amount of formula or milk is reported, the volume of intake can be estimated or verified in various ways: intake per feeding and feedings per day, cans of formula used per week or per month, frequency of formula or milk purchase, amounts discarded after feedings or at the end of the day, etc. Because the volume of breast milk cannot be directly measured, adequate intake must be measured by adequacy of growth. If growth is decelerating or faltering, referral to a dietitian or lactation consultant may be needed to support successful breast-feeding. Nutrient intake may be inadequate or inappropriate if one or more of the following patterns prevail:

- Formula intake for an infant is less than 24 oz in 24 hours; breast-fed infants are fed fewer than six times in 24 hours or have fewer than six wet diapers in 24 hours
- Milk intake for a child is less than 16 oz in 24 hours (unless cheese or other calcium-rich foods are included in the diet in adequate amounts)
- Formula or milk intake is greater than 32 oz in 24 hours. This may indicate that an older infant (9–12 months) or child is not eating a variety of other foods. Infants who weigh more than 11½ lb (5.2 kg) but are less than 4 to 6 months of age and are not ready for solid foods yet may need to ingest more than 32 oz of formula in 24 hours to continue their normal growth pattern.

If growth parameters are not within normal limits, formula preparation may be inaccurate. Parents should be able to describe formula preparation if cans, cups, scoops, and bottles are available to aid in their description. If they cannot describe or demonstrate formula preparation, they may not be giving infant formula or preparing it accurately. Overdilution of formula may provide inadequate nutrition. Sometimes families add extra water because they think the baby needs the extra water or they may be trying to make the formula last longer (so they won't run out before they can get more). In some infants, nutrient additives or supplements or adding less water when preparing formula may be needed as a means of enhancing nutrient intake. If this is done without adequate professional advice or supervision, nutrient intake may be excessive or imbalanced.

Mineral/Vitamin Supplements

General recommendations for formula-fed infants include iron fortification of the formula.[5] If an infant is receiving a formula that is not iron fortified, iron intake/status must be addressed to prevent the occurrence of iron deficiency anemia.[6,7] Although human milk contains only small amounts of iron, breast-fed infants should not need an iron supplement until solid foods are started.[8] Other vitamin or mineral supplements may be used to enhance intake, but may also provide excessive intake if incorrect dosage is given. Most commercial formulas contain fluoride at 0.1–0.3 mg/L. Recommendations for the upper limit of fluoride intake are 0.07 mg/kg/day. Fluoride supplementation is not needed for infants or toddlers if the water used for drinking, preparing foods or beverages, or diluting concentrated or powdered formula contains at least 0.3 ppm (0.3 mg/L) fluoride.[9] If water supplies contain fluoride at less than 0.3 ppm, a supplement of 0.25 mg/day may be given, provided that other dietary sources such as bottled water or other beverages would not contribute to excessive intake. Young toddlers may also ingest a significant amount of fluoride by swallowing toothpaste during brushing.[9]

Bottle Feeding

Propping a bottle or allowing a baby/child to take a bottle to bed can cause earache or choking. Once teeth have erupted, if milk, juice, or other liquids containing carbohydrate remain in contact with the tooth surface for prolonged periods, cariogenic bacterial action is enhanced and the incidence of dental caries increases.[10]

Feeding Progression and Behavior

Infants and children should follow a predictable pattern of feeding progression, enjoy eating, take feedings easily, and generally display signs of a good appetite. Questions about the kinds of utensils used, foods consumed, feeding frequency, hunger and satiety cues, and feeding behaviors can help provide information about the quality and quantity of an infant's/toddler's nutrition. These questions can also identify problems with the process in feeding or progression of feeding development and behaviors (see chapter 4).

Kinds of Foods

Breast milk or infant formula provides the best source of nutrition for infants up to 6 months of age. Although spoon feedings are usually started by 4 to 6 months of age, they may not provide a balanced source of nutrients needed for rapid growth and development until all food groups are included in the diet. As solid food becomes a significant source of total nutrition, providing more than one-third of total energy needs at 7 to 9 months of age, all food groups should be adequately represented in the diet as recommended in table 3-2. Because toddlers usually obtain less than one-third of their total nutrition from milk, food selection becomes more important. Table 3-3 provides food intake recommendations for children ages 1 to 3 years.

Schedule of Feedings

The frequency of feedings may be difficult to assess. If parents report that the infant eats every three to four hours, one might assume the infant is fed six to eight times a day. If the infant takes an hour to eat and sleeps from 8 p.m. to 5 a.m., the infant may only be receiving three to four feedings a day. Infants need to eat at least five to six times a day. Toddlers need to eat at least three to five times a day. Eating less often may not allow the opportunity to consume adequate amounts of food. Breast-fed infants may eat more frequently than formula-fed infants, at least in part because breast milk is more easily digested. To increase maternal milk supply during growth spurts, breast-fed infants nurse more frequently (the supply of breast milk is about 85–90% replenished within 2–2½ hours after each feeding). Feedings that occur more frequently than every 2–2½ hours for prolonged intervals, whether breast-feeding or bottle-feeding, may exhaust the parent as well as the infant or toddler, depending on the duration of feeding.

Feeding Cues

Although hunger and satiety cues are fairly universal in content, their expression may be obvious or subtle. Infants and parents must work out an individual form of communication in their responses to these cues. Problems may occur if the infant is sleepy or has difficulty achieving a quiet-alert state, is fretful and cries frequently before, during, and after feeding, or if the infant falls asleep or becomes easily distracted during feeding and seems to give signs of satiety before an adequate amount of food is taken. The parent may be preoccupied or distracted so that cues go unnoticed or are misread. Whatever the cue, it is important for parents to recognize and appropriately respond to feeding cues, so that the infant gradually learns to trust that food is available when he is hungry, and that food is not forced upon him when he is full.

Vomiting/Diarrhea/Constipation

Most young infants vomit small amounts of food and have changes in stool frequency or consistency at least occasionally. When intake does not correspond to growth, or parents identify a problem with vomiting, diarrhea, or constipation, the history must determine the presence of any of the following:

- A medical problem that requires referral to a physician for further assessment or treatment
- A feeding method problem that requires parent education for appropriate formula preparation and handling or feeding technique
- A formula problem which requires consultation with a registered dietitian and/or physician to identify the best formula alternative
- Parental misperception that requires education regarding normal expectations for spitting and vomiting, stool frequency, consistency, and color.

For detailed information about clinical assessment of vomiting, diarrhea, and constipation, see chapter 6.

Table 3-4. Medical Conditions Associated with Nutritional Problems During Infancy and Early Childhood

Anemia
Bronchopulmonary dysplasia
Chronic renal insufficiency
Congenital alimentary tract anomalies (cleft lip/palate, tracheoesophageal fistula, etc.)
Congenital heart disease
Cystic fibrosis
Failure to thrive
Gastroesophageal reflux
Human immunodeficiency virus infection
Inborn errors of metabolism
Large for gestational age at birth
Low birth weight:p
very low birth weight (< 1500 g)
extremely low birth weight (< 1000 g)
Malabsorption
Neurological impairment
Obesity
Osteopenia of prematurity
Parenteral nutrition required beyond hospital discharge
Poverty or low socioeconomic status
Short bowel syndrome
Small for gestational age at birth
Spina bifida (myelomeningocele)
Tracheostomy
Tube feeding required beyond hospital discharge

Adapted with permission from Groh-Wargo S, Thompson M, and Cox JH, eds. Nutritional care for high-risk newborns. rev. ed. Chicago: Precept Press, 1994; 377.

Chronic Illness/Medications

Table 3-4 provides a list of chronic illnesses and medical conditions that may increase an infant's or toddler's risk for developing nutritional problems. Chronic use of some medications may interfere with nutrient absorption or metabolism (see appendix J).

Questions

Although the place for parental questions or concerns is often last on most screening forms and questionnaires, parents may need to express their questions or concerns about growth or nutrition at the beginning, particularly if they perceive an aberration from the norm. Addressing their questions or concerns first may provide a shortcut to a problem for which parents are seeking help and allow parents to move on to other issues. This may also open the relationship between service provider and parent for teamwork in solving this and other problems in the future.

Criteria for Nutrition Referral

In some situations, a registered dietitian experienced in pediatric nutrition may be involved in the screening process to provide more extensive evaluation and/or intervention as nutritional risk is being identified. If a registered dietitian is not involved in the screening process, referral should be made if growth, clinical signs and symptoms, or feeding and dietary risk factors are present (as identified in Appendixes A and B).

Summary

Adequate dietary intake provides the process—the substance and substrates—for the ultimate outcome—growth and development. Assessment of dietary intake must be performed in concert with assessment of growth, development, and clinical findings to obtain a full and balanced understanding of nutritional status. Beyond assessment, the nutrition service provider must identify nutritional needs and develop a treatment plan that can be easily integrated into the family's overall plan for their infant/child in cooperation with other medical and/or community programs in which the family is involved.

References

1. Bayerl CT, Ries JD. Early start: Nutrition services in early intervention in Massachusetts. Zero to Three 12:29–31, 1992.
2. Campbell MK, Kelsey KS. The PEACH survey: A nutrition screening tool for use in early intervention programs. J Am Diet Assoc 94:1156–58, 1994.
3. Wolf LS, Glass RP. Feeding and swallowing disorders in infancy: Assessment and management. Tucson: Therapy Skill Builders, 1992.
4. American Academy of Pediatrics, Committee on Nutrition. Imitation and substitute milks. Pediatrics 73:876, 1984.
5. American Academy of Pediatrics, Committee on Nutrition. Iron-fortified infant formulas. Pediatrics 84:1114–5, 1989.
6. Reeves JD, Yip R. Lack of adverse side effects of oral ferrous sulfate therapy in 1-year old infants. Pediatrics 75:352–55, 1985.
7. Walter T, Dallman PR, Pizarro F, et al. Effectiveness of iron-fortified cereal in prevention of iron deficiency anemia. Pediatrics 91:976–82, 1993.
8. Pizarro F, Yip R, Dallman PR, et al. Iron status with different infant feeding regimens: Relevance to screening and prevention of iron deficiency. J Pediatr 118:687–92, 1991.
9. Schuman AJ. How much fluoride is too much? The new guidelines. Contemp Pediatr 12:65–74, 1995.
10. Lucas B. Normal nutrition from infancy through adolescence. In: Queen PM, Lang CE, eds. Handbook of pediatric nutrition. Gaithersburg, Md.: Aspen, 1993; 159.

Nutrition Manual for At-Risk Infants and Toddlers
Janice Hovasi Cox, editor

4

FEEDING ASSESSMENT

Karen Gray, OTR, and Wendy King, PT

Eating should be an easy, enjoyable experience. Much social interaction also takes place during a feeding, strengthening the bond between infant/child and parent. Difficult or unpleasant feedings may distress both the infant/child and the parent. The infant/child may become fussy or withdrawn, avoiding interaction with the parent at feeding times. Simple problems may become quite complex as the infant/child and parent develop compensatory feeding patterns.[1] Nutrition may become inadequate and growth may begin to lag. The parent may have feelings of failure or become tense as feeding times approach.

Feeding problems comprise a large portion of the parental concerns that arise with otherwise healthy infants and children, as well as those with specific medical conditions or diagnoses such as those listed in table 4-1. A specific diagnosis often may be associated with particular feeding problems, but interventions are more appropriately designed and implemented when attention is focused on the feeding problem, and its definition and underlying cause rather than on the medical diagnosis.[2]

Feeding problems generally fall into two categories: delayed development and dysfunctional feeding patterns. Either may cause parents much worry and may compromise nutrition. Delayed progress in feeding skills may be the result of premature birth, frequent or prolonged illness, decreased exposure to more advanced feeding techniques,

Table 4-1. Conditions or Diagnoses Associated with Feeding Problems

- Craniofacial anomalies—cleft lip, cleft palate, high-arched palate, micrognathia, hypertrophic tongue, etc.
- Arnold-Chiari malformation (myelomenigocele)
- Tracheo-esophageal fistula, esophageal strictures, or other conditions that require abdominal surgery or prolonged nonoral feedings
- Cardiopulmonary/respiratory/breathing problems—cyanotic congenital heart disease, bronchopulmonary dysplasia, asthma, allergy, aspiration, or recurrent pneumonia
- Neurologic problems—hypertonia, hypotonia, cerebral palsy, degenerative musculoskeletal disorders, etc.

parental misperceptions, or lack of information. Dysfunctional feeding behaviors may be the result of physical or neurological deficits. Many delayed development feeding problems can be managed with patience, parent education, and minor dietary manipulations. If progress is delayed for a prolonged period, or feeding behaviors are dysfunctional, an experienced feeding therapist may be needed to delineate the feeding problem and establish a plan of therapy. The experienced feeding therapist may be an occupational, physical, or speech therapist who has special training or experience in feeding infants and young children. Such individuals are usually available through local school systems or hospitals.

Feeding Development

The ability to progress in feeding skills is determined by developmental readiness rather than chronological age. Oral skills develop in concert with other skills, such as head and trunk control, speech, language, and fine motor development. A feeding problem is a feeding behavior that does not meet the expected performance for that infant/child. Normal feeding expectations and "red flags" signaling the need for detailed feeding assessment are given in table 4-2.

Some skills, even though they are normal at a young age, may signal problems if they persist at an older age. For example, suckling or "lick sucking" is an early oral skill. Suckling is characterized by rhythmic in and out (retraction and extension) movements of the tongue, marked opening and closing of the jaw, and frequently by loose lip closure.[3] Sucking is a more mature pattern featuring up-and-down tongue movements, less noticeable up-and-down jaw movements, and better lip closure. Negative pressure builds up in the mouth as a result of these changes, increasing feeding efficiency. When new skills, new foods, or new food textures are introduced, a suckling pattern may initially reappear, then progress to sucking as organization in the new skill increases. Another example is drooling. When drooling is copious enough to saturate clothing and is not expected at a certain developmental stage, further assessment of oral motor skills may be needed. When coughing and gagging occurs frequently, problems of aspiration or oral sensory defensiveness may be present.

Screening for Feeding Problems

Nutrition screening often includes questions such as those listed in table 4-3 that can identify the presence of feeding problems (see also chapter 3). If the infant/child has difficulty sucking or swallowing or is slow to progress or not progressing to spoon feedings or textured foods, a feeding therapist can teach the parent to provide oral stimulation or other therapies that can help the infant/child develop normal feeding patterns. Oral defensiveness or aversion may delay progression of feedings. Alterations in trunk tone and gross- or fine-motor development may also affect ability to progress with feedings. Therapy programs can be devised to overcome feeding aversions or fears and develop normal muscle tone or control of other muscles that support normal feeding abilities and behaviors.

Feedings that number less than 5 or more than 10 per day may signal a problem. Most infants and young children cannot consume large volumes of milk or food at one time. A rule of thumb is about 1 oz/kg (½ oz/lb) body weight per feeding up to a volume of 8–10 oz. The infant/child may not give frequent enough hunger cues—or the parent may not perceive hunger cues frequently enough—to allow adequate intake every day. Feedings may take too long and be too tiring to allow an adequate number of feedings every day. Infants should be able to take adequate volumes of milk or food if fed six to eight times per day. Feeding more often than every three to four hours may exhaust the caregiver as well as the infant, depending on feeding duration. If feeding is ineffective or volumes taken are too small, feeding intervals may be too frequent to allow adequate time for sleep or play. Toddlers may take large volumes of liquids that may be of limited nutritional value, leaving little room for other foods. Solving this problem may require helping the parent perceive hunger cues or helping the parent work out a schedule for feeding that better meets the infant's/child's needs. The parent may need to limit the amount of liquids offered to the toddler at mealtimes or to offer liquids after solid foods are eaten. Liquids given should be nutrient-rich, such as infant/toddler formula or whole milk. Juices and sugar-sweetened beverages should be given in limited amounts to allow appetite for other foods.

Table 4-2. Feeding Development in the Infant and Toddler

Age (mo)	Developmental stage	Oral-motor skills and suck/swallow/breathe coordination	Food type	Utensil	Drooling	Red flags
0–4	Held reclined ≈45° for feeding; may be held more upright with increased head control Hand to mouth Hand to breast or bottle Full term—dominated by physiologic flexion Prematurely born infant—may continue to be relatively hypotonic	Takes 2 or more sucks in sequence from breast or bottle before pause to breathe or swallow Changes from reflexive to voluntary control of oral-motor structures and eating behaviors; feeding cues become more obvious, e.g., turning away from breast or bottle to signal satiety	Breast milk Formula	Breast Bottle	Minimal when lying on back; more drooling when in other positions; more drooling with more mouth opening at 3-4 mo	Difficulty initiating sucking pattern Poorly sustained suck; weak suck Lacks strength to initiate let down Large amount of liquid loss Tongue or lip retraction; biting Arching Longer than 30 minutes to eat
4–6	Head erect and steady Sits with minimal support Both hands to bottle Accepts spoon and cup feeding By 6 mo may bring cracker to mouth and use munching motion More variety of sounds Less crying	Long sucking sequences at breast or bottle. Liquid loss at beginning of suck or when nipple removed Continuous sucks at cup followed by uncoordinated swallow. Choking or coughing with large amounts of liquid. Much liquid loss from cup Suckling or sucking; sucking or suckling pattern on spoon and soft or hard solid foods; may gag on new textures; scrapes hard solids on gums; uses munching pattern	Breast milk Formula Juice Pureed food Cereal Soft cookie	Breast Bottle Cup Spoon Fingers	Rarely, unless fingers in mouth May see when babbling, or when using hands for reaching, pointing or manipulating May see during or after feedings or with certain foods	As for 0–4 mo Consistently fussy with feedings
7–9	Sits unsupported with good head control Takes liquids from cup Assists with cup and spoon; holds own bottle Begins self-feeding Uses mouth, hands, eyes to explore objects; bites on objects when teething	Long coordinated sequences of suck/swallow/breathe with no liquid loss from breast or bottle; by 9 mo takes fewer sucks or suckles before pulling away from nipple or cup Suckles liquid from cup; loses liquid with cup removal or position change Uses upper lip to remove food from spoon; beginning chewing; diminished gag but may see with new textures	Breast milk Formula Juice Foods with different textures Mashed table foods	Breast Bottle Cup Spoon Fingers	Drools during teething By 9 mo no longer drools during gross motor activities	As for 0–4 and 4–6 mo Refuses strained foods consistently Gags, coughs, chokes with presentation of strained foods

Table 4-2. Feeding Development in the Infant and Toddler (continued)

Age (mo)	Developmental stage	Oral-motor skills and suck/swallow/breathe coordination	Food type	Utensil	Drooling	Red flags
10–12	Sits with increased ability to move or reach and maintain balance; moves in and out of sitting, hands and knees, and standing positions; creeps Finger feeding and cup drinking improve Uses spoon with minimal success May say single words; begins to use jargon	Long coordinated sequences of suck/swallow/breathe with no liquid loss from breast or bottle Tongue under cup to hold in mouth, upper lip comes down on cup; short suck/swallow sequences from cup with less liquid loss; may choke or cough if liquid flow is too fast Cleans off spoon with upper lip Sucking with some suckling to move food back in mouth; moves food with tongue from center to sides of mouth; chews with up-down and diagonal motion Controlled bite on soft cookie; breaks off pieces of hard solids	Breast milk Formula Table foods that are ground, mashed, or chopped, including easily chewed meats	Breast Bottle Cup Spoon Fingers	Rare except with teething May drool a little when trying new gross skills	Consistently upset or rejects presentation of lumpy or textured foods Presentation of lumpy or textured foods causes arching away, gagging or vomiting
15	Refines skills for self-feeding Picks up and drinks from cup with some spilling Feeds self from spoon with many spills Expressive jargon; may have 6 to 12 words	Swallowing follows sucking without pause when drinking from cup; sequence of at least 3 suck/swallows before pause Sucking pattern or mixture of sucking and suckling from spoon; may bite playfully on spoon; uses upper teeth to clean lower lip Chews with smooth coordinated diagonal rotary jaw movements.	Milk Juice Table foods that are ground, mashed, or chopped, including easily chewed meats	Cup Spoon Fingers	No longer drools with new gross motor skills Drools with teething May drool a little when trying new fine-motor skills	As for 10–12 mo

Table 4-2. Feeding Development in the Infant and Toddler (continued)

Age (mo)	Developmental stage	Oral-motor skills and suck/swallow/breathe coordination	Food type	Utensil	Drooling	Red flags
18	Sits unsupported at table; no longer needs high-chair Further refines skills for independent feeding May have up to 20 words; imitates new sounds and easy words	Bites on edge of cup; upper lip closes on edge of cup; uses suckling pattern to drink from cup Sustained bite on cookie Lip closure with chewing; may see food or saliva loss with chewing Elevates tongue tip to swallow; may see tongue protrusion when swallowing solids	Liquids Table foods coarsely chopped Most meats Some raw vegetables	Cup Spoon Fingers	No longer drools with fine-motor activities like self-feeding, undressing or random play Drools with teething	Gags or chokes when foods that require chewing are presented Pouches or stuffs food in mouth Thrusts or retracts jaw or tongue Retracts lips or has tonic bite when foods are placed in mouth for chewing
24	Uses spoon throughout meal without spilling Starts to use fork Drinks independently from cup Begins to combine 2 or more words	When drinking, holds cup between lips with up-down pattern; swallows liquid from cup with lip closure, more than 2 sucks, and no liquid loss Moves food side to side with tongue; swallows solids with no saliva or food loss No tongue protrusion with swallow	Same as 18 mo	Cup Spoon Fingers Fork	No longer drools with fine motor tasks or 2-3 word combinations	As for 18 mo Drools during or immediately after meals; drools with fine-motor activities; drools throughout day
24+	Further refines self-feeding skills Increase in 2-3 word combinations	Free sweeping motion of tongue to clean food from upper and lower lips; controlled jaw movements with biting; chews with combination of jaw movements	Same as 18 mo	Cup Spoon Fingers Fork	None	As for 18 and 24 mo

References: Wolf and Glass,[2] Morris and Klein,[3] Arvedson and Brodsk,[4] Alexander, Boehme, and Cupps,[5] and Morris.[6]

Table 4-3. Nutrition Screening for Feeding Problems

Does your baby/child eat: (circle all that apply)
Strained/pureed/baby foods: cereal juice fruit vegetable meat dinners egg yolk
Table foods: cereal bread pasta juice fruit vegetable meat poultry fish beans peanut butter cheese

How does your baby/child eat? (circle all that apply)
Breast Bottle Cup Spoon Fingers Fork Infant feeder Feeding tube

How often does your baby/child eat? every ______ hours; ______ times a day; ______ meals; ______ snacks

How do you know your baby/child is hungry? (circle all that apply)
Awakens Sucks on hands or fingers Fussy Cries Screams Says word/words that mean food Points

How do you know your baby/child is full? (circle all that apply)
Stops eating Falls asleep Spits out food or nipple Turns away from food/feeder Plays with food/easily distracted

What describes your baby's/child's usual feeding behavior?
[ ] Seems to enjoy eating, takes feedings easily, good appetite
[ ] Happy at beginning of feeding, then often gets fussy or distressed during feedings
[ ] Frequently has trouble breathing while eating
[ ] Often does not wake for feedings, tires easily with feedings, *or* often has difficulty finishing feedings
[ ] Eats slowly, usually takes more than 30 min (infant)/45 min (toddler) to eat (excluding time for diaper changes, play, etc.)
[ ] Frequently gags, coughs, *or* chokes during feedings
[ ] Refuses to eat, is difficult to feed, fussy throughout most of feeding, arches backward, *or* doesn't seem to enjoy eating
[ ] Picky eater, seems to eat very little, not interested in food or eating, *or* has poor appetite

Parents must learn to recognize cues for hunger and satiety, but these cues may not be clear.[7] Some infants may be sleepy or have difficulty achieving a quiet alert state. Others may be fretful and cry frequently before, during, and after feedings. Some infants may fall asleep or become easily distracted during feedings and seem to give signs of satiety before adequate amounts of milk are consumed. If the infant/child is fussing or crying much of the time, it may be difficult to distinguish hunger or satiety from other cues. When language skills are delayed, the toddler may have difficulty expressing specific needs. Parents who lead complicated and stressful lives may have needs that sometimes usurp the needs of their infant/child or make it difficult for them to perceive feeding cues.

Working hard to maintain a flexed position, block out distracting stimulation, or coordinate sucking with swallowing and breathing may exhaust the infant before an adequate amount of milk or food is consumed. Suck may be inefficient or ineffective due to position or placement of the tongue. Excluding breaks for diapering, playing, and so on, infants should be able to take in a full feeding in 10 to 20 minutes and toddlers in 30 to 45 minutes. Feeding for longer periods can exhaust both the infant/child and the parent. Premature infants may have decreased strength of flexor muscle groups, decreased strength of lip closure, and underdeveloped buccal pads that are important in developing sucking efficiency. A significant amount of milk or food may be lost due to inadequate lip closure in both the infant and toddler. The feeding therapist can help the parent achieve the best position and environment for feedings and identify appropriate therapy techniques and feeding equipment to enhance development of normal feeding skills.[7]

Inappropriate gag reflex may be due to neurological compromise or noxious stimulation such as endotracheal tubes, feeding tubes, and suctioning. The feeding therapist can identify feeding techniques or therapies that can help reduce or eliminate problems with hyperactive gag reflex. Inadequate gag reflex and/or frequent episodes of choking or coughing usually indicates an anatomical or neurological problem. A videofluoroscopic observation of sucking or chewing, formation of bolus, and swallowing may help identify a course of therapy.

Decreased development of flexor muscle groups and problems with airway maintenance may result in increased arching backward, making feedings difficult and frustrating for both infant/child and caregiver. This behavior may also be interpreted as a satiety cue, bringing feedings to an end before the infant/child has taken an adequate amount of food.

Toddlers who are picky eaters, seem to eat very little, or have little interest in food may just be responding to the normal decline in appetite that corresponds with the normal growth deceleration after the first year. Dental problems or difficulty chewing or swallowing may also contribute to poor appetites.

When nutrition screening shows that growth is falling below what is expected, careful evaluation of feeding behaviors becomes of greater importance. Screenings such as these can be used to identify infants/children who would benefit from a detailed evaluation by a feeding therapist.[2] Criteria for referral to a feeding specialist for more in-depth evaluation or treatment are given in table 4-4.

Table 4-4. Criteria for Referral to a Feeding Therapist

- Suck or swallow incoordination or weak suck
- Delayed or absent progress to spoon feedings or table foods within expected time
- Discomfort, increased fussiness, distressed, severe irritability, arching during feedings
- Disrupted breathing or apnea during feedings
- Lethargy, decreased arousal during feedings, tires easily and has difficulty finishing a feeding
- Feeding takes longer than 30 min for an infant or 45 min for a child
- Abnormal oral-motor anatomy or physiology: lips, tongue, jaw, or palate
- Choking, excessive gagging or recurrent coughing during feedings, toward the end of a feeding, or between feedings. This may signify a feeding problem or may be related to primary respiratory disease
- Recurrent vomiting during or after a feeding. This may signify a feeding problem or may be related to allergy or gastrointestinal disease
- Unexplained food refusal or inability to take adequate nutrition to support growth
- Physical symptoms or diagnoses such as dysphagia, recurrent pneumonia, aspiration, hypertonicity, hypotonicity, failure to thrive, or those listed in table 4-1.

Adapted with permission from Arvedson JC, Brodsky L.[4]

Feeding Assessment: History and Observation

Feeding assessment involves obtaining a detailed history and observing a feeding (see appendixes D and E). The goal in feeding assessment is to identify and define any feeding problems that may exist and to determine their underlying cause or constellation of causes.[2] Questions about feeding behaviors are more probing and require more time than those used for screening.

Historical information should be obtained from the caregiver who feeds the infant/child most frequently; their perceptions of the feeding problem can be invaluable. When feedings are not successful, caregivers may have feelings of failure or loss in self-confidence or control.[2] These feelings must be acknowledged. Given the sensitive nature of questions about feeding behaviors, it is extremely important to gather information in a supportive, nonthreatening manner. Building a strong, positive rapport with the caregivers sets the tone for future interactions and enlists their willingness to implement changes in feeding environment or techniques.[2]

After completing the feeding history, direct observation of feeding behaviors helps to better define a feeding problem and determine whether a referral to a feeding therapist is needed (see appendix E). The mental state of the infant/child, whether drowsy, quiet alert, or active alert, should be able to support the ability to consume an adequate amount of nutrients. Any signs of stress during feeding (table 4-5), extension motor patterns, abnormal oral-motor evaluation, suspect or abnormal findings, pouching food, frequent episodes of vomiting, rumination, excessive drooling, or loss of food from the mouth, are findings that may indicate the need for further evaluation and intervention by an experienced feeding therapist (see table 4-4).

Enhancing Development of Normal Behaviors

Infants/children are often seen at those times when new feeding skills are emerging. Parents may have questions or may need encouragement in supporting their infant/child through the different stages of feeding development. The tables in this section provide suggestions for choosing the right nipple (table 4-6), the transition from liquid to strained foods (table 4-7), the transition from strained to lumpy foods (table 4-8), choosing the correct cup (table 4-9), selecting the right spoon/fork (table 4-10), and determining readiness for self-feeding (table 4-11). Guidelines for enhancing nippling skills for prematurely born infants are given in chapter 7.

Table 4-5. Signs of Stress for Infants

Autonomic system	Motor system	State system	Self-regulatory system
Respiration: pauses, tachypnea gasping Color changes: paling around nares perioral duskiness mottled, cyanotic, gray, flushed, ruddy Visceral: hiccups, spitting up, straining as if actually producing a bowel movement Motor: seizures tremoring/startling twitching coughing sneezing yawning sighing	Fluctuating tone: flaccidity of trunk, extremities, face Hypertonicity: leg extensions salutes airplaning sitting on air arching finger splays tongue extension fisting Hyperflexions: trunk extremities fetal tuck Frantic, diffuse activity	Diffuse states: Sleep: twitches sounds jerky moves irregular respirations whimpers grimacing fussy in sleep Awake: eye floating glassy eyed strained fussy staring gaze aversion panicked, worried or dull look weak cry irritability abrupt state changes	May use the following to attempt to gain balance: Lowers state Postural changes Motoric strategies: leg/foot bracing hand clasping foot clasping finger folding hand to mouth sucking grasping hand holding tucking Good self-quieting and consolability Rhythmic, robust crying Clear sleep state Focused alertness with: shiny-eyed and focused attention animated expression frowning cheek softening "ooh" face cooing smiling

Adapted with permission from Als, H et al.[9]

Table 4-6. Choosing the Right Nipple for Bottle-Fed Infants

Size	Comfortable fit allows tongue to curl around it Does not trigger gag reflex Allows adequate space between nipple and tongue for effective tongue movements Provides greatest front-to-back contact for tongue to facilitate appropriate tongue movements on the nipple
Shape	Matches sucking skills and shape of mouth Standard shape fits tongue's central groove Flatter shape is similar to human nipple
Stiffness	Stays inflated during sucking If too soft, may collapse If too hard, infant may fatigue too quickly Softer nipples are helpful when infant has a weak suck or fatigues easily
Nipple hole	Allows flow that infant can handle easily without choking or sputtering Allows fast enough flow to prevent fatigue or frustration
Flow rate	Flow rates may be slow, medium, or fast: Too fast a rate may contribute to apnea/bradycardia, coughing or choking Too slow a rate may prolong feedings or cause fatigue or frustration Flow rates may be affected by: age of nipple thickness of liquid stiffness of nipple (softer nipples deliver faster flow)

Note: Try the same nipple for several feedings. Changing nipples frequently may cause nipple confusion. Match pacifier shape to shape of nipple (bottle or breast).

Suggested parent handouts: Klein and Delaney[10] p. 107.

References: Wolf and Glass,[2] Morris and Klein.[3]

Table 4-7. Facilitating Transition from Liquid to Strained Foods

Most babies start accepting strained foods from a spoon around 4 to 6 mo of age. Ways to prepare a baby for spoon feedings include:

- Encourage hand to mouth play
- Encourage toy to mouth play
- Provide toys that have a variety of textures to explore and cannot be swallowed
- Allow tastes of foods from the baby's fingers or from a clean toy or pacifier
- Use the spoon the baby will be using to give tastes of familiar liquids
- Gradually thicken liquids until they are baby food consistency

Suggested parent handouts: Klein and Delaney,[10] pp. 123–124.

Table 4-8. Facilitating the Transition from Strained Foods to Lumpy Foods

Most babies start accepting lumpy-textured foods around 7 to 9 mo of age. Ways to prepare a baby for lumpy foods include:

- Gradually thicken strained foods
- Gradually provide more texture in a familiar food, e.g., adding regular canned applesauce to strained applesauce or mixing graham cracker crumbs with strained food
- Offer mashed banana or mashed potato
- Mash other soft foods that require little chewing, such as scrambled egg
- Try foods that stick together easily, such as rice, spaghetti, or macaroni and cheese
- Provide soft cookies or graham crackers for finger-feeding

Suggested parent handouts: Morris and Klein[3] pp. 272–75; Klein and Delaney[10] pp. 131–35.

Table 4-9. Choosing the Correct Cup*

Cup characteristic	Comments
Cut-out lip	Useful for infants/toddlers who need to tuck the chin for drinking liquids
Flared lip	Useful for infants/toddlers who require extra jaw support
Wide-mouth	Useful for infants/toddlers who need to tuck the chin for drinking liquids
Lid	Allows independent drinking with fewer spills; allows for the feel of a regular cup and helps develop lip control; helpful in controlling flow rate
Spouted lid	Controls flow rate and helps get liquid from front to back of mouth for beginners; provides biting surface for child who needs to bite on edge of cup
Two handles	Assists the child who is beginning independent cup drinking skills or the child who may have difficulty with grasp
Weighted bottom	Useful if more controlled movements are needed for a child working on drinking from a cup independently
Straw	Straw drinking can be introduced as early as 11 mo, although this skill may not be fully developed until 2 to 2½ yr of age. Straw cups or cups with a straw hole in the lid are good starting tools for straw drinking

*Cup drinking with assistance can be initiated around 6 to 7 mo, although independent cup drinking may not occur until 24 mo. Consider the infant/toddler's individual needs and skill level when choosing a cup. Always use a cup that is shatterproof.

Suggested parent handouts: Klein and Delaney[10] pp. 175–83.

Table 4-10. Spoon and Fork Selection

- Always choose utensils made of shatterproof materials
- Short handles are easier for self-feeding
- Match the bowl of the spoon to the size of the child's mouth; the child should be able to cup tongue slightly at the edges of the spoon
- The shallower the bowl of the spoon, the easier the removal of food from the spoon

Suggested parent handouts: Klein and Delaney[10] p. 137.

Table 4-11. Determining Readiness for Self-Feeding*

- Swallows food of varying textures without problems
- Understands the feeding process
- Anticipates next bite when being fed
- Reaches for food when being fed
- Finger-feeds self
- Plays with food
- Shows food preferences
- Stable enough in sitting position to have arms free

*When positioning a child for self-feeding, be sure that the child can see the plate, bowl, or cup. Feet should be flat on a surface. Make sure the child can bring hands to mouth comfortably.

Suggested parent handouts: Klein and Delaney[10] pp. 145–54.

Summary

Many techniques are available to help parents overcome problems they may have with feeding their infant/child. It is important to identify and treat feeding problems as early as possible, before adversive or inappropriate compensatory behaviors begin to develop. If nutritional adequacy is a concern, a pediatric dietitian should be consulted. If medical problems such as gastroesophageal reflux or aspiration are suspected, the infant's/child's pediatrician should be contacted.

References

1. Humphry R. Impact of feeding problems on the parent-infant relationship. Infants Young Child 3: 30–38, 1991.
2. Wolf LS, Glass RP. Feeding and swallowing disorders in infancy: Assessment and management. Tucson: Therapy Skill Builders, 1992.
3. Morris SE, Klein MD. Pre-feeding skills: A comprehensive resource for feeding development. Tucson: Therapy Skill Builders, 1987.
4. Arvedson JC, Brodsky L. Pediatric swallowing and feeding: Assessment and management. San Diego: Singular Publishing Group,1993.
5. Alexander R, Boehme R, Cupps B. Normal development of functional motor skills. Tucson: Therapy Skill Builders, 1993.
6. Morris S. The normal acquisition of oral feeding skills: Implications for assessment and treatment. Meyer Palmer M, ed. Santa Barbara, Calif.: Therapeutic Media, 1982.
7. Coyner AB, Zelle RS. Habilitative approaches to facilitate more adaptive oral patterns related to eating and expressive language. In: Developmentally disabled infants and toddlers: Assessment and intervention. Philadelphia: Davis, 1983; 443–74.
8. Morgan AM et al. Neonatal neurobehavioral exam: A new instrument for quantitative analysis of neonatal neurological status. Phys Ther 68:1357, 1988.
9. Als H et al. Manual for assessment of preterm infant behavior (APIB). In: Fitzgerald HE, Lester BM, Yogman MW, eds. Theory and research in behavioral pediatrics, vol 1. New York: Plenum Press, 1982; 65–132.
10. Klein MD, Delaney TA. Feeding and nutrition for the child with special needs: Handouts for parents. Medvescek, CR, ed. Tucson: Therapy Skill Builders, 1994.
11. Aspen Reference Group, Caregiver education guide for children with developmental disabilities. Rockville, Md.: Aspen, 1994.

Nutrition Manual for At-Risk Infants and Toddlers
Janice Hovasi Cox, editor

5

GROWTH ASSESSMENT

Janice Hovasi Cox, MS, RD

Evaluation of growth is often considered the hallmark of nutrition assessment for infants and children. Weight for age and weight for length have long been used to help identify infants with varying degrees of undernutrition and obesity,[1,2] but aberrant growth is not always caused solely by inadequate or inappropriate nutrition. Growth is the ultimate outcome—the culmination of myriad interrelated processes including genetic potential; general health and development; presence of disease or disability; adequate shelter; a safe, loving, and nurturing environment; and adequate nutrition. This chapter is a review of the established norms for growth and general guidelines for using these norms when evaluating or interpreting an individual infant's or toddler's growth.

Growth assessment for infants and children under 3 years of age generally includes measurement of weight, supine length, head circumference, incremental growth, and comparison of these measurements to established norms. Weight is the most commonly used measure of growth, being relatively simple to determine accurately, and weight quickly reflects changes in diet or health. Standing height may be measured in children over 2 years of age, but care must be taken to compare this measurement to norms for standing height. Although length and height are closely correlated, they are not equal, differing by 0.6 to 2.2 cm (0.25-0.9 in.).[3] Although a sitting height index is available for children 2 years of age and older,[4] measurement of length is preferred in this age group.

Weight-for-length or weight-for-height norms allow evaluation of body size independently of age. This is particularly helpful in third-world countries where age may be uncertain. Weight divided by length or height squared (g/cm^2 or kg/m^2) is commonly called body mass index (BMI), whereas weight divided by length or height cubed (gm/cm^3) is usually called the ponderal index (PI).

Triceps and subscapular skin folds and arm muscle area are not used in the routine assessment of growth because accurate measurements are difficult to obtain, percentile ranges differ by only a few millimeters, and body fat stores may normally decrease during later infancy and early toddler years.[1] These measurements may be useful beyond infancy to further define the nutritional status of children whose other measurements of growth vary significantly from the norm.[5] Mid-arm circumference and triceps skin fold measurements are used to calculate upper arm muscle area and fat area (appendix N). These values may be compared with norms, although there is some controversy over whether young children can be identified as having excessive or inadequate body fat stores or being "muscle wasted" using these norms.[4, 5] Relative contribution of fat and muscle mass to overall weight may at least be identified.

Standard techniques for measurement of infants and young children are described in detail elsewhere.[1, 4-6] To enhance their validity and usefulness, all measurements must be (1) made using standard methods and equipment, (2) performed by adequately trained personnel, (3) monitored at regular intervals, and (4) accurately recorded.[7-9] Measurements of prematurely born infants and toddlers up to 24 months of age should be plotted at their age calculated from term rather than birth, often called "corrected age." (See chapter 7 for a more complete discussion of growth assessment in the prematurely born infant.)

Growth Charts and Tables

Various growth charts are available (see appendixes F through I). Each chart has been developed using different data sets and may be presented in a slightly different format. An understanding of the benefits and drawbacks of each chart provides a basis for its use in the interpretation or evaluation of growth for the individual infant or toddler.

National Center for Health Statistics (NCHS) percentiles (appendix F)[10]

Approximately 240 infants and toddlers of each sex were measured between 1930 and 1978 at The Fels Research Institute in Yellow Springs, Ohio, to provide the data for the NCHS percentile charts for boys and girls, from birth to 36 months of age. Infants were measured at 1, 3, 6, 9, and 12 months of age, and children were measured at six-month intervals. It is important to note that lengths were measured in the supine position.

More than 20,000 subjects ages 2 to 18 years were measured during the Health Examination Survey and the Health and Nutrition Examination Survey between 1963 and 1975 to provide the data for the NCHS percentile charts for boys and girls ages 2 to 18. Standing heights were measured in this population. Both data sets have statistically smoothed curves to generate the percentile charts for weight, length or height, head circumference, weight for length, and weight for height.

The benefits of using the NCHS charts are that (1) they are widely used and readily available, (2) they include weight-for-length and weight-for-height percentiles, and (3) they include subjects with a wide range of socioeconomic backgrounds. The drawbacks of using the NCHS charts are that (1) they do not address changes in rates of gain, (2) data were collected from a relatively small number of infants at wide time intervals, and (3) the majority of infants were formula-fed rather than breast-fed, with early introduction of solid foods.

Oregon Health Science Center Growth Record for Infants (appendix G)[11]

Birth measurements of infants of known gestational age provide the data for 26 to 40 weeks' gestation.[12] These do not represent postnatal growth, but rather fetal growth to term. Data beyond term were adapted from measurements in more than 4,000 children followed through the first year of life.[13]

The benefits of using the Oregon Growth Record for Infants are (1) the juxtaposition of birth data and early growth for infants who are born prematurely, (2) the large sample size from term to 1 year, and (3) all three parameters of growth are on the same side of the page. The drawbacks of using this chart are that (1) data for boys and girls are combined, (2) weight for length is not included, (3) it ends at 1 year, and (4) measurements are plotted on a logarithmic scale using only the metric system.

Infant Health and Developmental Program Growth Percentiles (appendix H)[14]

These charts were developed to describe the growth observed in very low birth weight (birth weight ≤ 1500 g) and low-birth-weight (birth weight 1501–2500 g) prematurely born (≤ 37 weeks' gestation) boys and girls from term age to 36 months "corrected age." Although percentiles for the low-birth-weight infants are quite similar to standard charts for infants born at term, growth percentiles for the very low birth weight infants are significantly lower than standard charts. The investigators admit that these charts do not necessarily represent ideal growth, and that infants whose growth parameters fall below the *mean* may require further analysis of medical, nutritional, and genetic factors.[15] The advantage of using these charts is the comparison of prematurely born infants to other prematurely born infants of similar birth weight. The disadvantages are that (1) growth data prior to term are not included, (2) the charts do not necessarily represent ideal growth, and (3) weight-for-length grids are not included. (See chapter 7 for a more complete discussion of growth in the prematurely born infant.)

Gairdner and Pearson Growth Charts (appendix I)[16, 17]

Data from 24 to 40 weeks' gestation represent measurements taken at birth of infants of known gestational age. Data from term to 24 months represent measurements of infants who were born at term.

The advantages of using the Gairdner/Pearson charts are (1) the juxtaposition of preterm growth to growth through 24 months' "corrected age"; (2) weight, length, and head circumference are on the same side of the page; and (3) ample space is available for recording growth velocity in addition to specific measurements and percentile ranking. Disadvantages include (1) weight for length is not included, (2) measurements are plotted on a logarithmic scale using only the metric system, and (3) lack of widespread availability and use in the United States.

Incremental Growth Tables

Incremental growth assessment requires that two measurements be taken at an adequate interval of time and averaged over the elapsed days, weeks, or months (see tables 5-1 through 5-5).[17, 19, 20] Although this is more cumbersome and perhaps unnecessary for every infant or child, incremental growth assessment may be useful to identify or evaluate:

Table 5-1. Incremental Weight Gain of Infants

Age (mo)	Weight gain (g/day)*	Weight gain (oz/wk)†
0–1	30 ± 9.4 (15)	3½–9
1–2	35 ± 8.5 (22)	5–10
2–3	27 ± 7.9 (15)	3½–8
3–4	20 ± 3.6 (15)	3½–4½
4–5	17 ± 3.4 (12)	3–5
5–6	16 ± 3.5 (11)	3–4
6–8	13 ± 2.4 (10)	2–4
8–10	12 ± 2.4 (9)	2–3
10–12	10 ± 2.3 (7)	2–3

*Mean ± 1 SD (5th percentile)
†Range is 5th to 95th percentile

Adapted with permission from Guo S, Roche AF, Fomon SJ, et al. Reference data on gains in weight and length during the first two years of life. J Pediatr 119:355, 1991.

Table 5-2. Incremental Weight Gain of Children

Age (yr)	kg/6 mo*	lb/6 mo*
1.0–1.5	1.32 (0.52–2.29) ♂	2.9 (1.1–5.0) ♂
	1.33 (0.43–2.08) ♀	2.9 (0.9–4.6) ♀
1.5–2.0	1.13 (0.46–1.81) ♂	2.5 (1.0–4.0) ♂
	1.21 (0.50–1.97) ♀	2.7 (1.1–4.3) ♀
2.0–2.5	1.03 (0.33–1.74) ♂	2.3 (0.7–3.8) ♂
	0.97 (0.36–1.87) ♀	2.1 (0.8–4.1) ♀
2.5–3.0	0.97 (0.41–1.64) ♂	2.1 (0.9–3.6) ♂
	1.02 (0.37–1.83) ♀	2.2 (0.8–4.0) ♀
3.0–3.5	0.98 (0.27–1.71) ♂	2.2 (0.8–3.6) ♂
	1.00 (0.42–1.80) ♀	2.2 (0.9–4.0) ♀
3.5–4.0	0.95 (0.36–1.63) ♂	2.1 (0.6–3.8) ♂
	0.98 (0.30–1.73) ♀	2.2 (0.8–3.8) ♀

*Values represent the mean (range 5th to 95th percentile).

Adapted from Baumgartner RN, Roche AF, Himes JH.[18] Used with permission of the publisher, © 1986, American Society for Clinical Nutrition.

Table 5-3. Incremental Linear Growth of Infants and Toddlers (Supine)

Age (mo)	Linear growth (mm/day)*	Linear growth (in./mo)†
0–3	1.07 ± 0.11 (0.89) ♂	1–1.5 ♂
	0.99 ± 0.13 (0.80) ♀	1–1.25 ♀
3–6	0.69 ± 0.08 (0.56) ♂	0.75–1 ♂ ♀
	0.67 ± 0.08 (0.55) ♀	
6–9	0.52 ± 0.05 (0.46) ♂	0.5–0.75 ♂ ♀
	0.52 ± 0.05 (0.45) ♀	
9–12	0.43 ± 0.04 (0.36) ♂	0.5 ♂ ♀
	0.44 ± 0.04 (0.36) ♀	
12–18	0.37 ± 0.09 (0.25) ♂	0.25–0.5 ♂ ♀
	0.38 ± 0.09 (0.25) ♀	
18–24	0.30 ± 0.08 (0.20) ♂	"
	0.31 ± 0.07 (0.22) ♀	
24–30	0.26 ± 0.06 (0.17) ♂	"
	0.26 ± 0.08 (0.18) ♀	
30–36	0.23 ± 0.06 (0.14) ♂	0.2–0.4 ♂ ♀
	0.23 ± 0.06 (0.15) ♀	

*Mean ± 1 S.D. (5th percentile) for males (♂) and females (♀).
†Range is 5th to 95th percentile for males (♂) and females (♀).

Adapted with permission from Guo S, Roche AF, Fomon SJ, et al.[19]

Table 5-4. Incremental Gains in Standing Height for Preschool Children

Age (yr)	cm/6 mo*	in./6 mo*
3.0–3.5	3.81 (2.64–5.00) ♂	1.5 (1–2) ♂
	3.79 (2.84–5.24) ♀	1.5 (1–2) ♀
3.5–4.0	3.59 (2.49–4.77) ♂	1.5 (1–1.75) ♂
	3.65 (2.72–4.97) ♀	1.5 (1–2) ♀

*Mean (range 5th to 95th percentile) for males (♂) and females (♀)

Adapted from Baumgartner RN, Roche AF, Himes JH.[18] Used with permission of the publisher, © 1986, American Society for Clinical Nutrition.

Table 5.5. Increments in Head Circumference During Infancy in Centimeters Per Month

	Boys		Girls	
Age interval (mo)	50th percentile cm/mo	5th–95th percentile cm/mo	50th percentile cm/mo	5th–95th percentile cm/mo
1–2	2.5	1.87–3.30	2.34	1.66–2.35
2–3	1.5	1.21–1.88	1.42	1.12–1.77
3–4	1.09	0.92–1.32	1.04	0.86–1.24
4–5	0.86	0.73–1.01	0.83	0.70–0.96
5–6	0.71	0.61–0.84	0.69	0.59–0.80
6–7	0.61	0.52–0.71	0.59	0.51–0.69
7–8	0.54	0.45–0.63	0.52	0.44–0.62
8–9	0.48	0.39–0.57	0.47	0.39–0.56
9–10	0.43	0.35–0.52	0.43	0.35–0.51
10–11	0.39	0.32–0.48	0.39	0.32–0.48
11–12	0.36	0.29–0.45	0.36	0.29–0.44

Reprinted with permission from Guo S, Roche AF, Moore WM.[20]

- Catch-up or lag-down growth when subject's measurements are above or below normal percentiles
- Significant shifts in percentile ranking
- Growth response to changes in nutrition over specific intervals of time (although accuracy of measurement and timing of feeding, urination, or stooling with respect to measurement become more important, especially for infants over short intervals of time[1]).

The most commonly used incremental growth tables are those generated from data collected at the University of Iowa during studies of infant growth and nutrition and from the Fels Longitudinal Study.[18–20] Growth data from more than 1,500 normal, term infants including those breast-fed and formula-fed were reported from these studies combined.

Intervals of measurement grow wider with age due to increased variation in daily weight gains and smaller daily or weekly increments in weight and length. Normal fluctuations in weight with feeding, urination, and defecation make more frequent assessment difficult beyond the first few months of life. The differences between monthly 5th and 50th percentile linear increments beyond 6 months of age are less than the margin of error for measurement, so that increments over 2 to 3 months are used. Data collected monthly are used for measurement of head circumference. Although daily or weekly gains have been calculated from these data, incremental growth for weight, length, and head circumference should be assessed over adequate periods of time to be clinically useful and valid.

Triceps Skin Fold, Arm Circumference, and Arm Muscle Area

Standards are available for comparison of triceps skin fold, upper-arm circumference, and arm muscle area from data collected on more than 20,000 subjects ages 2 to 18 years during the Health Examination Survey and the Health and Nutrition Examination Survey between 1963 and 1975.[4] Although use of these standards in the assessment of the individual child may be useful in determining relative leanness or fatness, these standards do not necessarily identify health risk nor should they be used to label children as "too fat" or "too lean." Most sources do not recommend that these measurements be used in the routine nutrition assessment of infants and young children.[5]

Growth Assessment/Interpretation

One of the most fascinating aspects of nutritional assessment in the pediatric population is the dynamic nature of growth. Nutrition is not the sole determinant of growth outcome, but it certainly plays an important role. Most screening tools include growth assessment as a measure of health, well-being, and nutritional adequacy. Although care must be taken in applying observations of postnatal growth from groups of children (growth charts) to the individual infant or child, guidelines for the identification of growth patterns that may warrant further investigation are summarized in table 5-6. When growth falls outside the norm, referral to a registered dietitian may be indicated to evaluate the processes that support growth:

- Genetic background
- Dietary intake (see chapter 3)
- Feeding skills (see chapter 4)
- Clinical condition (see chapter 6)
- Physical environment
- Emotional environment.

Growth During the First Month

Size at birth may be categorized as (1) appropriate for gestational age (AGA), with weight, length, and head circumference plotting within two standard deviations from the mean, or between the 10th and 90th percentiles on the Lubchenco Intrauterine Growth Chart[21]; (2) small for gestational age (SGA), with weight, length, and/or head circumference plotting below these established norms; and (3) large for gestational age (LGA), with weight, length, and/or head circumference plotting above these established norms. It is generally believed that size at birth is determined by length of gestation, maternal size, and the intrauterine environment, whereas subsequent growth reflects

Table 5-6. Criteria for Referral or Further Nutrition Evaluation

1. Weight loss or no weight gain evaluated at monthly intervals in infants and six-month intervals in children
2. Significant decline in percentile ranking (≥ 25 percentile shift)
3. Rate of weight gain for "corrected age" in infants:
   < 20 g/day (< 5 oz/wk) term–3 mo
   < 15 g/day (< 3½ oz/wk) 3–6 mo
   < 10 g/day (< 2 oz/wk) 6–9 mo
   < 7 g/day (< 1½ oz/wk) 9–12 mo
4. Rate of gain < 5th percentile in children
5. Weight for length, weight for height or body mass index < 5th or ≤ 10th percentile
6. Disproportional head growth in infants
7. Head circumference growth for corrected age:
   < 0.5 cm/wk term–3 mo
   < 0.25 cm/wk 3–6 mo*
   > 1.25 cm/wk any time during infancy*
8. Triceps skin fold (or triceps + subscapular skin fold) < 5th percentile or > 85th percentile for age
9. Arm muscle area < 5th percentile for age or height

Note: Growth assessment is but one parameter of overall nutritional assessment of the pediatric patient. Nutritional intake, feeding behaviors and skills, and clinical and laboratory components must also be included to provide a comprehensive assessment of nutritional status.

*Manser JJ. Growth in the high-risk infant.[40]

genetic determinants of both parents and postnatal environment, including access to adequate nutrition.[22, 23] Weight changes during the first few weeks of life reflect developmental maturity and physiological changes that occur during the transition from intrauterine to extrauterine life. In general, these changes may be described as follows:

- Infants initially lose 7–10% (up to 15–20% if born prematurely) of their birthweight during the first 4-8 days of life.[24-26]
- Birth weight is usually regained by 10–14 days of age, although infants born prematurely may not regain birth weight until 22 days of age.
- Infants born SGA may lose less and regain faster because their body composition and extracellular fluid volume reflects more their gestational maturity than size alone.[27]
- Subsequent weight gain generally is in the range of 21–36 g/day or 5–8 oz/week. Many factors can affect each of these generalizations. These parameters are particularly useful for assessing newborns who have been discharged from the hospital within 24 hours of birth, before they have reached their lowest weight and, for breast-fed infants, before the mother's milk supply has been fully established.

Growth During the First Year

When infants continue along growth channels present at birth, there is usually no cause for concern, provided that the channel of growth is between the NCHS 10th and 90th percentiles.[10] When infants' growth parameters fall outside established norms, or deviate significantly from their expected channel of growth, (1) measurements should be carefully checked for accuracy, (2) referral to a registered dietitian to evaluate the processes that support growth may be considered, and (3) a medical examination may be required to further investigate growth deviation and evaluate general health. Size at birth and its relationship to subsequent growth has been studied and reported in various ways.[22, 23, 28-36] Although a review of these reports may reveal findings that seem contradictory and confusing, several observations recur or are in close agreement:

- Most growth charts are composed of cross-sectional measurements of large numbers of children at various identified ages and do not necessarily represent an individual child's pattern of growth.
- Rates of growth during the first few months or years may vary widely as genetic and environmental factors replace maternal and intrauterine effects on growth.
- Infants born at the extremes of the distribution for growth are likely to experience catch-up or lag-down growth toward the mean during the first 6 months of age, with some continuing to shift channels of growth up to 2 years of age.[23, 28-36]
- *On average*, infants who are longer and heavier at birth remain longer and heavier throughout childhood, and infants who are shorter and lighter at birth remain shorter and lighter throughout childhood.[28] *Average* measurements for each group tend to approach the mean but do not converge.[28] *Individual* infants and children within these groups may shift growth channels as *rates* of gain among smaller infants may actually exceed those for larger infants.[31, 33-35]
- Of those infants whose growth shifts percentile ranking, 75% achieve a stable growth channel by 5 months of age and 95% achieve this by 13 months of age.[23, 36, 37]
- Excluding infants with well-defined causes of intrauterine growth retardation such as chromosomal disorders, severe malformations, intrauterine viral infections, or cerebral palsy, nearly 75% of infants SGA at birth achieve normal percentile rankings within the first year of life, and 85–90% do by 4 years of age. Linear catch-up growth is more gradual than weight catch-up.[34]
- Macrosomic infants born LGA due to hyperglycemia and hyperinsulinemia associated with maternal diabetes mellitus may have an increased incidence of obesity during late childhood and adolescence.[32]
- When growth parameters do not plot at similar percentile rankings, weight and head circumference may be observed in relationship to length and compared to norms.[10, 38]
- Although head circumference is not useful for nutrition screening,[10] a strong correlation exists between head circumference and length during the first year of life.[37] Ninety-five percent of the population have measurements within the ranges established by the following equations:

$$\text{head circumference (cm)} = [0.5 \text{ length} + 9.5] \pm 2.5 \text{ cm}$$
$$\text{head circumference (in.)} = [0.5 \text{ length} + 3.75] \pm 1 \text{ in.}$$

  Infants with head-circumference-to-length discrepancies greater than these calculated limits or head circumference outside established norms for age may require careful monitoring or further investigation for medical abnormalities.[10, 38]
- If weight for length falls below the NCHS 5th percentile, acute or subacute illness or nutritional deficiency may be suspected.[10]
- If weight for length falls above the NCHS 95th percentile, obesity may be suspected, although some infants and children may have a greater proportion of muscle tissue, which contributes to a high weight-to-length ratio.
- When linear growth parameters fall outside the normal range, parental size-specific adjustments can be used to further evaluate linear growth, although adjustments are not more than 2–3 cm (¾–1¼ in.) unless mid-parental height is less than 160 cm (63 in.) or more than 180 cm (70¾ in.).[39]

Typical Variations of Growth Patterns

Preemie catch-up growth. Head circumference shows catch-up growth first, then weight, then length.[14, 15, 40-43] See figure 5-1 for an example of catch-up growth following premature birth. Calorie intakes may average as much as 165 kcal per kilogram per day.[44] Weight for length may be difficult to assess until length is 50 cm (19½ in.), although weight for length at various gestational ages may be plotted using the Lubchenco Intrauterine Growth Chart.[21] Weight in grams multiplied by 100 and divided by length in centimeters cubed should fall within the range of 2.3 to 3.1 g/cm^3. For example, an infant who weighs 2700 g and is 48 cm long has a weight-for-length ratio of: $[2700 \text{ g} \times 100] \div [48]^3 = 270{,}000 \div 110{,}592 = 2.44$, which roughly corresponds with the 25th weight-for-length percentile for 40 weeks' gestation.

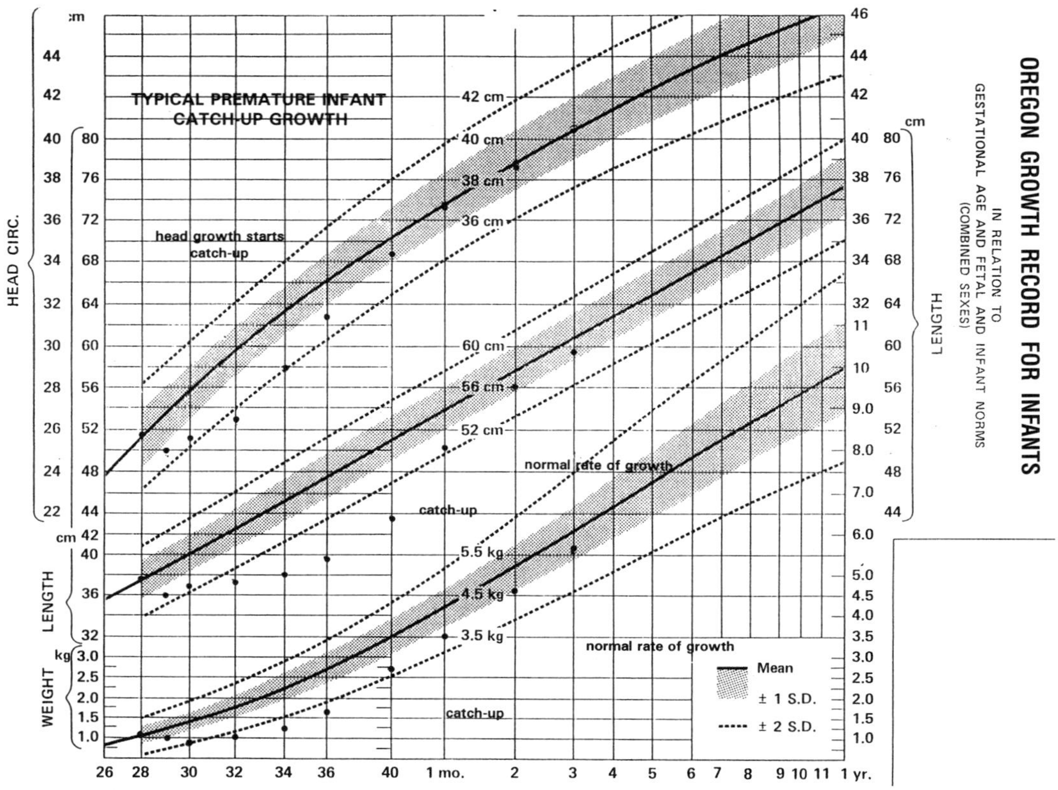

Figure 5-1. Typical premature infant catch-up growth. Growth chart used is the Oregon Growth Record. Used with permission.[11]

Term catch-up growth. Weight and head growth often catch up first, then length.[23] Weight for length usually plots within the NCHS 10th to 90th percentiles (see figure 5-2 for an example of catch-up growth). Growth recovery from protein-calorie malnutrition or other illness depends upon the timing and duration of the adverse conditions. Catch-up weight gain in infants and toddlers may average over 60 g (2 oz) per day until weight for length achieves a normal status, with calorie intakes averaging as much as 160 cal/kg/day.[1, 45]

Obesity. Weight gain generally accelerates first, with weight for length/height often exceeding the NCHS 95th percentile (or 130% of average weight for length/height). Weight for length/height between the NCHS 90th and 95th percentiles (or a weight at least 110% of average weight for length/height) may be classified as overweight.[1, 45] Accelerated linear growth and increased lean body mass may also accompany obesity, although weight for length/height remains high.[47] Obesity may be distinguished from catch-up growth in that head growth does not accelerate or "catch up" first or before length; head growth may or may not accelerate later (see figure 5-3 for an example of accelerated weight gain characteristic of obesity). Although often difficult to measure in infants and young children, triceps and subscapular skin folds and upper arm fat area greater than the 95th percentile may help distinguish children with high weights due to increased adiposity from those with increased muscularity.[1, 5]

Lag-down growth. Most commonly, lag-down growth is characterized by weight, length, and head growth decelerating simultaneously.[48] Weight and head circumference may decelerate simultaneously, with length decelerating earlier or later.[23, 31] Although not as common, weight may be the only parameter of growth to decelerate. The latter pattern of growth is sometimes difficult to distinguish from the growth of an infant or child who is failing to thrive. In lag-down growth, weight for length usually meets or exceeds the NCHS 5th percentile, and growth proceeds at a normal *rate* once a new channel of growth has been determined. This pattern of growth, also called "constitutional growth delay," may be accompanied by delayed skeletal age, but it is characterized by normal nutritional status, psychosocial status, and physical examination, also normal thyroid and endocrine function studies.[48] Growth should be monitored at regular intervals to identify subsequent changes in growth pattern. Further medical evaluation may be indicated (1) if growth continues to drift downward because the rate of growth continues to lag, (2) weight for length is below the NCHS 5th percentile, or (3) any parameter of growth falls below three standard deviations from

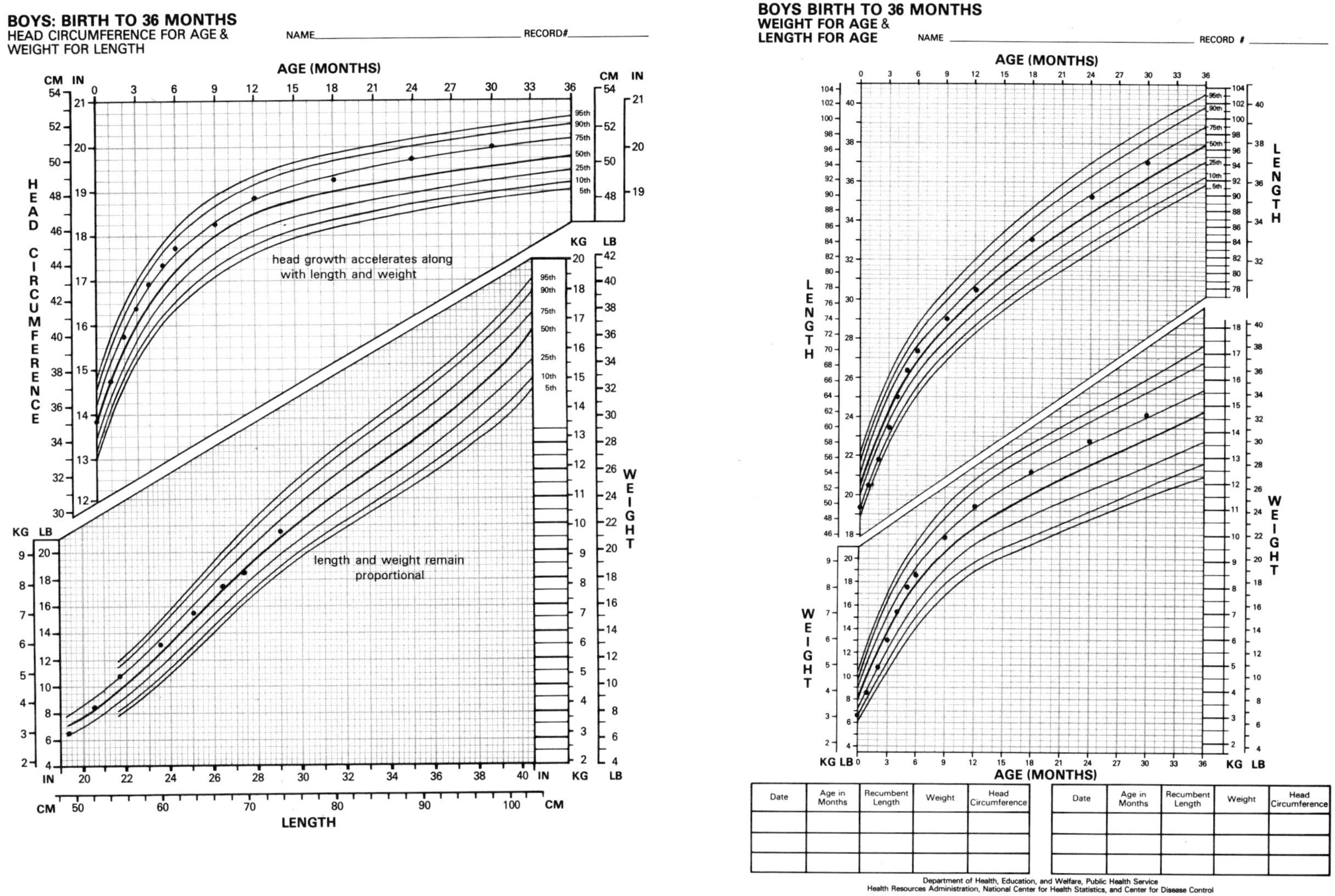

Figure 5-2. Term infant catch-up growth. Growth chart used is the National Center for Health Statistics growth chart. Used with permission of Mead Johnson Nutritionals.

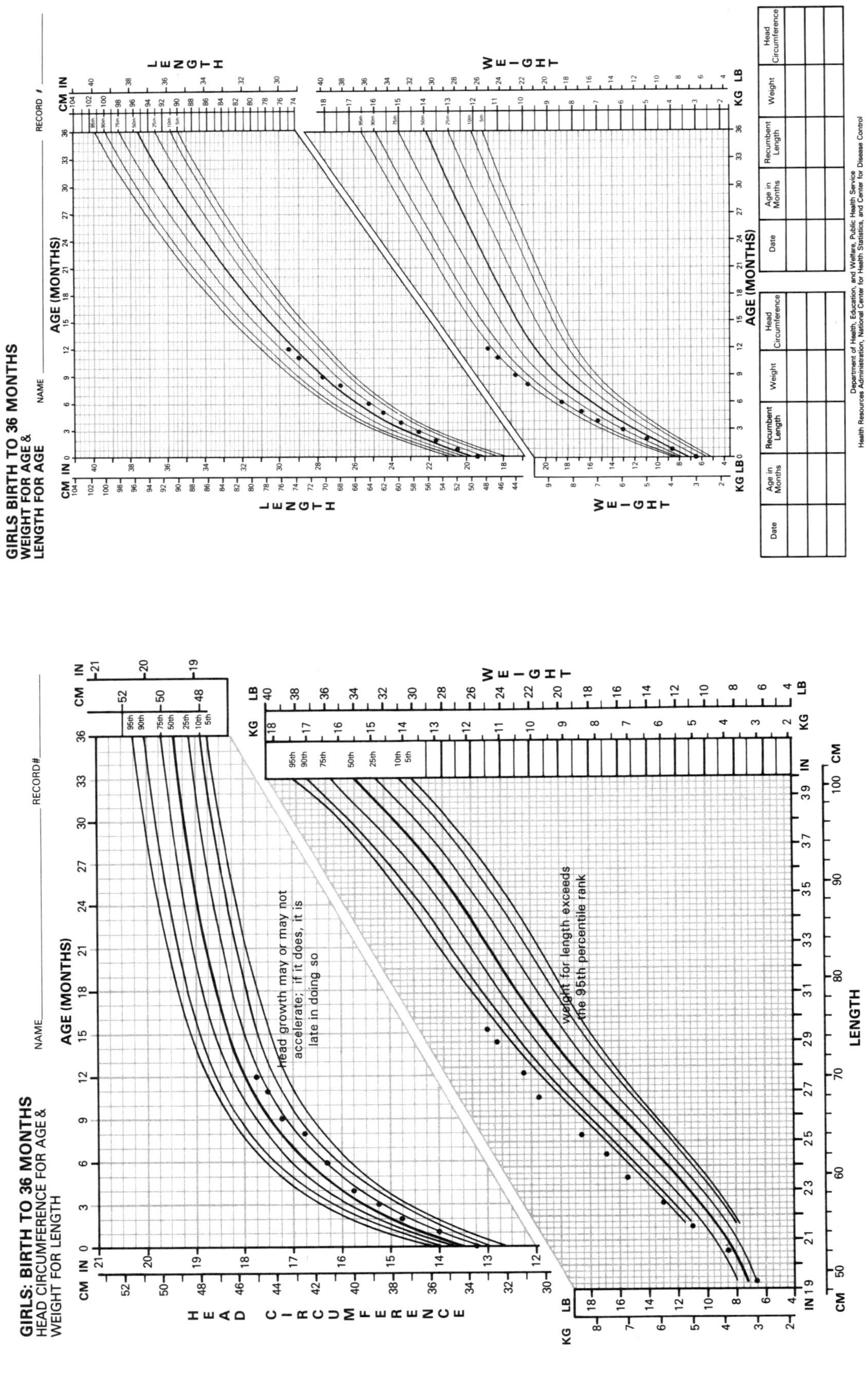

Figure 5-3. Obesity growth pattern. Growth chart used is the National Center for Health Statistics growth chart. Used with permission of Mead Johnson Nutritionals.

the mean (roughly 150% of the distance between the NCHS 50th and 5th percentiles).[48] (See figures 5-4 and 5-5 for examples of lag-down growth.)

Failure to thrive. A pattern of weight loss or a *rate* of gain less than two standard deviations below the mean for a period of at least two months duration characterizes failure to thrive during early infancy. Beyond 6 months of age, a faltering of growth for three or more months duration characterizes failure to thrive.[1] The faltering of weight generally precedes changes in other parameters of growth, so that weight for length or body mass index often falls below the NCHS 5th percentile. Recovery depends upon the severity, duration, and cause of growth faltering, but weight gain during recovery may proceed at a rate several times the normal rate for age (see figure 5-6 for an example of growth characteristic of an infant who is failing to thrive). Arm muscle area that falls below the 5th percentile for age or height may indicate low muscle mass; sum of skin folds or arm fat area less than the 5th percentile for age may indicate low adiposity and/or energy reserves.[4] Failure to thrive is a term that encompasses inadequate nurturing as well as nutritional parameters. (See chapter 9 for a more complete description and management recommendations concerning failure to thrive.)

Malnutrition. Beyond the initial stages of failure to thrive are the more severe states of malnutrition. Classifications are generally arbitrary, thus may not be consistent. Mild malnutrition is defined as a weight of 80–89%[1] (or 85–89%[2]) of expected weight for length/height; this roughly corresponds to a weight for length from below the 5th to at or above the 10th NCHS percentiles. Moderate malnutrition is defined as a weight that is 70–79%[1] (75–84%[2]) of expected weight for length/height. Severe malnutrition is defined as a weight less than 70%[1] (75%[2]) of expected weight for length/height. Both of these last classifications correspond to weight for length/height that is well below the NCHS 5th percentile.

Marasmus/kwashiorkor. If malnutrition is present for prolonged periods, linear growth may also decline. Prolonged semistarvation may result in marasmus, which is characterized by low length/height for age and low weight for length/height. Kwashiorkor is characterized by the presence of edema due to nutritionally induced hypoalbuminemia. Length/height may be somewhat low for age, but weight for length/height may be only slightly below the 5th percentile, or within the normal range, the latter primarily due to the presence of edema.[1]

Disproportional head growth. If head circumference is high or normal, but high relative to weight and length, this may represent abnormal head growth. The rate of head growth should be monitored (see above text and tables 5-5 and 5-6). This may also represent failure to thrive due to chronic illness or poor psychosocial environment if weight, length, and weight for length fall below normal parameters, even though head circumference falls within the normal range. If head circumference is low but weight and length are normal, this may represent abnormal head growth. The rate of head growth and its proportion to linear growth should be evaluated. Infants who have experienced intrapartum hypoxic-ischemic encephalopathy are at particular risk of microcephaly and neurological impairment. Identification of decelerating head growth during the first four months of life may help in the early identification of infants at greatest risk for neurologic sequelae.[49] If head circumference is normal but weight and length are high, the infant or child may be overweight or obese, particularly if weight for length is greater than the NCHS 95th percentile, although overfeeding can also cause accelerated linear growth, somewhat diminishing weight for length disproportion.

Growth in breast-fed versus formula-fed infants. Although many studies show no significant differences in growth between breast-fed and formula-fed infants during the first 12–18 months of life,[50-52] this has been a somewhat difficult aspect to study. Infants may be weaned, started on supplemental foods, or withdraw from the study at various ages. Slower velocities of linear growth and weight gain have been observed in separate studies, although growth remains within the limits of established norms.[53, 54] Because most growth charts are based primarily on formula-fed infants, the overall nutritional status of the breast-fed infant or child should be considered, and growth should be followed over a period of time before conclusions about inadequate growth and breast-feeding can be drawn.

Summary

Although growth evaluation is a routine component of nutrition assessment, aberrations in growth may be difficult to interpret. Parents are generally very interested in their child's growth. It is a measure of success in feeding and parenting. When growth does not fall within normal ranges, parents may become anxious and worried. Care should be taken to accurately measure, record, and interpret growth to avoid unnecessary parental concern. When growth parameters vary significantly from established norms and expectations based on genetic history, examination

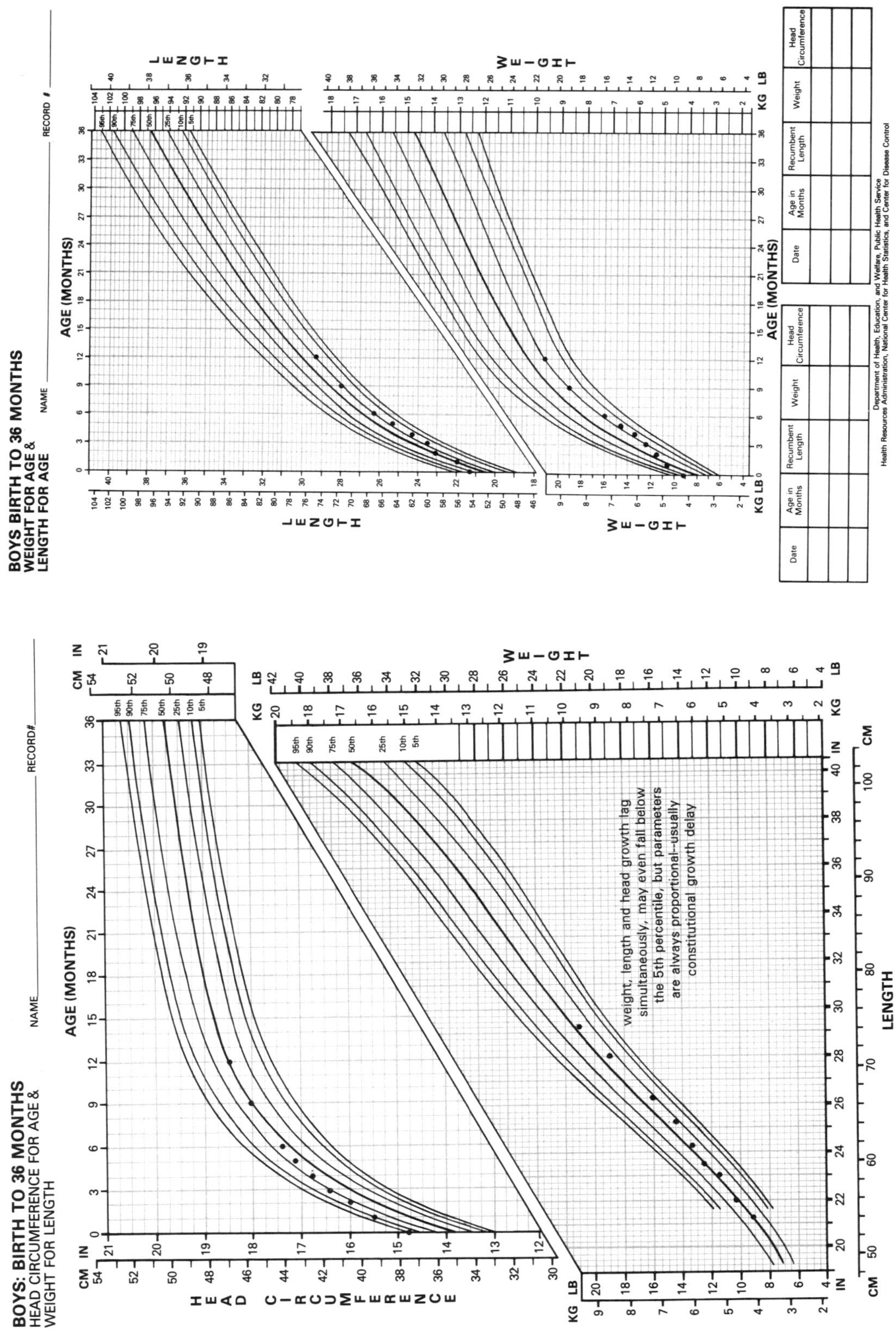

Figure 5-4. Typical lag-down growth pattern. Growth chart used is the National Center for Health Statistics growth chart. Used with permission of Mead Johnson Nutritionals.

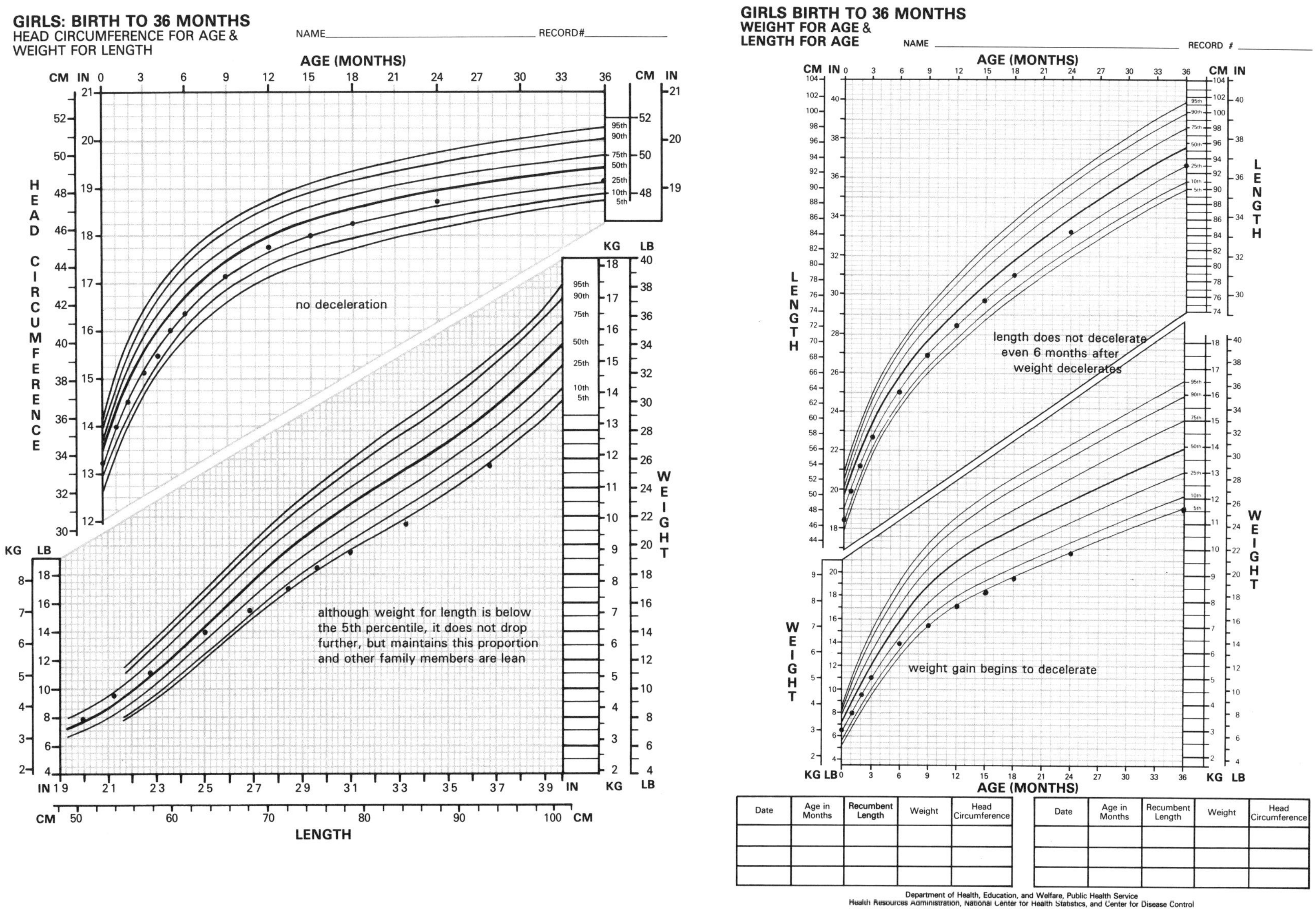

Figure 5-5. Alternate lag-down growth pattern. Growth chart used is the National Center for Health Statistics growth chart.[10] Used with permission of Mead Johnson Nutritionals Division, Mead Johnson and Company, Evansville, Indiana.

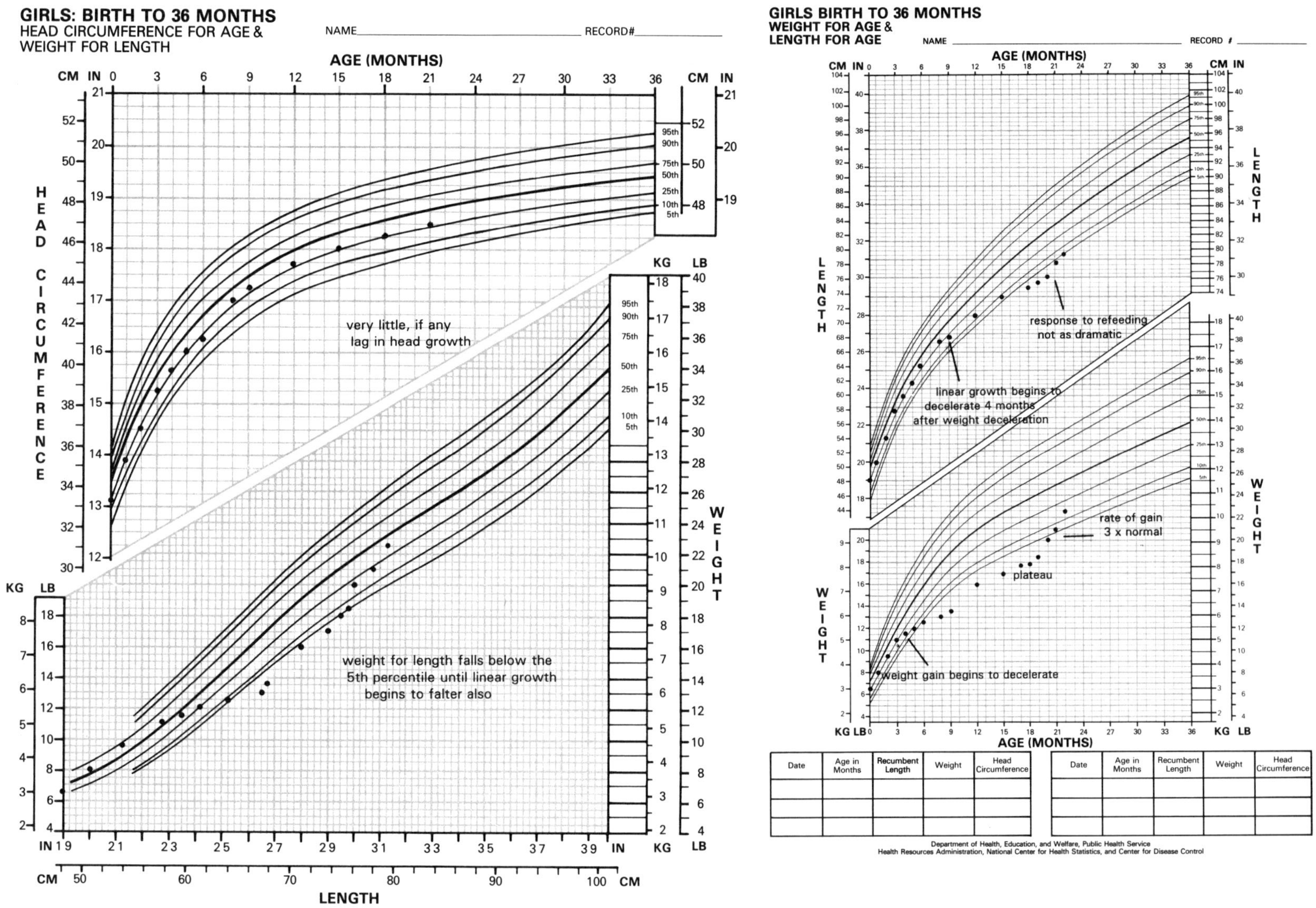

Figure 5-6. Growth pattern of an infant who is failing to thrive. Growth chart used is the National Center for Health Statistics growth chart.[10] Used with permission of Mead Johnson Nutritionals Division, Mead Johnson and Company, Evansville, Indiana.

of factors that contribute to growth should be evaluated by an experience registered dietitian to provide comprehensive information for the parents as well as for the physician who will be further evaluating growth.

References

1. Fomon S. Nutrition of normal infants. St. Louis: Mosby, 1993.
2. McLaren DS, Read WWWC. Classification of nutritional status in early childhood. Lancet 2:146–48, 1972.
3. Roche AF, Davis GH. Differences between recumbent length and stature within individuals. Growth 38:313–20, 1974.
4. Frisancho AR. Anthropometric standards for the assessment of growth and nutritional status. Ann Arbor: University Press, 1990.
5. Owen GM. Measurement, recording, and assessment of skinfold thickness in childhood and adolescence: report of a small meeting. Am J Clin Nutr 35:629–38, 1983.
6. U.S. Department of Health, Education, and Welfare, Public Health Service, Center for Disease Control, Atlanta. Evaluation of body size and physical growth of children. 1976.
7. Cooney K, Patyhak U, Watson A. Infant growth charts. Arch Dis Child 71: 159–60, 1994.
8. Doull IJM, McCaughey ES, Bailey BJ, et al. Reliability of infant length measurement. Arch Dis Child 72: 520–21, 1995.
9. Voss LD, Bailey BJR. Equipping the community to measure children's height: the reliability of portable instruments. Arch Dis Child 70:469–71, 1994.
10. Hamill PVV, Drizd TA, Johnson CL, et al. Physical growth: National Center for Health Statistics percentiles. Amer J Clin Nutr 32:607–29, 1979.
11. Babson SG, Benda GI. Growth graphs for the clinical assessment of infants of varying gestational age. J Pediatr 89:814–20, 1976.
12. Usher R, McLean F. Intrauterine growth of liveborn Caucasian infants at sea level. Standards obtained in seven dimensions of infants born between 25 and 42 weeks of gestation. J Pediatr 74:901, 1969.
13. Wingerd MA, Schoen EJ, Solomon IL. Growth standards in the first two years of life based on measurements of white and black children in a prepaid health care program. Pediatrics 47:81, 1971.
14. Casey PH, Kraemer HC, Bernbaum J, et al. Growth status and growth rates of a varied sample of low birth weight, preterm infants. A longitudinal cohort from birth to three years of age. J Pediatr 119:599–605, 1991.
15. Casey PH, Kraemer HC, Bernbaum J, et al. Growth patterns of low birth weight preterm infants: A longitudinal analysis of a large, varied sample. J Pediatr 117:298-307, 1990.
16. Gairdner D, Pearson J. Growth and development record, girls: preterm—2 years, length/weight/head circumference. Welwyn Garden City, Hertfordshire, England: Castlemead Publications, 1988.
17. Gairdner D, Pearson J. Growth and development record, boys: preterm—2 years, length/weight/head circumference. Welwyn Garden City, Hertfordshire, England: Castlemead Publications, 1988.
18. Baumgartner RN, Roche AF, Himes JH. Incremental growth tables: supplementary to previously published charts. Am J Clin Nutr 43: 711–22, 1986.
19. Guo S, Roche AF, Fomon SJ, et al. Reference data on gains in weight and length during the first two years of life. J Pediatr 119:355, 1991.
20. Guo S, Roche AF, Moore WM. Reference data for head circumference and 1-month increments from 1 to 12 months of age. J Pediatr 113:490–94, 1988.
21. Lubchenco LO, Hansman C, Boyd E. Intrauterine growth in length and head circumference as estimated from live births at gestational ages from 26 to 42 weeks. Pediatrics 37:403, 1966.
22. Pomerance HH, Krall JM. The relationship of birth size to the rate of growth in infancy and childhood. Am J Clin Nutr 39:95–99, 1984.
23. Smith DW, Truog W, Rogers JE, et al. Shifting linear growth during infancy: Illustration of genetic factors in growth from fetal life through infancy. J Pediatr 89:225–30, 1976.
24. Fanaroff AA, Martin RJ. Neonatal-perinatal medicine. Diseases of the fetus and infant. 4th ed. St. Louis: Mosby, 1987; 343, 364, 374–75.
25. Moya FR. Nutritional requirements of the term newborn. In: Suskind RM, ed. Textbook of pediatric nutrition. 2d ed. New York: Raven Press, 1993; 9.
26. Aherne W, Hall D. Brown adipose tissue and heat production in the newborn infant. J Pathol Bacteriol 91:233, 1966.
27. Bauer K, Cowett RM, Howard GM, et al. Effect of intrauterine growth retardation on postnatal weight change in preterm infants. J Pediatr 123:301–6, 1993.
28. Binkin NJ, Yip R, Fleshood L, et al. Birth weight and childhood growth. Pediatrics 82:828–34, 1988.
29. Davies DP, Beverley D. Changes in body proportions over the first year of life: Comparisons between 'light-for-dates' and 'appropriate-for-dates' term infants. Early Hum Dev 3:263–65, 1979.

30. Davies DP, Platts P, Pritchard JM, et al. Nutritional status of light-for-date infants at birth and its influence on early postnatal growth. Arch Dis Child 54:703–6, 1979.
31. Davies DP. Size at birth and growth in the first year of life of babies who are overweight and underweight at birth. Proc Nutr Soc 39:25–33, 1980.
32. Vohr BR, Lipsitt LP, Oh W. Somatic growth of children of diabetic mothers with reference to birth size. J Pediatr 97:196–99, 1980.
33. Wright CM, Matthews JNS, Waterston A, et al. What is a normal rate of weight gain in infancy? Acta Pædiatr 83:351–6, 1994.
34. Albertsson-Wikland K, Wennergren G, Wennergren M, et al. Longitudinal follow-up of growth in children born small for gestational age. Acta Pædiatr 82:438–43, 1993.
35. Hokken-Koelega ACS, De Ridder MAJ, Lemmen RJ, et al. Children born small for gestational age: Do they catch up? Pediatr Res 38: 267–71, 1995.
36. Jaffe M, Tal Y, Hadad B, et al. Variability in head circumference growth during the first 2 years of life. Pediatrics 90:190–2, 1990.
37. Tanner JM. Regulation of growth in size in mammals. Nature (London) 199:845, 1963.
38. Dine MS, Gartside PS, Glueck CJ. Relationship of head circumference to length in the first 400 days of life: A mnemonic. Pediatrics 67:506–07, 1981.
39. Himes JH, Roche AF, Thissen D, Moore WM. Parent-specific adjustments for evaluation of recumbent length and stature of children. Pediatrics 75:304–13, 1985.
40. Manser JJ. Growth in the high-risk infant. Clin Perinatol 11:19–40, 1984.
41. Ernst JA, Bull MJ, Rickard KA, et al. Growth outcome and feeding practices of the very low birth weight infant (less than 1,500 grams) within the first year of life. J Pediatr 117:S156, 1990.
42. Brandt I. Growth dynamics of low-birth-weight infants with emphasis on the perinatal period. In: Faulkner F, Tanner JM, eds. Human growth. vol. 2. Postnatal growth. New York: Plenum Press, 1978; 557–617.
43. Hack M, Breslau N, Weissman B, et al. Effect of very low birth weight and subnormal head size on cognitive abilities at school age. N Engl J Med 325:231, 1991.
44. European Society for Paediatric Gastroenterology and Nutrition (ESPGAN), Committee on Nutrition of the Preterm Infant. Nutrition and feeding of preterm infants. Acta Pædiatr Scand (suppl) 336:1, 1987.
45. Ashworth A, Millward DJ. Catch-up growth in children. Nutr Rev 44:157–163, 1986.
46. Dietz WH. Nutrition and obesity. In: Grand RJ, Sutphen JL, Dietz WH, eds. Pediatric nutrition: theory and practice. Boston: Butterworths, 1987.
47. Forbes GB. Lean body mass and fat in obese children. Pediatrics 34:308, 1964.
48. Underwood LE, Rosenfeld RG, Hintz RL. Human growth and growth disorders: An update. South San Francisco, Calif.: Genentech, Inc., 1985.
49. Cordes I, Roland EH, Lupton BA, et al. Early prediction of the development of microcephaly after hypoxic-ischemic encephalopathy in the full-term newborn. Pediatrics 93:703–07, 1994.
50. Köhler L, Meeuwisse G, Mortensson W. Food intake and growth of infants between six and twenty-six months of age on breast milk, cow's milk formula, or soy formula. Acta Pædiatr Scand 73:40–48, 1984.
51. Jung E, Czajka-Narinf DM. Birthweight doubling and tripling times: An updated look at the effects of birthweight, sex, race, and type of feeding. Am J Clin Nutr 42:182–89, 1985.
52. Saarinen UM, Siimes MA. Role of prolonged breast feeding in infant growth. Acta Pædiatr Scand 68:245–50, 1979.
53. Salmenparä L, Perheentupa J, Siimes MA. Exclusively breast-fed healthy infants grow slower than reference infants. Pediatr Res 3:307–12, 1985.
54. Dewey KG, Heinig MJ, Nommsen LA, et al. Growth of breast-fed and formula-fed infants from 0 to 18 months: The DARLING study. Pediatrics 89:1035–41, 1992.

Nutrition Manual for At-Risk Infants and Toddlers
Janice Hovasi Cox, editor

6

CLINICAL ASSESSMENT

Dena Goldberg, PhD, RD

Introduction

Thorough nutritional assessment of the infant or toddler with special health care needs involves an evaluation of anthropometric measurements (see chapter 5), biochemical indexes, clinical parameters, dietary intake (see chapter 3), eating concerns and behaviors, and oral motor development and feeding skills (see chapter 4). Clinical assessment is of particular importance in the presence of one or more of the following:

- Reported dietary intake does not seem to correspond to observed growth.
- The parent identifies a problem of diarrhea, constipation, vomiting, or other clinical symptom.
- Oral-motor dysfunction is present.
- Chronic use of prescription or over-the-counter medications or multiple drug therapy is present.

This chapter reviews the components of clinical assessment, including elimination, vomiting, drug/nutrient interactions, oral health, and nutrient deficiency. Each infant or child must be assessed individually with respect to individual physical, emotional, cultural, and socioeconomic circumstances. A particular clinical finding may be barely a nuisance for one family but an insurmountable problem for another. Thorough and practical clinical assessment should determine if an identified problem is among the following:

- A medical concern that requires referral to a physician for further assessment or treatment
- A feeding method issue requiring education of the parent for appropriate formula preparation, handling, or feeding
- A formula concern calling for consultation with the physician to identify the best formula or nutrition supplement alternative
- Not a concern, which requires education of the parent for appropriate perceptions of clinical parameters.

Elimination

Although stool frequency is often used to distinguish between normal and abnormal elimination, stool volume and consistency characteristics are usually of greater importance. Normal stool characteristics for the infant, which vary with the type of milk feeding, are described in table 6-1.[1]

Table 6-1. Normal Stool Characteristics

Human milk	Pasty, yellow, soft, seedy
Casein predominant	Formed, greenish brown, very little free water
Whey predominant	Small volume, pasty yellow, seedy, some free water
Hydrolyzed casein (with MCT oil)	Green, some mucous, small volume
Soy protein	Soft, yellow-green

Adapted from Hendricks KM, Walker WA. Manual of pediatric nutrition. Philadelphia: Decker, 1990. Used with permission of Mosby-Year Book.

The normal size, frequency, and consistency of bowel movements changes from birth through the preschool years. Although the frequency of bowel movements can be higher among breast-fed than formula-fed infants in early infancy, by 4 months of age most infants have two bowel movements a day.[2] After infancy, the frequency of stools decreases to one per day in the preschool child. Eighty-five percent of 1- to 4-year-old children have one bowel movement per day, with 96% in the range of once every other day to three times per day.[3] The rest of this section provides descriptions, causes, and treatments for acute diarrhea, chronic diarrhea, and constipation.

Acute Diarrhea

Diarrhea refers to an increase in the frequency, fluidity, or volume of stool compared to the individual's normal pattern.[4] Longitudinal studies indicate that children under 5 years of age experience between 1.3 to 2.3 episodes of diarrhea per year,[5] accounting for about 9–10.6% of all hospitalizations for this age group.[5, 6] Diarrhea accounts for 10% of all preventable postnatal deaths.[5, 7] These deaths are more related to social issues such as the race, age, and education of the child's mother and access to health care than the medical problems of the child.[5] Acute diarrhea can cause fluid and electrolyte losses and decreased nutrient absorption.[6] Fluid and electrolyte losses can lead to dehydration and acidosis, while decreased nutrient absorption can lead to malnutrition and impaired growth.[6, 8–10]

Causes. Acute diarrhea is caused by bacterial, viral, or parasitic infection in 50-75% of cases.[11] Other causes include infections outside the gastrointestinal tract, food poisoning, and side effects of medication.[7]

Treatment. Guidelines for the treatment of acute diarrhea are based on the presence and severity of dehydration. It is essential that the infant or child be rehydrated appropriately to prevent the dangers of prolonged acidosis and protracted vomiting with rapid refeeding.[12] The signs and symptoms of the various degrees of dehydration and recommended rehydration, fluid replacement, and dietary therapy are summarized in table 6-2.[6, 7] Recommendations for treatment of acute diarrhea include reestablishing hydration quickly, using oral rehydration solutions (ORS), and feeding a normal diet as soon as possible.[10, 12–20] Appropriate feeding practices during and after acute diarrhea minimize damage to the intestinal mucosa due to food restriction and the nutritional impact of the illness.[8, 9]

ORS are formulated to replace the composition and quantity of fluids lost. ORS solutions improve water and sodium chloride absorption from the intestine into the circulation because glucose and sodium absorption are coupled in the intestine.[7] According to the World Health Organization and the American Academy of Pediatrics (AAP), ORS used for rehydration should contain 75–90 mEq/L of sodium and a carbohydrate:Na ratio of 1-3:1.[6, 7, 13, 16] The 40–60 mEq/l of sodium contained in ORS in the United States is appropriate for prevention of dehydration and maintenance of hydration in infants and toddlers in this country.[6, 7, 21] Appendix C gives information on ORS solutions available in the United States. Carbonated beverages, coconut water, fruit juices, tea, sports beverages, and chicken broth should not be used for rehydration because they do not contain appropriate amounts of sugar and sodium to replace stool losses and can exacerbate the diarrhea.[6, 16]

If vomiting accompanies diarrhea, ORS may be given in minute doses of 5 ml (1 tsp) by spoon, syringe, or cup

Table 6-2. Diarrhea with Dehydration Treatment Chart

Degree of dehydration	Signs and symptoms	Rehydration therapy (within 4–6 hr)	Replacement of stool fluid losses	Dietary therapy
Mild (3–5% of body weight)	Slightly dry mouth and tongue, ↑ thirst	ORS* 50 ml/kg	10 ml/kg or ½ to 1 cup of ORS* for each diarrhea stool	Human milk or ½ to full-strength lactose-containing formula or undiluted lactose-free formula
Moderate (6–9% of body weight)	Sunken eyes, no tears, skin pinch retracts slowly, dry mouth and tongue, restless, irritable, ↑ thirst	ORS* 100 ml/kg	Same as above	Same as above
Severe (≥10% of body weight)	Drinks poorly or is unable to drink; signs of moderate dehydration with one of the following: rapid weak pulse, cyanosis, cold extremities, rapid breathing, lethargy, coma	Intravenous fluids (Ringer's lactate), 20 ml/kg/hr until pulse, perfusion, and mental status return to normal; then 50–100 ml/kg of ORS*	Same as above	Same as above

*ORS=Oral rehydration solutions such as Pedialyte or Infalyte.

Adapted with permission from Centers for Disease Control and Prevention.[6]

every one to two minutes until rehydration is accomplished.[6, 16, 21, 22] Feedings should be discontinued only if the infant or child is not alert, or intestinal obstruction is suspected (presence of marked abdominal distention or severe vomiting).[9, 16] As vomiting subsides, dose frequency may be decreased while volume is increased as tolerated. The usual diet should be started as soon as possible.

Advantages of continued feeding during diarrhea include faster recovery and prevention of (1) protein/calorie deficits, (2) damage to or delayed repair of the intestinal mucosa, (3) fasting-induced decrease in disaccharidase activity, (4) and disruption of breast-feeding.[8, 10, 12] Margolis et al reported that whether infants with mild diarrhea were fed their regular diet or a treatment diet did not affect the outcome or symptoms.[23] Infants on the restricted diet were hungrier, and parental compliance with the treatment diet was poor despite daily telephone contact. Studies reporting that early reintroduction of formula worsens diarrhea were completed in tertiary care centers, where infants were more likely to be malnourished or severely ill.[23]

The AAP recommendation regarding only gradual reintroduction of milk-based infant formula has been recently revised based on recent data indicating that after adequate rehydration, most infants and children (80% or more) tolerate full-strength milk-based formula.[6, 16] In spite of decreased lactase levels, few children have clinical signs or symptoms of malabsorption, and it is not necessary to restrict lactose.[9, 12, 13, 15, 16, 24, 25] Infants who are malnourished before the onset of diarrheal illness may have a prolonged duration of symptoms and are more likely to experience lactose intolerance. However, even malnourished infants should be fed using standard recommendations (table 6-2) unless evidence of intolerance occurs.

Appendix C lists lactose-free formulas for use with the small number of infants or children who continue to have loose, watery stools with increased flatulence and abdominal cramping, suggesting lactose intolerance. Formulas that have been marketed during the past several years for "management" of diarrhea are described in table 6-3.[26, 27] Isomil-DF changes only the consistency of the stool, not stool weight, nutrient absorption, or the duration of diarrhea.

Table 6-3. New Formulas Useful in the Treatment of Diarrhea

Lacto-free (Mead Johnson)

1. Differentiates lactose from protein intolerance
2. Allows change in carbohydrate without changing protein

Isomil-DF (Ross Laboratories*)

1. Does not affect volume or weight of stool output
2. Does not affect macronutrient absorption
3. Does not affect nutritional status during acute watery diarrhea
4. Does decrease duration of *liquid* stools

*Isomil-DF changes only the consistency of the stool—a rather "cosmetic" effect. Fiber in the mixed diets of older infants can effect the same result. Effects on long-term use, especially in the young infant, are not known (e.g., stool flora).

Reference: Brown KH, Perez F, Peerson JM, et al.[26]

However, the improved consistency of the stool may lead to greater infant comfort and may decrease the number of soiled diapers and linens. Fiber in the mixed diets of older infants can have the same result. The effects of long-term use—changes in intestinal microflora, especially in the young infant, for example—are not known.[26] Frequent formula changes can complicate diagnosis and management of diarrhea and should be made only after a specific food intolerance has been diagnosed.[10]

Solid foods usually consumed should be introduced within one day after rehydration in older infants and children.[8, 12–14] Foods high in complex carbohydrates (e.g., infant cereal for babies and rice, potatoes, pasta, crackers, and cereal) and foods containing fiber (e.g., beans, vegetables, and fresh fruit) for the toddler may decrease the duration of the diarrhea.[7, 28] Oral feedings that provide stool bulk also help restore normal bowel motility.[10] The traditional BRAT (banana, rice, applesauce, toast) diet is often recommended, although its efficacy has not been proven.[6, 7, 10] This diet, which includes starches and fruit, may seem to be a reasonable recommendation, but prolonged use does not meet calorie and protein needs.[6] Foods high in simple sugars, such as sweetened tea, juices, soft drinks, dilute gelatin, and presweetened cereals, should be avoided, because they can cause osmotic diarrhea.[6, 12] Because foods high in fat can delay gastric emptying, they may not be well tolerated initially.[6]

In summary, in almost all cases, children with acute diarrhea can continue their normal diet. Infants can continue to consume their usual milk feedings. Formulas do not need to be diluted. Infants and children should resume an appropriate diet for their age that is nutrient dense and easily digested.[7, 16]

Chronic Diarrhea

Diarrhea may be considered chronic if it lasts longer than 10 to 14 days.[16, 29, 30] Chronic nonspecific diarrhea (CNSD), the most common form in young children, typically occurs between ages 6 and 24 months.[31, 32] It is transitory; health and nutritional status are not affected.[32, 33] Chronic diarrhea may also occur in cystic fibrosis, pancreatic insufficiency, hepatobiliary disease, short bowel syndrome, celiac disease, and inborn errors of metabolism. Identification of the underlying cause facilitates effective treatment (see table 6-4).

Causes. Postulated causes of CNSD are disordered intestinal motility, food intolerance, excessive fluid intake, and restricted dietary fat intake.[4, 7, 31, 34] Because inadequately diluted formula is hyperosmolar, it can lead to diarrhea. Adding too much water when mixing formula can result in excessive fluid intake, thus leading to diarrhea. If a feeding is low in fat and inadequate in calories, the infant may consume excessive fluid while attempting to ingest adequate calories. Malabsorption of the carbohydrate in apple, pear, and grape juice has also been associated with CNSD.[34–38]

Chronic protracted diarrhea of infancy often is linked with mucosal injury, which causes malabsorption.[4, 19, 30, 31, 34] Signs and symptoms indicating that chronic diarrhea is due to protein, fat, or carbohydrate malabsorption or allergy and the appropriate dietary management are described in table 6-5.

Table 6-4. Chronic Diarrhea

Signs and symptoms	Causes	Dietary treatment
Carbohydrate		
Gas, bloating, cramps, loose watery stools Stool reducing substances > 0.5%; stool pH <6.0 Dehydration may or may not be present	Lactose intolerance most common: primary or secondary Secondary causes may be acute (Rotavirus) or chronic gastroenteritis, parasitic infestation, or antibiotic therapy Gluten or protein intolerance	Treat dehydration If primary cause, use alternate carbohydrate If secondary, 1–2 wk course lactose-free formula (breast feeding, no change) Yogurt with active culture or over-the-counter lactobacillus to reintroduce normal flora after course of antibiotics
Protein		
After starting foods containing wheat, stools become larger, softer, more frequent; abdominal distension, irritability, vomiting, poor weight gain	Gluten sensitivity enteropathy or celiac disease	Remove gluten from diet
Diarrhea usually with vomiting one to several hours after ingestion of offending food Atopic dermatitis and/or rhinoconjunctivitis or wheezing may be present Stool may contain blood Infant may have slow or poor weight gain	Allergy, sensitivity or intolerance to specific protein	Formulas with completely hydrolyzed protein: Alimentum (Ross Laboratories), Nutramigen (Mead Johnson), Pregestimil (Mead Johnson) Formulas containing amino acids as protein source, e.g., Neocate (SHS) Formulas with incompletely hydrolyzed protein such as Carnation Good Start are *not* suitable for management of allergy
Fat		
Large, bulky, oily, foul-smelling stools Usually with poor weight gain or unusually large intake with normal or less than normal weight gain	Fat malabsorption as seen in cystic fibrosis or pancreatic insufficiency or as seen in hepatobiliary disease Normal fat absorption ranges from 77 to 92%	Formulas with part of the fat content as MCT oil: Pregestimil (Mead Johnson), Alimentum (Ross Laboratories) Formula with only 3% of total calories as linoleic acid: Portagen, (Mead Johnson) may require linoleic acid supplement May need water-miscible form of vitamin A and E supplement; vitamin D and K supplement
Grey, white, or pale-colored stools	Hepatobiliary disease; bile salts may be reduced or absent, decreasing emulsification and absorption of fat	As above

Treatment. Inasmuch as CNSD is not associated with health changes, treatment involves providing parents reassurance, and helping them focus on the normal aspects of their child's health, such as growth.[32, 33] A high-fiber diet or psyllium compounds may relieve the symptoms.

In chronic protracted diarrhea, lactase is the first enzyme whose production decreases and the last to return to normal.[31] Problems with malabsorption may require the use of lactose-free or semielemental formulas until the intestinal mucosa has healed. If diarrhea is caused by chronic disease or is accompanied by malabsorption, diminished growth, or compromised nutritional status, the offending nutrient must be altered or omitted from the diet. Table 6-5 describes indications for protein hydrolysate formulas.

Table 6-5. Protein Hydrolysate and Amino Acid-Based Formula

Protein Hydrolysates: Alimentum (Ross Laboratories)
Nutramigen or Pregestimil (Mead Johnson)
NOT Carnation Good Start (Carnation)

Amino Acids: Neocate (SHS)

Indications:
- Sensitivity to intact protein(s)
- Pancreatic insufficiency, e.g., cystic fibrosis (Alimentum or Pregestimil)
- Severe malabsorption, short bowel syndrome
- Gastrointestinal tract immaturity
- Cholestasis (Pregestimil or Alimentum, although Portagen may be needed)
- Severe malnutrition (with small bowel atrophy)
- Lactose and sucrose intolerance

Constipation

In an infant or young child, constipation may be a transient problem that is easily resolved or may become a chronic problem that requires medical or surgical treatment.[2] Although normal frequency of stool passage encompasses a wide range, constipation is usually defined by the passage of hard, dry stools. Stool passage may be extraordinarily difficult[39, 40] and often contributes to discomfort, inconvenience, and family discord.[39, 41]

Causes. Constipation is commonly caused by insufficient fluid intake or increased fluid losses due to fever or diuresis. Inadequate dilution of powdered or concentrated liquid infant formulas can produce a high renal solute load, pulling all available free water for renal excretion and decreasing the amount of water available in the colon. Young infants, particularly those born prematurely, may have decreased intestinal motility due to gastrointestinal tract immaturity. Medications that slow peristalsis (e.g., tranxene, phenytoin, and lioresal) or diuretics that deplete fluids may also cause constipation.

Constipation may be associated with several structural, metabolic, and neurological disorders that influence gastrointestinal motility, distal colonic retention, and ease of defecation.[41] In most cases, constipation is not caused by an organic problem.[41] However, presence of an organic problem may be signaled by onset of constipation in the first few days of life, severe constipation that is not responsive to dietary or medical intervention, or constipation associated with abdominal distention and failure to thrive.[40, 42]

When stools are chronically hard and difficult to pass, a child may withhold stool to prevent pain or discomfort, causing stool to accumulate in the rectum and stretching the rectal wall. Encopresis may occur when the rectum is stretched maximally, allowing softer stool to leak out involuntarily.

Constipation is a common complaint in children with developmental disabilities due to generalized hypotonia, limited bowel muscle function, inadequate fluid intake, low fiber intake, or limited physical activity.[43] Although the prevalence of constipation and encopresis is high among individuals with mental retardation, even those with severe or profound mental retardation can be toilet-trained.[44]

Treatment. Dietary modification can control mild symptoms of acute constipation.[41] Young infants may benefit from assurance of appropriate formula dilution and adequate fluid intake. Inclusion of such laxative fruits as prunes, apricots, and plums or high-fiber vegetables such as peas, corn, potatoes, carrots, broccoli, and spinach in the diet of the older infant may be helpful.[45] The addition of corn syrup to infant formula is often recommended, although its efficacy has not been proven. Prune juice is a better alternative from a nutritional point of view. Occasionally, a laxative, preferably a malt-barley extract, is needed to increase stool softness.[41, 46]

The AAP recommends that except in very rare cases of altered iron metabolism,[47,48] all infants who are given formula receive iron-fortified formula throughout the first year to prevent iron-deficiency anemia. However, mothers may feel that the iron causes constipation or other gastrointestinal distress, having associated these side effects with iron supplements they took during pregnancy. Unlike in adults, adverse side effects from iron supplementation are rare in infants.[49] Research does not indicate that gastrointestinal problems such as colic, constipation, diarrhea, or regurgitation are more common among infants receiving a iron supplement or fed iron-fortified formulas compared to low-iron formulas.[48–52] However, when parents are trying to manage their infant's gastrointestinal distress, they may choose to avoid formula with iron. The "low-iron formula" may be perceived as containing enough iron, whereas standard formula may be perceived as a "high-iron formula" that contains too much iron. Because iron stores are generally adequate for the first 4–6 months of life, a *short-term* "therapeutic" trial of low-iron formula in the young infant should not be harmful, although it is not likely to be helpful. However, it is *imperative* that iron-fortified formula or an iron supplement be restarted before 4–6 months of age, when iron stores are becoming depleted.[47,53] Premature infants, who have smaller iron stores, should receive iron supplementation by 2 months of age.[53,54] Infants whose laboratory indexes reveal the presence of anemia may require additional iron supplements.

Increasing dietary fiber is an important component of the treatment of constipation in children.[55-57] The typical diet of American children is low in fiber.[58,59] The intake of fruits, vegetables, and whole grains recommended in the USDA Food Pyramid guide will help ensure a healthy level of dietary fiber intake for children.[57] Table 6-6 describes recommended intakes from these food groups. Children with constipation may need additional fiber. Dried beans and peas and bran cereals may be included in the diet of the toddler to provide additional fiber. Unprocessed bran can be added to such foods as cereals, applesauce, peanut butter, casseroles, and ground meats or used in preparation of baked goods, gradually increasing to 1–2 tbsp/day.[60] Dietary changes to increase fiber should be initiated slowly to increase acceptance and prevent such gastrointestinal side effects as bloating and flatulence.[56] Making the increase in dietary fiber a permanent dietary change for the whole family will make compliance for the child easier.[56]

It is imperative that children drink enough fluid when dietary fiber is increased. Guidelines for fluid intake on a high-fiber diet are presented in table 6-7. These guidelines are based on minimum requirements given in appendix K.[61,62] The recommended amount of fluid may need to be adjusted based on the child's usual fluid intake.

Table 6-6. Recommended Daily Fiber Intake Based on Food Guide Pyramid for Children Aged 1 to 3

Food group	Serving size	Number of servings
Fruit	1.2 or 1 small	2
Vegetable	¼ cup	3
Grain (whole grain foods provide more fiber than refined products)	½ slice bread ¼ cup cooked cereal ½ cup dry cereal ¼ cup rice or pasta	6

Increasing physical activity is another recommended treatment for constipation. For infants who are not yet very active, abdominal massage and moving the infant's legs while dressing and changing diapers or after bathing can help.[46]

Prevention. Prevention and treatment of constipation during infancy and toddler years is important to prevent stool retention and eventual encopresis.[41,63] Critical issues during infancy are (1) an awareness of normal variation in stooling patterns; (2) an understanding that straining is normal; and (3) avoiding unwarranted interventions such as formula changes, which may confirm the parents' perception of a problem when none exists. Avoidance of pain and issues of control during toilet training are important during the toddler years. Other contributing factors at all age levels may include family stress or dysfunction or the presence of hyperactivity/attention deficit disorder.[42]

Table 6-7. Guidelines for Fluid Intake on a High-Fiber Diet*

Weight lb (kg)	Fluid consumption per 24 hr oz (ml)
12 (5.5)	22 (660)
21 (9.5)	38 (1140)
26 (11.8)	44 (1320)
35 (15.9)	54 (1620)
44 (20.0)	64 (1920)

*Fluid recommendations given here are 20-30% higher than minimum fluid recommendations. See Appendix K for minimum fluid recommendations for infants and children.

Vomiting

Benign Vomiting

Infants commonly regurgitate small amounts of feedings.[64–66] In most cases this reflects physiological immaturity and resolves by 6 to 18 months of age. Health and growth are not affected. Factors contributing to this benign "spitting up" and suggestions for management are described in table 6-8. Although volume is used to differentiate spitting up from vomiting, the presence of other health problems is generally of greater importance.[66]

Vomiting that Affects Growth and/or Health

Vomiting can be serious and may be the result of the conditions described in table 6-9. If choking, respiratory problems, increased irritability, poor weight gain, or sudden refusal of feeding are present, a diagnostic workup is indicated.[66] Because infant stress and poor maternal-infant interaction can contribute to vomiting and failure to thrive, assessment of the problem may need to include an evaluation of the mother-infant relationship.[64]

Illness. Vomiting due to illness may be accompanied by other symptoms such as fever, diarrhea, dehydration, and electrolyte imbalance. The child should be evaluated for signs of dehydration. ORS may be given in small doses of 5 ml (1 tsp) by spoon, syringe, or cup every 1–2 minutes.[6, 16, 21, 22] Feedings should be discontinued only when the infant or child is not alert, or intestinal obstruction is suspected (presence of marked abdominal distention or severe vomiting).[9, 16] As vomiting subsides, dose frequency may be decreased while volume is increased as tolerated. The usual diet should be started as soon as possible. Formula preparation and storage techniques should be evaluated if food-borne illness is suspected.

Gastroesophageal reflux. Gastroesophageal reflux (GER) is the movement of stomach contents back into the esophagus.[65] In infants, GER is due to transient spontaneous relaxation of the lower esophageal sphincter or an increase in intra-abdominal pressure.[65, 67–69] At 2 months of age, about 50% of infants regurgitate at least twice daily, decreasing to 1% by 1 year of age. Most infants who develop GER will have symptoms by 6 weeks of age, and 60% will be free of symptoms by 18 months of age without intervention.[65, 68, 70] The greatest improvement is noted between 8–10 months of age when the infant sits upright. In addition to chronological age, factors affecting the incidence of GER include gestational age, state (awake, sleeping, crying), positioning, feeding, and caregiving activities.[69] GER is more common among premature than term infants. Infants are most likely to have GER when awake, compared to sleeping or crying, or in a supine versus prone position.[69] Caregiving activities such as diaper changes and oral, nasal, or pharyngeal suctioning tend to increase GER.[69]

GER is considered pathologic if it is associated with recurrent vomiting, failure to thrive, reactive airway disease or aspiration (especially in premature infants and children with neuromuscular disorders), or esophagitis.[69–71] Infants experiencing pain from GER may limit their food intake or refuse to eat.[65]

Treatment of gastroesphageal reflux is described below.[68, 72–78]

- *Size and frequency of feedings.* Many young infants cannot consume large volumes of milk or food at one time. A rule of thumb is about 1 oz/kg (about ½ oz/lb) body weight per feeding (at each of six feedings per day). Every-three-hour feedings would require 0.75 oz/kg (⅓ oz/lb) per feeding. If volume is still too great,

Table 6-8. Benign Vomiting or 'Spitting Up' Caused by Physiological Immaturity (Growth and Health Unaffected)

Overfeeding: Decrease feeding volume; may increase feeding frequency or formula density if overall intake is insufficient when decreasing volume

Swallowing air before or during feeding:
- Start feeding before infant reaches cries for prolonged time
- Support cheeks for good lip closure on nipple
- Position infant so that nipple can be easily and completely grasped
- Position bottle so that nipple is filled with milk
- Burp more frequently

Excessive stimulation: Create a calm, relaxed feeding environment by:
- Avoiding excessive handling or jostling during or after feedings
- Providing a quiet atmosphere
- Avoiding bright lights or other distracting visual stimulation

Reflux (may be present in 40-60% of all newborns, more common in prematurely born infants). The following measures may reduce reflux:
- Prone positioning after feedings
- Smaller, more frequent feedings
- Avoiding diaper changes immediately after feedings

Delayed gastric emptying:
- Avoid hyperosmolar formulas
- Avoid feedings with added fat which may further delay gastric emptying

Table 6-9. Causes/Characteristics of Vomiting that Affects Growth and/or Health

Illness, accompanied by diarrhea, dehydration, or electrolyte imbalance, may be caused by:
- Food-borne pathogens
- Inappropriate dilution of formula
- Outdated formula
- Inappropriate rehydration solutions

Gastroesophageal reflux may become a serious problem, causing:
- Regurgitation-malnutrition syndrome (growth failure)
- Esophagitis
- Respiratory symptoms (frequent upper respiratory tract illness, reactive airway disease, or aspiration pneumonia)

Allergy/intolerance, usually accompanied by:
- Diarrhea
- Atopic dermatitis
- Wheezing

Inborn error of metabolism, usually accompanied by:
- Failure to thrive
- Neurologic symptoms such as hypotonia, seizures, developmental delay, abnormal electroencephalogram (EEG)

Stricture/obstruction/ileus is often characterized by emesis that:
- Contains bile
- Contains blood or "coffee grounds"
- Is projectile
- Is accompanied by weight loss and dehydration or failure to thrive

using a concentrated formula (e.g., 24 cal/oz) will allow smaller volume feedings while maintaining adequate intake. Continuous tube feedings or transpyloric tube feedings may be required in extreme cases.

- *Positioning.* Horizontal or elevated (30°) prone positioning is recommended. Although the AAP recommends placing all healthy infants in the supine position for sleeping due to the association of the prone position with sudden infant death syndrome (SIDS), the prone position is appropriate for infants with GER.[79]
- *Thickening feedings.* Adding cereal (1 tbsp dry rice cereal/oz formula) is controversial. This technique may not work; it decreases emesis and crying, but not reflux; it increases sleep time and coughing and can make feedings difficult to manage.
- *Changing formula.* Unless vomiting is due to allergy, changing formulas is usually not effective. Smaller curd of elemental formulas may be effective; increasing osmolality of feeding may increase reflux. Although increasing the caloric density of formula can slightly increase osmolality, it can improve caloric intake with decreased volume.
- *Other dietary measures.* For children, weight reduction may be indicated if obesity is present; avoid high-fat foods, which may delay gastric emptying; avoid high-acid foods such as orange juice and tomato products; and avoid carbonated beverages.
- *Other conservative measures.* Avoid tight clothing, exposure to second-hand smoke, and unnecessary use of drugs that worsen GER.
- *Medication.* Medications may be given to enhance gastric emptying, increase sphincter pressure, decrease acid secretion, or neutralize gastric acid.
- *Surgery.* Nissen fundoplication (wrapping gastric fundus around distal esophagus) and pyloroplasty (loosening pyloric sphincter to enhance gastric emptying) may be indicated in extreme cases.

GER is more prevalent in the child with neurological impairment. These children are less likely to respond to medical management and more likely to require surgery. Aggressive nutritional therapy in these children can augment medical therapy and make surgery less risky.[68]

Allergy. Gastrointestinal symptoms are the most common signs of food sensitivity. Food protein–induced enteritis can cause delayed growth, although the diarrhea is less severe.[80] The most common causes during the first year of life are cow's milk and soy protein.[80] Other foods that commonly cause allergic reactions in children are eggs, peanuts, filberts, cashews, and fish.[81] The food antigen can be passed on to the infant in breast milk and cause a reaction.[80, 81] In most cases, adverse food reactions resolve by 3 years of age.[80]

Inborn errors of metabolism. Vomiting is one of the clinical symptoms in the newborn period of several inborn errors of metabolism, including methymalonic acidemia, phenylketonuria, and tyrosinemia.[82] These conditions respond to dietary management that includes restriction of the essential amino acid that can not be metabolized. Special formulas are available that allow the child to meet protein needs for growth and development and prevent the detrimental effects on brain development and physical growth of the accumulation of the essential amino acid that can not be degraded.

Drug/Nutrient Interactions

Prescription drugs can have a negative impact on nutritional status by interfering with nutrition absorption, utilization and excretion, or influencing appetite. Conversely, food and specific nutrients can impair the effectiveness of some drugs.[83]

Drug/nutrient interactions can be significant concerns for children with special health care needs because at least one of the following risk factors is often involved:

- Drugs used for more than six months at a time
- Multiple medications given at one time
- Marginal or poor nutritional intake
- Medications prescribed by different health care providers with no one coordinating all prescriptions.[84]

An evaluation of possible drug/nutrient interactions should be a part of the nutrition assessment of an infant or child with special health care needs. Information should include:

- All medication, vitamin/mineral supplements, and other supplements the child is taking
- Length of time each has been used
- Timing of drug administration in relation to meals and snacks
- Intake of any specific nutrients known to interact with current drugs.[84]

Multiple drug regimens, especially when the drugs are taken with meals, can cause gastrointestinal distress and lead to decreased food intake. Changing the timing of medication can alleviate the symptoms and improve food intake. It is important to remember that when medications are administered through a feeding tube, they can adhere to the plastic feeding bag or tube, resulting in a decreased dosage.[84]

Information on nutrition-related side effects of medications commonly given to children with special health care needs is given in appendix J.[85] Suggestions for alleviating these side effects are described in table 6-10.

Oral Health

Children with special health care needs are at high risk for caries (tooth decay) and periodontal (gum) disease. Due to the complex medical, psychosocial, and feeding problems a child with special health care needs may experience, oral hygiene is an area often overlooked. A program of regular oral hygiene is essential, because poor dental health can impair chewing, make eating painful or unpleasant, and decrease food intake.[87] Oral dental health concerns are summarized in table 6-11.[87, 88]

Nutrient Deficiency

Included in a comprehensive nutrition assessment is a physical examination for clinical signs of nutrient deficiency.[89, 90] These clinical signs, which represent an advanced state of nutrient depletion, are described in table 6-12.[90] Although some physical symptoms of nutrient deficiency are characteristic of a deficiency of one nutrient, most indicate deficiency of more than one nutrient.[89] Presence of any of these physical findings should be followed by a medical referral and laboratory tests or other studies to confirm the deficient state.[89] Suggested laboratory tests to confirm nutrient deficiencies are included in table 6-12.

Gastrointestinal disease

Gastrointestinal disease encompasses a broad range of congenital or medical conditions that may interfere with normal gastrointestinal functions of ingesting and transporting food, then digesting and absorbing nutrients in adequate amounts to support normal growth and development. Table 6-13 provides a list of the more commonly encountered gastrointestinal diseases that are associated with nutritional problems.

Table 6-10. Dietary Suggestions to Aid in the Relief of Nutrition-Related Side Effects of Drugs

Nausea
- Honor food references. Disliked foods may aggravate nausea
- Offer small quantities of easily digestible foods at frequent intervals. Eat slowly
- Reduce food volume at meals. Serve liquids after meal or limit liquid intake with meals
- Eat toasted dry enriched white bread, crackers, or graham crackers, cooked or dry ready-to-eat cereals early in the morning or before rising
- Serve cold, clear or carbonated liquids or juices. Avoid lukewarm beverages
- Avoid fried, greasy or fatty foods
- Cold foods may be better tolerated than hot foods, as hot aromas may aggravate nausea
- If nausea occurs at consistent times each day, reschedule meal and snack times

Epigastric Distress
- After drug administration, remain upright for 15-30 minutes
- Evaluate dietary habits for specific foods or beverages that may contribute to epigastric distress
- Offer small quantities of food at frequent intervals in a relaxed environment. Avoid overeating
- Avoid extremely hot or extremely cold foods or liquids (may stimulate acid secretion)
- Limit caffeine, decaffeinated coffee, colas, peppermint, chocolate, pepper, chili powder, and spicy food
- Limit citrus juices, tomato products, and other highly acidic foods
- Avoid greasy, fried fatty foods (may delay gastric emptying)
- Evaluate the intake of milk or cream (may stimulate acid secretion)
- Avoid eating at least one hour before bedtime

Loss of Appetite
- Create a pleasant environment for eating. If possible, eliminate distractions and time pressure
- If early satiety occurs or meals are not well tolerated, offer small, frequent attractive meals or snacks
- Enhance flavors by using seasonings. Marinate meat in sauces or fruit juice
- Encourage weakened patients to select foods that require minimal eating effort

Appetite Stimulation
- Educate caregiver that certain drugs may increase appetite and desire for sweets
- Encourage slow eating
- Encourage intake of low-calorie foods, condiments, beverages, and snacks
- Incorporate high-fiber foods or snacks that may contribute to early satiety
- Instruct caregiver to control access to specific high-calorie foods, snacks, or beverages

Adapted with permission from Pronsky ZM. Powers and Moore's food-medication interactions. 9th ed. Pottstown, Pa.: Food-Medication Interactions, 1995.

Table 6-11. Oral Health Concerns

Problem	Comments and examples
Oral sensitivity	Often seen in children who have been mechanically ventilated or on tube feedings. May cause delays in feeding progression from tube to nipple, from nipple to spoon, or from pureed foods to foods with greater texture; hyperactive gag reflex associated with increased oral sensitivity may contribute to vomiting and poor oral intake. Makes tooth brushing and other aspects of oral hygiene difficult
Medications	Dilantin can cause gingival overgrowth that can impair mastication or trap food debris. Some medications can cause dry mouth. The decreased saliva can impair chewing and swallowing and increase susceptibility to dental caries and other oral infections. Adequate saliva is essential to oral health
Poor oral musculature coordination	Movement of the tongue, cheek, and lip muscles aids in cleaning the oral cavity by removing food particles that become lodged on the teeth
Prolonged dependence on the bottle	Frequent exposure of the teeth to sugar-containing beverages such as milk, fruit juice or drink, and formula can lead to "baby bottle tooth decay," the leading cause of caries among children under age 3
Chewing and swallowing difficulties	Chewing and swallowing difficulties may require the consumption of soft and/or pureed foods that stick to the teeth and take a long time to remove. Firm-textured foods are needed to stimulate the oral facial musculature

Reprinted with permission from Faine M. Dental nutrition concerns of children with special health care needs. Nutr Focus July/Aug 1992. Nutrition Section, CHDD, University of Washington, Seattle.

Table 6-12. Clinical Signs/Symptoms of Nutrient Deficiency

Clinical sign	Suspect nutrient	Laboratory findings
Epithelial		
Skin		
Xerosis, dry scaling	Essential fatty acids	Triene/tetraene ratio >0.4
Hyperkeratosis, plaques around hair follicles	Vitamin A	↓ plasma retinol
Ecchymoses, petechiae	Vitamins K and C	Prolonged prothrombin time ↓ serum ascorbic acid
Acrodermatitis enteropathica	Zinc	↓ plasma/serum zinc
Hair		
Easily plucked, dyspigmented, dull	Protein/energy	↓ total serum protein, albumin and transferrin
Nails		
Thin, spoon-shaped	Iron	↓ serum iron, ↑ TIBC
Mouth, lips, and tongue		
Angular stomatitis (inflammation at the corners of the mouth)	Riboflavin	↓ RBC glutathione reductase
Cheilosis (reddened lips with fissures at angles)	Riboflavin Vitamin B_6	↓ RBC glutathione reductase ↓ pyridoxal phosphate
Glossitis (inflammation of tongue)	Riboflavin, Vitamin B_6, Niacin	As above ↓ plasma tryptophan ↓ urinary N-methyl nicotinamide
Magenta tongue	Riboflavin	See above
Tongue edema or fissures	Niacin	See above
Spongy, bleeding gums	Vitamin C	↓ plasma ascorbic acid
Ocular		
Pale conjunctivae due to anemia	Iron Folic acid Vitamin B_{12} Copper	↓ serum iron, ↑ TIBC ↓ serum or RBC folic acid ↓ serum B_{12} ↓ serum copper or ceruloplasmin
Bitot's spots (grayish, yellow or white foamy spots on the whites of the eye); conjunctival or corneal xerosis, keratomalacia (softening of part or all of cornea)	Vitamin A	↓ plasma retinol
Musculoskeletal		
Rickets: craniotabes (thinning of the inner table of the skull); palpable enlargement of the costochondral junctions (rachitic rosary); thickening of wrists and ankles; bowing of legs if weight-bearing	Vitamin D	↓ 25-OH vitamin D ↑ alkaline phosphatase ± ↓ serum calcium ± ↓ serum phosphorus X-ray of long bones

Table 6-12. Clinical Signs/Symptoms of Nutrient Deficiency (continued)

Clinical sign	Suspect nutrient	Laboratory findings
Osteopenia: Decreased bone density on x-ray	Calcium	↓ serum calcium, ↑ PTH ↑ 1,25 $(OH)_2$ D_3
	Phosphorus	↓ urinary phosphorus ↑ urinary calcium
Bone pain	Phosphorus	As above
Skeletal lesions	Copper	↓ serum copper or ceruloplasmin X-ray changes similar to scurvy
Scurvy (tenderness of extremities, hemorrhages under periosteum of long bones; enlargement of costochondral junction; cessation of osteogenesis of long bones)	Vitamin C	↓ serum ascorbic acid Abnormal long bone x-rays due to abnormal collagen formation
Muscle wasting, prominence of body skeleton, poor muscle tone	Protein/energy	↓ arm muscle circumference, area ↓ serum protein
Generalized hypotonia; cardiomyopathy	Carnitine	↓ serum carnitine; nonketotic hypoglycemia during periods of stress or high fever
General		
Edema	Protein	↓ serum protein, albumin
Pallor due to anemia	Iron Vitamin E (premature infants) Folic acid Vitamin B_{12} Copper	↓ serum iron; ↑ TIBC Hemolysis on blood smear ↓ serum folic acid; macrocytosis ↓ serum B_{12}; macrocytosis ↓ serum copper
Poor growth	Zinc Carnitine	↓ serum/plasma zinc ↓ plasma acyl carnitine/free carnitine ratio
Poor wound healing; increased susceptibility to infection	Zinc	As above
Internal Systems		
Nervous system		
Mental confusion	Protein Thiamin	↓ serum proteins ↓ RBC transketolase
Cardiovascular: beriberi (enlarged heart, congestive heart failure, tachycardia)	Thiamin	As above
Tachycardia due to anemia	As above	As above
Gastrointestinal		
Hepatomegaly	Protein/energy Carnitine	↓ serum proteins ↓ serum carnitine; nonketotic hypoglycemia during stress or high fever
Glandular		
Thyroid enlargement	Iodine	↓ total serum iodine: inorganic PBI

Adapted with permission from Kerner Jr. JA. Manual of pediatric parenteral nutrition. New York: Churchill Livingstone, 1983; 22–23. Used with permission of Churchill Livingstone, © 1983.

Table 6-13. Gastrointestinal Anomalies, Diseases, and Conditions that Often Require Nutrition Intervention

Disease/condition	Common nutrition-related problems	Nutrition intervention
Cleft lip/palate	Inadequate lip seal on nipple; inefficient sucking; regurgitation of fluid through the nose; choking and/or gagging during feedings; decreased endurance with oral feedings; difficulty chewing if malocclusion present; slow weight gain	For breast-feeding with cleft lip, hold infant so that the side with cleft is against the breast, allowing breast to fill the cleft; for cleft lip or palate, initiate let-down before putting infant to breast; massage breast and manually express milk during feeding to help infant empty breast; when bottle-feeding, use elongated nipple with large base, cross-cut hole, or variable flow-rate nipple; hold infant in a semiupright position (45–60°); use flexible plastic bottle, squeezing small amounts rhythmically to assist feeding; limit feeding sessions to 20–30 min to avoid fatigue; supplement with high-calorie formulas or tube feedings if necessary to support normal growth; consult with feeding therapist; may require videofluoroscopy if choking persistent or life threatening
Micrognathia	Small lower jaw may not allow adequate closure on nipple; tongue may fall back and occlude airway if infant is placed on back	Jaw and chin support during feedings; feed in prone position, lying down for breast-feeding or with angled bottle; use high-calorie formulas or tube feedings if necessary to support normal growth; consult with feeding therapist if growth is slow or feeding sessions are prolonged
Esophageal atresia (and/or tracheoesophageal fistula)	Esophagus may be narrow or lack patency; after surgical repair, complications may include anastomosis leakage, strictures, dysmotility, gastroesophageal reflux, vomiting, and poor weight gain due to inadequate intake or vomiting; movement of liquids or food from the mouth to the stomach may be slow or difficult; foods may become stuck in the esophagus and block other foods or liquids from getting to the stomach	Frequent small feedings of high nutrient density; feedings of pureed food or foods with greater texture should not be started without approval of the physician (usually the surgeon); infant foods that are more likely to become stuck are junior foods, food with lumps, foods that require chewing, and stringy foods; feed infants or toddlers in an upright position to let gravity help move food down the esophagus to the stomach; before starting solids, give infants heavier liquids such as peach or pear nectar; progress to strained or pureed foods thinned with a little breast milk, formula, juice, or milk; melted ice cream or custard-style yogurt may also work well; progress to thicker pureed foods and junior foods as tolerated; some thicker pureed foods such as peas or meats may always require thinning with a little liquid; swallowing may take longer—allow enough time between each mouthful; frequent sips of liquid may help "wash down" solid foods; table foods that are more likely to become stuck are dry foods and foods that require chewing or are difficult for the young child to chew, including nuts, seeds, skins, hulls, bread, raw fruits and vegetables, and meats
Gastroesophageal reflux	See table 6–9	See text

Table 6-13. Gastrointestinal Anomalies, Diseases, and Conditions that Often Require Nutrition Intervention (continued)

Disease/condition	Common nutrition-related problems	Nutrition intervention
Gastroschisis	Congenital protrusion of abdominal contents through the abdominal wall, usually at the right of the umbilicus, rarely associated with other congenital anomalies, but may include gastrointestinal defects such as atresia, volvulus, or perforations requiring resection and anastomoses of small bowel with resultant malabsorption syndrome	Human milk, standard or enriched infant formulas usually well tolerated; if lactose intolerance is significant, lactose-free formulas may be indicated; if malabsorption is significant, elemental formulas containing hydrolyzed protein, glucose polymers, and medium-chain triglycerides may be indicated. See appendix C
Omphalocele	Often associated with other congenital anomalies that may involve nutrition, such as congenital heart disease, trisomy syndromes, or Beckwith-Wiedemann syndrome; intra-abdominal contents (loops of small intestine, large intestine, liver, pancreas, spleen, and/or bladder) herniate into the base of the umbilical cord; function of the gastrointestinal tract is usually normal; complications may include adhesive obstructions of the gastrointestinal tract	As for gastroschisis
Biliary atresia/cholestasis/chronic liver disease	Anorexia; decreased presence of bile acids in the intestine causing decreased absorption of fat, essential fatty acids, and fat-soluble vitamins; decreased absorption of calcium, magnesium, zinc, and iron; decreased losses of copper and manganese due to decreased enterophepatic circulation of these trace minerals; hypoproteinemia; growth failure (both wasting and stunting)	If growth is slow, may require formula that contains 40–60% of the fat as medium-chain triglycerides; essential fatty acid intake should well exceed minimal requirements to ensure absorption of adequate amounts to prevent deficiency; 5000–25,000 IU vitamin A (water miscible)/day 5000–8000 IU vitamin D_2 (or 3–5 mcg/Kg 25-OH vitamin D)/day 15–25 IU/kg/day vitamin E (water-soluble D-α-tocopherol)/day or 50–400 IU vitamin E (α-tocopherol)/day 2.5–5.0 mg vitamin D, 2 to 7 times/week 2 times the RDA for water-soluble vitamins; optimal intake of calcium, phosphorus, magnesium, iron, and zinc
Pancreatic insufficiency	See chapter 13	See chapter 13
Pyloric stenosis	Decreased gastric emptying; gastroesophageal reflux; projectile vomiting	Small frequent feedings; whole milk or casein-predominant formulas may form too large a curd to pass through pylorus; human milk or hydrolyzed protein formula may be indicated
Diarrhea/constipation	See text and table 6–4	See text and table 6–4

Table 6-13. Gastrointestinal Anomalies, Diseases, and Conditions that Often Require Nutrition Intervention (continued)

Disease/condition	Common nutrition-related problems	Nutrition intervention
Short bowel syndrome	Normal small bowel length at birth is 5 times crown-heel length; small bowel length of 15 cm with ileocecal valve or 40 cm without ileocecal valve can usually adapt, in time, to support normal growth and development without parenteral nutrition; shorter lengths associated with malabsorption and growth failure	Human milk protein or protein hydrolysates (di- and tri-peptides) usually well tolerated Lactose may be least well tolerated carbohydrate; glucose polymers usually tolerated well
	Loss of proximal small bowel associated with ↓ fat digestion/absorption, ↓ fat-soluble vitamin absorption, ↑ losses of water-soluble vitamins, ↓ mineral absorption, ↓ disaccharide absorption	Medium-chain triglycerides usually tolerated better than long-chain triglycerides, although intake of long-chain triglycerides should be adequate to prevent essential fatty acid deficiency, allowing for some malabsorption
	Loss of terminal ileum associated with vitamin B_{12} deficiency and increased losses of zinc, copper, and calcium and decreased absorption of fat and fat-soluble vitamins due to decreased reabsorption of bile salts	Fat-soluble vitamin requirements may be increased with all oral or enteral feeding if steatorrhea or cholestasis is present; parenteral vitamin B_{12} may be needed if terminal ileum is absent
	Loss of ileocecal valve may be associated with decreased transit times, bacterial overgrowth of small bowel, and frequent, watery stools	Zinc, copper, and calcium intake should meet at least the RDA if terminal ileum is absent; sodium needs may be increased if colon is absent Iron needs may be greater than normal if duodenum is absent
Hirschsprung's disease	Decreased motility of large intestine, which may lead to impaction, ulceration, perforation, and peritonitis; surgical resection and colostomy may be associated with decreased fluid and electrolyte absorption; normal length of colon in term newborn is 40 cm	Enhanced fluid and electrolyte intake if losses are greater than normal

References:

Sokol RJ. Fat-soluble vitamins and their importance in patients with cholestatic liver diseases. Gastroenterol Clin North Am 23:673-705, 1994.

Wessell JJ. Short bowel syndrome. In: Groh-Wargo SL, Thompson M, Cox JH, eds. Nutritional care for high-risk newborns. rev. ed. Chicago: Precept Press, 1994.

References

1. Hendricks KM, Walker WA, eds. Manual of pediatric nutrition. Philadelphia: Decker, 1990.
2. Weaver LT. Constipation: diagnosis and treatment: Introduction. Semin Pediatr Gastroenterol Nutr 3(4):1–4; 1992.
3. Weaver LT, Steiner H. The bowel habits of young children. Arch Dis Child 59:649–52, 1984
4. Fitzgerald JF, Clark JH. Chronic diarrhea. Pediatr Clin North Am 29:221–231, 1982.
5. Glass RI, Lew JF, Gangarosa RE, LeBaron CW, Ho M. Estimates of morbidity and mortality rates for diarrheal diseases in American children. J Pediatr 118:S27–S33, 1991.
6. Center for Disease Control and Prevention. The management of acute diarrhea in children: oral rehydration, maintenance, and nutritional therapy. MMWR 41/No. RR-16, Oct. 16, 1992.
7. Kleinman R, Sack D, Dale C. Diarrheal management with oral rehydration therapy. Pediatr Basics 67(Winter):10–16, 1994.
8. Brown KH, MacLean WC. Nutritional management of acute diarrhea: An appraisal of the alternatives. Pediatrics 73:119–25, 1984.
9. Lifschitz CH, Shulman RJ. Nutritional therapy for infants with diarrhea. Nutr Rev 48:329–38, 1990.
10. Lifshitz F, da Costa Ribeiro H. Diarrheal diseases. In: Paige DM, Jacobson HN, Sherwin R, Solomons NW, Young VR, eds. Clinical nutrition. St. Louis: Mosby, 1988; 447–62.
11. Cohen MB. Etiology and mechanisms of acute infectious diarrhea in infants in the United States. J Pediatr 118:S34–S39, 1991.
12. Conway SP, Ireson A. Acute gastroenteritis in well nourished infants: comparison of four feeding regimens. Arch Dis Child 64:87–91, 1989.
13. Bezerra JA, Stathos TH, Duncan B, Gaines JA, Udall JN. Treatment of infants with acute diarrhea: What's recommended and what's practiced. Pediatrics 90:1–4, 1992.
14. Brown KH. Dietary management of acute childhood diarrhea: Optimal timing of feeding and appropriate use of milks and mixed diets. J Pediatr 118:S92–S98, 1991.
15. Chew F, Penn FJ, Peret Filho LA, et al. Is dilution of cows' milk formula necessary for dietary management of acute diarrhea in infants aged less than 6 months? Lancet 341:194–97, 1993.
16. Provisional Committee on Quality Improvement, Subcommittee on Acute Gastroenteritis. Practice parameter: The management of acute gastroenteritis in young children. Pediatrics 97:424–34, 1996.
17. Dugdale A, Lovell S, Gibbs V, Ball D. Refeeding after acute gastroenteritis: a controlled study. Arch Dis Child 57:76-78. 1982.
18. McDowell HP, Evans-Jones G. Is gradual reintroduction of milk feeds in gastroenteritis necessary? Lancet I:690, 1985.
19. Jelliffe B. Dietary management of young children with acute diarrhea: manual for managers of health. 2d ed. Geneva: World Health Organization, 1991.
20. Lanata CF, Black RE, Greed-Kanashiro H, et al. Feeding during acute diarrhea as a risk factor for persistent diarrhea. Acta Pediatr Suppl 361:98–103, 1992.
21. Santosham M, Greenough WB. Oral rehydration therapy: A global perspective. J Pediatr 118 (4 part 2): S44–S51, 1991
22. Santosham M, Duggam C, Brown KH, Greenough WB. Management of acute diarrhea. In: Wyllie R, Hyams JJ, eds. Pediatric gastrointestinal disease pathophysiology, diagnosis, management. Philadelphia: Saunders, 1993; 1157–66.
23. Margolis PA, Litteer T. Hare N, Pichichereo M. Effects of unrestricted diet on mild infantile diarrhea. Am J Dis Child 144:162–64, 1990.
24. Davidson GP, Goodwin D, Robb TA.. Incidence and duration of lactose malabsorption in children hospitalized with acute enteritis: study in a well-nourished urban population. J Pediatr 105:587–90, 1984.
25. Groothuis JR, Berman S, Chapman J. Effect of carbohydrate ingested on outcome in infants with mild diarrhea. J Pediatr 108:903–06, 1986.
26. Brown KH, Perez F, Peerson JM, et al. Effect of dietary fiber (soy polysaccharide) on the severity, duration, and nutritional outcome of acute, watery diarrhea in children. Pediatrics 92: 241–47, 1993.
27. Mead Johnson Pediatrics: Pediatric products handbook, 1993.
28. Alarcon P, Montoya R, Rivera J, Perez F, Peerson JM, Brown KH. Effect of inclusion of beans in a mixed diet for the treatment of Peruvian children with acute watery diarrhea. Pediatrics 90:58–65, 1992.
29. Avery GB, Villavicencio O, Lilly JR, Randolph JG. Intractable diarrhea in early infancy. Pediatr 41:712–22, 1968.
30. World Health Organization. The treatment and prevention of acute diarrhea: Practical guidelines. Geneva: WHO, 1989.
31. Reif S, Lebenthal E. Nutritional considerations in the treatment of acute and chronic diarrhea. In: Suskind RM, Lewinter-Suskind L, eds. Textbook of pediatric nutrition. New York: Raven Press, 1993; 325–39.
32. Walker-Smith JA. Toddler's diarrhea. Arch Dis Child 55:329–30, 1980.
33. Bass DM, Walker WA. Acute and chronic nonspecific diarrhea syndromes. In: Gellis SS, Kagan BM, eds. Current pediatric therapy 13. Philadelphia: Saunders, 1990; 186.
34. Hyams JS, Leichtner AM. Apple juice: An unappreciated cause of chronic diarrhea. Am J Dis Child 139:503–05, 1985.

35. Hoekstra JH, van Kempen AAMW, Kneepkens CMF. Apple juice malabsorption: fructose or sorbitol? J Pediatr Gastroenterol Nutr 16:39–42, 1993.
36. Hyams JS, Etienne NL, Leichtner AM, Theuer RC. Carbohydrate malabsorption following fruit juice ingestion in young children. Pediatrics 82:64–68, 1988.
37. Lifshitz F, Ament ME, Kleinman RE, et al. Role of apple juice carbohydrate malabsroption in chronic nonspecific diarrhea in children. J Pediatr 120: 825–29, 1992.
38. Smith MM, Davis M, Chasalow FI, Lifshitz F. Carbohydrate absorption from fruit juice in young children. Pediatrics 95:340–44, 1995.
39. Levine MD. Constipation and encopresis. In: Gellis SS, Kagan BM, eds. Current pediatric therapy 13. Philadelphia: Saunders, 1990; 183–86.
40. Murphy MS. Organic causes of constipation: Diagnosis and management. Semin Pediatr Gastroenterol Nutr 3(4):4–8, 1992.
41. Pettei MJ. Chronic constipation. Pediatr Annals 16:796, 798, 800, 804, 806, 811, 813, 1987.
42. Rappaport LA. The prevention of constipation and encopresis: a developmental model and approach. Pediatr Clin North Am 33:859–869, 1986.
43. Cloud HH. Developmental disabilities. In: Queen PM, Lang C, eds. Handbook of pediatric nutrition. Gaithersburg, Md.: Aspen, 1993; 400–21.
44. Groves JA. Interdisciplinary treatment of encopresis in individuals with developmental disorders: need and efficacy. Monogr Am Assoc Mental Deficiency 5:279–327, 1982.
45. Agostoni C, Riva E, Giovannini M. Dietary fiber in weaning foods of young children. Pediatrics 96:(suppl):1002–05, 1995.
46. Klein MD, Delaney TA. Feeding and nutrition for the child with special needs. Tucson: Therapy Skill Builders, 1994.
47. Fomon, SJ. Recommendations for feeding normal infants. In: Fomon SJ, ed. Nutrition of normal infants. St. Louis: Mosby, 1993; 456.
48. Committee on Nutrition American Academy of Pediatrics. Iron-fortified formulas. Pediatrics 84:1114–15, 1989.
49. Reeves JD, Yip R. Lack of adverse side effects of oral ferrous sulfate therapy in 1 year old infants. Pediatrics 75:352–55, 1985.
50. Nelson SE, Zeigler EE, Copeland AM, Edwards BB, Fomon SJ. Lack of adverse reactions to iron-fortified formula. Pediatrics 81:360–64, 1988.
51. Bradley CK, Hillman L, Pennridge Pediatric Associates; Sherman AR, Leedy D, Caylor-Nickel Research Institute; Cordano A. Evaluation of two iron-fortified, milk-based formulas during infancy. Pediatrics 91:908–914, 1993.
52. Oski FA. Iron-fortified formulas and gastrointestional symptoms in infants: A controlled study. Pediatrics 66:168–70, 1980.
53. Oski FA. Iron deficiency in infancy and childhood. New Engl J Med 329:190–93, 1993.
54. Olivares M, Llaguno S, Marin V, Hertrampf E, Mena P, Milad M. Iron status in low-birth-weight infants, small and appropriate for gestational age. A follow-up study. Acta Paediatr 81:824–28, 1992.
55. McClung HJ, Boyne L, Heitlinger L. Constipation and dietary fiber intake in children. Pediatrics 96(suppl):999–1001, 1995
56. Durschlag R. Dietary management of constipation in children. Semin Pediatr Gastorenterol Nutr 3(4):11–14, 1992.
57. Dwyer JT. Dietary fiber for children: how much? Pediatrics (suppl)96:1019–21, 1995.
58. Saldanha LG. Fiber in the diet of US children: Results of national surveys. Pediatrics 96(suppl):994–97, 1995.
59. American Academy of Pediatrics, Committee on Nutrition. Plant fiber intake in the pediatric diet. Pediatrics 67:572–75, 1981.
60. Olness, KO, Tobin, J. Chronic constipation in children. Can it be managed by diet alone? Postgrad Med 72(4)149–54, 1982.
61. Lingard CD. Enteral nutrition. In: Queen PM, Lang CE, eds. Handbook of pediatric nutrition. Gaithersburg, Md.: Aspen, 1993; 249–78.
62. Davis A. Indications and techniques for enteral feeds. In: Baker SB, Baker RD, eds. Pediatric enteral nutrition. New York: Chapman & Hall, 1994; 67–94.
63. Hatch TF. Encopresis and constipation in children. Pediatr Clin North Am 35:257–80, 1988.
64. Fleisher DR. Functional vomiting disorders in infancy: Innocent vomiting, nervous vomiting, and infant rumination syndrome. J Pediatr. 125:S84–S94, 1995.
65. Hyman PE. Gastroesphageal reflux: One reason why baby won't eat. J Pediatr 125:S103–S109, 1994.
66. Keller G.Clinical assessment. In: Groh-Wargo S, Thompson M, Cox JH, eds. Nutritional care for high-risk newborns. rev. ed. Chicago: Precept Press, 1994; 15–22.
67. Werlin SL, Dodds WJ. Hogan WJ, Arndorfer RC. Mechanism of gastroesophageal reflux in children. J Pediatr 97:244–49, 1980.
68. Orenstein SR. Gastroesphageal reflux. Curr Prob Pediatr. May/June, 1991.
69. Thompson M. Gastroesphageal reflux. In: Groh-Wargo S, Thompson M, Cox JH, eds. Nutritional care for high-risk newborns. rev. ed. Chicago: Precept Press, 1994; 308–14.
70. Herbst JJ. Gastroesophageal reflux. J Pediatr 98:859–70, 1981.
71. Black DD, Haggitt RC, Orenstein SR, Whitington PF. Esophagitis in infants. Gastroenterol 98:1408–14, 1990.
72. Orenstein SR, Magill HL, Brooks P. Thickening of infant feedings for therapy of gastroesophageal reflux. J Pediatr 110:181–86, 1987.

73. Orenstein SR. Controversies in pediatric gastroesphageal reflux. J Pediatr Gastroenterol Nutr 14:338–48, 1992.
74. Meyer WF. Herbst JJ. Effectiveness of positioning therapy for gastroesophageal reflux. Pediatr 69:768–72, 1982.
75. Bailey DJ, Andres JM, Danek GD, Pineiro-Carrero VM. Lack of efficacy of thickened feeding as treatment for gastroesophageal reflux. J Pediatr 110:187–89, 1987.
76. Vanderplas Y, Sacre L. Milk-thickening agents as a treatment for gastroesophageal reflux. Clin Pediatr 26:66–68,1982.
77. Orenstein SR. Prone positioning in infant gastroesophageal relux: Is elevation of the head worth the trouble? J Pediatr 117:184–87, 1990.
78. Orenstein SR, Whitington, PF. Positioning for prevention of infant gastroesophageal reflux. J Pediatr. 103:534–37, 1983.
79. AAP Task Force on Infant Positioning and SIDS. Pediatr 89:1120–26, 1992.
80. Bock SA, Sampson HA. Food allergy in infancy. Pediatr Clin North Am 41:1047–65, 1994.
81. Bukus, SN, Mahan LK. Food allergies: Immunological reactions to food. J Am Diet Assoc 86:601–08.
82. Hereditary metabolic disorders. In: Ekvall SW. Pediatric nutrition in chronic diseases and developmental disorders., New York: Oxford University Press, 1993.
83. Miller MJS. Nutrient-drug interactions in children. In: Suskind RM, Lewinter-Suskind L, eds. Textbook of pediatric nutrition. New York: Raven, 1988.
84. Brizee L. Drug-nutrient interaction concerns for children with special health care needs. Nutr Focus Nov./Dec. 1992.
85. Pronsky ZM. Powers and Moore's food-medication interactions. 8th ed. Pottstown, Pa.: Food-Medication Interactions, 1993.
86. Smith CH, Bidlack WR. Dietary concerns associated with the use of medications. J Am Diet Assoc 84:901–14, 1984.
87. McKinney LA, Palmer CA, Dwyer JT, Garcia R. Managing dentally related nutrition concerns of children with special health care needs: parts 1 and 2. Top Clin Nutr 6:70–85, 1991.
88. Faine MP. Dental nutrition concerns of children with special health care needs. Nutr Focus. July/Aug. 1992.
89. Owen GM. Physical examination as an assessment tool. In: Simko MD, Cowell C, Gilbride JA. Nutrition assessement: A comprehensive guide for planning intervention. 2d ed. Gaithersburg Md.; Aspen, 1995; 85–92.
90. Krug-Wispe S. Nutritional assessment. In: Queen PM, Lang CE. Handbook of pediatric nutrition. Gaithersburg, Md.: Aspen, 1993; 26–82.

SECTION III

MEDICAL/SURGICAL PROBLEMS

Nutrition Manual for At-Risk Infants and Toddlers
Janice Hovasi Cox, editor

7

PREMATURELY BORN INFANTS

Sharon Groh-Wargo, MS, RD, LD, and Janice Hovasi Cox, MS, RD

In the United States, 9.7% of live births are premature.[1] Low birth weight (LBW) (< 2500 g) occurs in 7.1% of live births.[2] These infants experience a disproportional share of neonatal and infant mortality and have higher rates of major morbidity than their term, normal-weight contemporaries.[2–4]

The need for appropriate follow-up is underscored by the younger ages and lower weights at which high-risk newborns are currently discharged from the hospital as compared to a few years ago. It is not uncommon for premature infants to go home at 1800 g (4 lb). Table 7-1 lists those infants at highest risk for nutrition problems after discharge from the neonatal intensive care unit (NICU). These infants are singled out because they may have one or more of the following:

- Decreased nutrient reserves
- Increased nutrient needs
- Increased nutrient losses
- Feeding difficulties related to immaturity and/or abnormal neurodevelopmental progression
- Require special nutritional support products.

This chapter includes growth and feeding assessment guidelines as well as feeding recommendations for prematurely born infants from hospital discharge through 3 years of age. A glossary of terms appears as appendix O.

Growth Assessment

Interpreting the growth of infants and children born prematurely requires a combination of knowledge and clinical experience. Well-accepted norms are lacking. The varied methods of reporting growth data and the use of the

Table 7-1. Infants at Highest Risk for Nutritional Problems after Discharge from Neonatal ICU

- Very low birth weight infants (<1500 g birth weight)
- Extremely low birth weight infants (<1000 g birth weight)
- Small-for-gestational-age infants
- Breast-fed infants
- Infants on special formulas
- Infants on parenteral nutrition >4 weeks during hospitalization
- Infants on parenteral nutrition after hospital discharge
- Infants with a determination of any of the following:
  —Bronchopulmonary dysplasia
  —Chronic renal insufficiency
  —Congenital alimentary tract anomalies
  —Cyanotic congenital heart disease
  —Inborn errors of metabolism
  —Malabsorption
  —Osteopenia of prematurity
  —Poverty or low socioeconomic status
  —Severe neurological impairments
  —Short bowel syndrome
- Infants with gastrostomies or tracheostomies
- Infants who require tube feedings at home
- Infants who fail to gain at least 20 g/day prior to discharge

Reprinted by permission from Groh-Wargo S, Thompson M, Cox JH, eds. Nutritional care for high-risk newborns. rev. ed. Chicago: Precept Press, 1994.

term *catch-up* make comparison of data difficult[5–16] (see appendix O). Some observations on growth summarized in a recent publication[17] are given below:

- Better postnatal growth occurs in infants who also have good developmental outcome. This group of infants also tends to have a shorter, more benign neonatal course, lower incidence of chronic disease, and lower incidence of rehospitalization.[5–8]
- During 38 to 48 weeks postconceptual age, the prematurely born infant may show rates of weight gain similar to the rapid weight gain that normally occurs during 32 to 36 weeks gestation in utero.[9–12] This period of catch-up growth seems to correlate with calorie intake and absence of continued medical compromise.[12, 18] Ad libitum nutritional intake during this time may exceed that normally expected at this age, in the range of 135–165 kcal/kg/day.[12, 19–21]
- Mean values for weight and length for children with birth weights less than 2000 g may be within the normal range, but may continue to fall below the mean for postconceptual age-matched children up to 8 years of age.[9, 10, 12–16, 22] Children with weight and height below the 10th percentile at 2 years of age are more likely to remain below the 10th percentile at 5 and 8 years of age.[12, 15]
- Whether or not early catch-up growth has occurred, the rate of gain beyond 4 months postterm for weight and length of infants born prematurely is not strikingly different from term infants of similar postconceptual age.[12, 13, 19–21]
- Head circumference shows the least difference between low-birth-weight preterm infants and normal term infants. Catch-up growth measured by increasing head circumference (reflecting brain growth) is usually better and earlier than catch-up weight gain or linear growth.[9, 10, 12, 13, 18, 23] This must be differentiated from excessive growth due to intracranial hemorrhage, infection, or hydrocephaly.[18, 24] Head circumference growth that has not achieved normal percentile ranking by 8 months postterm date has been associated with poor cognitive function, academic achievement, and behavior at 8 years of age.[23]

Excluding infants with known chromosomal or congenital causes for intrauterine growth failure, infants born small for gestational age (SGA) have the following characteristics:

- Disproportionality (linear and head growth sparing) increases with decreasing birth weight percentile ranking. Body mass index (BMI) scores, ponderal index, and weight-to-head circumference ratios decrease with decreasing birth weight percentile ranking.[25]
- From 65 to 85% of SGA infants are above -2 SD for weight by 1 year of age. Seventy-five percent of SGA infants are above -2 SD for length by 1 year of age; this increases to around 85% at 2.5 years.[26, 27]

Follow-up of large-for-gestational-age (LGA) infants reveals that although the growth of some LGA infants continues to plot > +2 SD, many show a growth lag-down and a weight for length that approaches the mean by 1 year of age.[25, 28] Also, LGA infants of diabetic mothers may show an increased incidence of obesity during late childhood and adolescence.[29]

Various charts are available for growth assessment[13, 30–32] (see chapter 5). When plotting weight, length, or head circumference on any of the available growth charts, the premature infant's age is usually "corrected" to account for premature birth (see appendix O). Corrected age is generally used until at least 18 months and often until 3 years of age. Beyond 3 years of age, the weeks or months of prematurity become less significant in growth assessment. The most widely available growth charts in the United States are likely those of the National Center for Health Statistics (NCHS)[30] (see appendix F). Although these charts represent growth data for term infants, they may be used for growth assessment of prematurely born infants. The corrected age of the premature infant must be used and should be labeled so that others interpret the plotted growth appropriately. Other growth charts available include:

The Oregon Growth Record for Infants,[31] also referred to as the Babson Intrauterine and Postnatal Growth Chart (see appendix G). This chart represents cross-sectional data from a small group of newborns born from 26 to 40 weeks of gestation along with longitudinal data from over 4,000 *term* infants through the first year of life. An advantage of this chart is that growth from the time of preterm birth through 12 months postterm can be plotted on the same chart. Two standard deviations (SD) above and below the mean roughly correspond with the 97.5 percentile; 2.5 percentile; 1 SD above and below the mean roughly correspond to the 84th and 16th percentiles. Only one chart is available for both males and females.

The Gairdner and Pearson Growth and Developmental Records[32] include separate charts for boys and girls from 24 weeks' gestation to 2 years postterm (see appendix I). Data from 24–40 weeks' gestation represent measurements taken at birth of infants of known gestational age. Data from term to 2 years represent measurements of infants born at term. These charts closely match the Oregon chart with the following exceptions:

- The mean lengths on the Gairdner and Pearson charts are generally lower between 26 and term than on the Oregon chart, though the range is similar.
- The lower percentiles for weight are higher on the Gairdner and Pearson charts than on the Oregon chart from 38 weeks' gestation to 6 weeks postterm.

The Gairdner and Pearson charts are similar to the NCHS charts for weight, length, and head circumference from term to 24 months.

The Infant Health and Development Program (IHDP) Charts[13], also known as the Casey Charts (see appendix H). Separate charts are available for very low birth weight (VLBW) and low-birthweight (LBW) infants born prematurely—≤37 weeks' gestational age (GA):

- VLBW premature boys ≤ 37 weeks GA, ≤ 1500 g birth weight (BW)
- VLBW premature girls ≤ 37 weeks GA, ≤ 1500 g BW
- LBW boys ≤ 37 weeks GA, 1501–2500 g BW
- LBW premature girls ≤ 37 weeks GA, 1501–2500 g BW

The growth of the VLBW infants studied, both boys and girls, differs from the NCHS percentiles for the same postconceptual age term-born infants. The 25th percentile (roughly 1 SD below the mean) for the VLBW infants corresponds with the 5th percentile (nearly 2 SD below the mean) for term infants. The 75th percentile (roughly 1 SD above the mean) for the VLBW infants corresponds with the mean for term infants. The growth of the LBW infants studied more closely parallels the standard NCHS and Oregon charts. The benefit of using these charts over others is that the growth of an individual premature infant is compared to other premature infants. However, some words of caution include:

- These grids do not determine "normal" or "abnormal" growth for LBW or VLBW infants, although SGA and other infants who would be known to have altered growth patterns were omitted from the sample. They merely represent what actually occurred in the group of infants studied.[9]
- Growth should be plotted at corrected age. Further investigation of nutrition may be indicated when measurements are markedly different from the *50th percentile* (not the 10th percentile, as with the NCHS charts), or when growth percentile changes rapidly.
- These charts do not contain weight-for-length grids or body mass index charts, which are helpful for interpreting growth, particularly when parameters fall outside the norm.
- The growth record prior to 40 weeks' gestational age is not included on the same graph for comparison as it is on the Oregon and Gairdner/Pearson charts. This is important because many infants are discharged prior to term.

Assessment of growth velocity may be helpful for premature infants whose growth parameters are not within expected percentiles, who are crossing percentile ranks, or who are being evaluated at closer intervals than the

Table 7-2. Velocity of Growth, 28–40 Weeks' Gestation*

	Weight (g/day)	Length (cm/wk)	Head circumference (cm/wk)
28–32 wk	24.0	1.2	0.9
32–36 wk	30.0	1.2	0.8
36–40 wk	28.0	0.6	0.4

* Values are mean figures calculated from Babson SG. Growth of low-birth infants. J Pediatr 77:11, 1970.

Table 7-3. Growth Rates of Weight, Length, and Head Circumference by Birth Weight, Group, and Sex

	Group I*		Group II†		Group III‡	
	Male (no.)	Female (no.)	Male (no.)	Female (no.)	Male (no.)	Female (no.)
Weight	65	67	200	226	168	155
Growth rate (g/day)						
12 mo	9.3±1.6	8.9±1.8	9.0±1.6	9.0±1.7	9.1±1.6	8.9±1.9
24 mo	5.7±1.3	5.6±1.4	5.6±1.3	5.9±1.6	5.9±1.5	6.0±2.0
36 mo	4.2±1.2	4.3±1.3	4.2±1.2	4.6±1.5	4.6±1.5	4.7±2.2
Length	64	67	200	224	168	154
Growth rate (mm/mo)						
12 mo	13.0±1.1	13.0±1.3	12.3±1.1	12.4±1.1	12.0±1.0§	12.0±1.0§
24 mo	8.0±1.0	8.4±1.0	8.0±0.9	8.4±1.0	8.0±0.9	8.2±0.9
36 mo	6.0±1.0	6.5±0.9	6.1±0.8	6.6±1.0	6.3±0.9	6.6±0.9
Head Circumference	65	66	198	226	169	165
Growth rate (mm/mo)						
12 mo	3.1±0.3	3.0±0.4	3.0±0.4	3.0±0.4	3.0±0.3	3.0±0.3
24 mo	1.3±0.2	1.3±0.2	1.4±0.3	1.4±0.3	1.5±0.2§	1.5±0.2§
36 mo	0.7±0.1	0.8±0.2	0.9±0.2	0.9±0.2	0.9±0.2§	0.9±0.2§

Values (except no.) are expressed as mean ±SD.
*Birth weight ≤1250 g
†Birth weight ≥1251 but ≤2000 g
‡Birth weight ≥2001 but <2500 g
§p <0.001
Adapted with permission from Casey et al.[13]

chart allows.[12, 13, 18, 30, 33–37] Tables 7-2 and 7-3 provide weight, length, and head circumference standards for preterm and postterm growth velocity (see chapter 5 for additional postterm growth velocity data). Corrected age of the premature infant should be used any time values from term newborns are used for comparison. *Rate* of gain, not just percentile ranking, is an important parameter to monitor. Catch-up growth occurs primarily during weeks 38–48, with subsequent growth rates falling into the normal range.

Growth is affected by overall health, genetic, nutritional, and environmental factors. Criteria for referral for further nutrition evaluation based on growth assessment are listed in table 7-4. Those assessing the growth of prematurely born infants should (1) consider the corrected age of the infant, (2) choose the most appropriate growth chart, and (3) calculate the velocity of growth, when appropriate. Figure 7-1 includes a sample growth assessment of a prematurely born infant.

Table 7-4. Criteria for Referral for Further Nutrition Evaluation

- Infant sustains a weight loss or fails to gain weight after discharge
- When plotted for corrected age, weight, length or head circumference, falls below previous percentile ranking
- Infant is not gaining at least: [32, 35, 36]
  - 20 g/day from term to 3 mo corrected age
  - 15 g/day from 3–6 mo corrected age
  - 10 g/day from 6–9 mo corrected age
  - 6 g/day from 9–12 mo corrected age
- Infant's weight for length falls below the 5th percentile
- Infant's head circumference is not maintaining a growth pattern that is proportional to weight gain and linear growth, or is less than:[18]
  - 0.5 cm/wk from term to 3 mo corrected age
  - 0.25 cm/wk from 3–6 mo corrected age
- Infant's head circumference is growing more than 1.25 cm/wk[18].

Reprinted by permission from Groh-Wargo S, Thompson M, Cox JH, eds. Nutritional care for high-risk newborns. rev. ed. Chicago: Precept Press, 1994.

Feeding Assessment

Every visit to the clinic should include some assessment of the infant's dietary intake. Use of a nutrition screening tool such as those given in appendixes A and B facilitates history taking. Growth that does not proceed as expected may signal a problem in one or more of these areas. The focus of the feeding assessment is largely determined by the adequacy of growth. When growth parameters are satisfactory, the feeding assessment may be more "qualitative," as it focuses on the quality rather than the quantity of food in the infant's diet. If growth parameters are not normal or the qualitative evaluation reveals problems, a quantitative evaluation is indicated. This quantitative evaluation should probe more carefully into the amounts of all foods consumed. The estimated intake of calories and grams of protein per kilogram of ideal body weight can then be calculated. Calculation of the intake of other nutrients such as calcium, phosphorus, or vitamin D may also be appropriate. These values are compared to the Recommended Dietary Allowance (RDA) for the corrected age of the infant. See a sample nutrition assessment in figure 7-2.

Infants born prematurely are at risk for feeding problems. Understanding the reasons for these problems can aid in treatment and result in improved nutrition status. Table 7-5 lists the common causes of feeding problems in prematurely born infants.

The following guidelines for improving the feeding skills of infants born prematurely are summarized from materials by Morris and Klein.[38]

- Create the best mealtime environment. Minimal amounts of light and noise, plus appropriate room temperature, can help decrease distracting stimulation.
- Observe the infant's cues for stress and relaxation. The infant should be calm when feedings are started. Feeding should stop if stress signals are observed (see table 4-5).

Sample Growth Assessment for a Prematurely Born Female

Birth through discharge:
- Gestational age (GA) at birth: 27 wk on 1/1/96 (40 wk–27 wk = 13 wk premature).
- Chronological age at discharge: 7 wk on 2/19/96.
- Gestational age at hospital discharge: 34 wk

Follow-up:

1st visit:	Gestational age	36 wk on 3/4/96
	Chronological age	9 wk (2 wk following discharge)
	Corrected age	9 wk–13 wk = –4 wk (not term yet)
2nd visit:	Gestational age	53 wk on 7/1/96
	Chronological age	6 mo (26 wk)
	Corrected age	26 wk–13 wk = 13 wk or 3 mo
3rd visit:	Gestational age	55 wk on 7/15/96
	Chronological age	6½ mo (28 weeks)
	Corrected age	28–13 wk = 15 wk or 3½ mo

Summary of Anthropometrics

	Weight (g)	Length (cm)	Head circumference (cm)
Date of birth 1/1/96) 27 wk GA	1000	36	25.0
Date of discharge (2/19/96) 34 wk GA	1800	44	31.5
1st clinic visit (3/4/96) 36 wk GA	2750	48	33.0
2nd clinic visit (7/1/96) 3 mo corrected age	4500	58	40.0
3rd clinic visit (7/15/96) 3½ mo corrected age	4900	59.5	40.5

Calculated Rates of Gain

Time interval	Weight (g/day)	Length (cm/wk or mo)	Head circumference (cm/wk or mo)
Discharge to 1st visit:			
Calculation	(2750–1800) ÷ 14 days =	(48–44) ÷ 2 wk =	(33–31.5) ÷ 2 wk =
Actual rate	67.9	2.0	0.75
Expected rate*	30.0	1.2	0.80
1st to 2nd visit:			
Calculation	(4500–2750) ÷ 119 days =	(58–48) ÷ 4 mo =	(40–33) ÷ 4 mo =
Actual rate	14.7	2.5	1.75
Expected rate†	23.2	2.8	1.40
2nd to 3rd visit:			
Calculation	(4900–4500) ÷ 14 days =	(59.5–58) ÷ ½ mo =	(40.5–40) ÷ ½ mo =
Actual rate	28.6	3.0	1.0
Expected rate†	23.2	2.8	1.4

*From table 7-2
†From table 7-2 and table 5-1

Evaluation of Growth

Discharge to 1st visit:
- Exhibiting catch-up growth for weight and length
- Oregon chart: plots around the mean for corrected age
- Gairdner - Pearson chart: plots similar to Oregon chart
- IHDP chart: plots around the 75th percentile for corrected age

1st to 2nd visit:
- Faltering of weight and length growth rate; thorough nutrition assessment warranted; head circumference growth maintained
- Oregon chart: weight has fallen off chart
- Gairdner - Pearson chart: weight plots at about the 3rd percentile
- IHDP chart: weight plots at 5-25th percentile
- NCHS chart: plots similar to IHDP

2nd to 3rd visit:
- Rate of weight and length growth improved; response to nutritional intervention apparent; overall head circumference growth 1st to 3rd visit acceptable
- Growth charts: difficult to assess over short observation period of 2 wk

Figure 7-1. Sample growth assessment for a prematurely born female.

Sample Nutritional Assessment for a Prematurely Born Female

Time interval	Assessment	Instructions
Discharge (34 wk GA)	Premature formula 24 kcal/oz w/Fe ad lib on demand providing ≈ 135 kcal/kg/day. Weight gain past week averaging 38 g/day	Continue premature formula 24 kcal/oz w/Fe plus Fer-In-Sol 0.2 cc QD. Return for follow-up in 2 wk
DIscharge to 1st visit (36 wk GA)	Formula and supplement intake as prescribed at discharge. Exhibiting catch-up growth	Change to Similac NeoCare 22 kcal/oz w/Fe Discontinue Fer-In-Sol when 50 ml bottle given at discharge is finished. Schedule routine child care with primary care provider; return to special follow-up clinic at 3 mo corrected age
1st to 2nd visit (3 mo corrected age)	Infant receives standard formula 20 kcal/oz and significant solid foods (cereal and fruit) Estimated intake: 100 kcal/kg, 1.8 g protein/kg, 300 mg calcium/day, and < 2 mg iron/kg. Infant eats poorly from a spoon so solids are given in the bottle. Faltering of weight and length growth rate	Change back to Similac NeoCare 22 kcal/oz w/Fe to improve calorie, protein, and mineral intake. (If Similac NeoCare not available, recommend 24 kcal/oz standard formula w/Fe). Encourage solid food intake to stop until 4–6 mo corrected age, or at most, to consist of small amounts of infant cereal from a spoon Schedule follow-up for weight check in 2 wk
2nd to 3rd visit ($3\frac{1}{2}$ mo corrected age)	Formula intake as prescribed at previous visit. Infant cereal from a spoon once daily Rate of weight and length growth improved	Continue formula feeding. Advance solid foods from a spoon slowly, based on acceptance and corrected age. Reevaluate continued need for Similac NeoCare (or increased caloric density formula) in 3 mo based on growth and other medical problems. Return to special follow-up clinic at 6 mo corrected age; continue routine child care with primary care provider

Figure 7-2. Sample nutritional assessment for a prematurely born female, based on the assumption that care is provided in a special neonatal ICU follow-up clinic setting. For complete anthroponetric assessment, see figure 7-1.

Table 7-5. Causes of Feeding Problems in Prematurely Born Infants

- Neurological immaturity
- Abnormal muscle tone
- Lack of proximal stability of the neck, shoulders, and trunk
- Exaggerated extensor patterns of movement
- Weakened and irritable state
- Insufficient energy to consume sufficient quantity of food
- Poor weight gain
- Dislike of mealtimes
- Depressed oral-motor reflexes; weakened suck
- Decreased tongue mobility and lip seal
- Decreased sucking pads; poor cheek stability
- Oral hypersensitivity due to tube feedings
- Disorganization of the suck-swallow-breathe pattern
- Prolonged use of endotracheal tubes, resulting in increased hyperextension
- Insufficient jaw stability for maintaining good suck
- Inadequate hunger and thirst signals

Adapted from Morris and Klein.[38]

- Choose the correct nipple in terms of softness and ease of flow (see table 4-6).
- Be sure the taste and temperature of the formula are acceptable.
- Create a rhythmic foundation for feeding. Walking or rocking the baby before feeding may help.
- Select a comfortable position. The baby's body should be flexed, the chin tucked, and the shoulders and arms forward.
- Provide cheek or jaw support, as needed.
- Provide more frequent meals if the baby is unable to take large amounts at a time.
- Record intake and times so that realistic goals can be set.

Feeding development in the infant and toddler normally progresses in predictable ways (see table 4-2). For the infant born prematurely, this progression should be observed if the corrected age of the infant is used. Referral to an occupational, speech, or physical therapist is indicated if the child fails to accomplish feeding skills as expected for corrected age or exhibits any of the abnormal feeding behaviors listed in the glossary (see table 4-4).

Feeding Recommendations

Using corrected age, feeding progression recommendations for most premature infants are the same as for infants born at term (see table 3-2). For example, human milk or iron-fortified infant formula is recommended until 1 year corrected age, with solid foods introduced at 4 to 6 months corrected age. Early feeding recommendations may require special considerations for infants who may be at increased risk for nutritional problems due to:

- Extremely low birth weight (ELBW)
- $\leq$ 36 weeks' gestational age or weight of < 2000 g at discharge
- Osteopenia at discharge (serum phosphorus < 4 mg/dl, alkaline phosphatase > 600 IU/L between 36 and 42 weeks gestational age, or evidence of bone demineralization on x-ray)
- Protein deficiency at discharge (prealbumin < 10 mg/dl)
- Significant residual medical problems at discharge (e.g., bronchopulmonary dysplasia, necrotizing enterocolitis, gastroesophageal reflux, neurological impairment, or continued need for tube feeding)

Breast Milk

Breast-feeding after premature birth is recommended and encouraged whenever possible. The separation of mother and infant during the infant's hospitalization and the immaturity of the infant's suck often present challenges to successful breast-feeding. At discharge, breast-feeding evaluation focused on the following points can identify nutritional adequacy or the need for individualized support or supplementation:

- What is the approximate milk supply of the mother?
- How closely does the milk supply match the infant's estimated fluid and nutrient needs?
- How effectively does the infant latch on?
- What is the estimated volume of intake?

Intake can be estimated from infant weight before and after nursng, the amount of time the infant is effectively sucking, or the infant's satisfaction between feeding intervals. Suggestions for increasing the success of breast-feeding after premature birth are offered in figure 7-3. Resources for parents are listed at the end of this chapter, and several good reviews on the subject are published elsewhere.[39, 40]

Breast-feeding the Prematurely Born Infant

- Feed the infant at breast on demand every 1½ to 3 hours, or at least 8–12 times/day
- Evaluate adequacy as you would other breast-fed infants (see text)
- Express some milk to encourage latching-on; a few minutes of hand expression or use of a pump can facilitate this
- Support the baby's head and body with generous use of pillows—be comfortable!
- Support and position the mother's breast using the C-cup hold so that the infant can fully and easily grasp the nipple. The mother's thumb and index finger can come forward to support the jaw, if necessary (see figures 7-4 and 7-5 on p.90)
- Continue pumping after most breast feedings for the first 2 or 3 weeks at home to ensure that breasts are being emptied and to further stimulate adequate milk supply. Consider cup, syringe, or bottle-feeding hind milk to ensure adequate caloric intake
- Supplement as suggested in table 7-6. Supplements should be decreased and eliminated as soon as possible after discharge based on weight gain and other nutrient needs
- Suggest feeding the infant on alternate breasts (one breast per feeding) for the mother whose supply is greater than the infant's need to ensure that the baby gets hind milk

---

Figure 7-3. Suggestions for increasing the success of breast-feeding after premature birth.

Infants at increased risk for nutrition problems after hospital discharge may benefit from fortification of their mother's milk. Recommendations for supplementation are given in tables 7-6 and 7-7 (also see appendix C). The purpose of continued fortification is to provide adequate protein, calorie, and mineral intake to support rapid growth.[41–43]

Infant Formula

In practice, premature infants who do not receive maternal breast milk/breast-feeding are fed standard formula, premature infant formula, or enriched infant formula after hospital discharge (see appendix C for the nutrient composition of these products). Although premature infants' nutrient needs may be higher during a rapid catch-up growth phase,[44] prolonged use of premature infant formula has been associated with vitamin D toxicity and may supply several times the daily RDA for vitamin A at intakes > 500 ml per day.[45,46] The enriched infant formula presently available is Similac NeoCare (Ross Laboratories, Columbus, Ohio). Its calorie, protein, vitamin, and mineral content is about midway between standard and premature infant formulas.

In a study reported by Lucas et al., premature infants fed enriched infant formula for nine months grew better than matched controls fed standard formula.[44] This difference appeared to be due to increased protein and mineral intake; the calorie intake was similar in both groups. Although the difference in daily weight gain between the groups was relatively small (about 3–4 g/day), this accelerated weight gain sustained over three to six months allows achievement of a higher percentile ranking, thus significant catch-up growth, for infants fed enriched formula. Another study showed significantly better initial weight gain and a trend toward an improved rate of growth in length in infants receiving enriched formula.[47] Improved bone-mineral content at 9 months' corrected age has also been shown in premature infants fed an enriched formula following hospital discharge.[48] Further studies are needed to better define the effectiveness of continued use of premature infant formulas for a defined period beyond discharge versus a longer course of enriched formula.

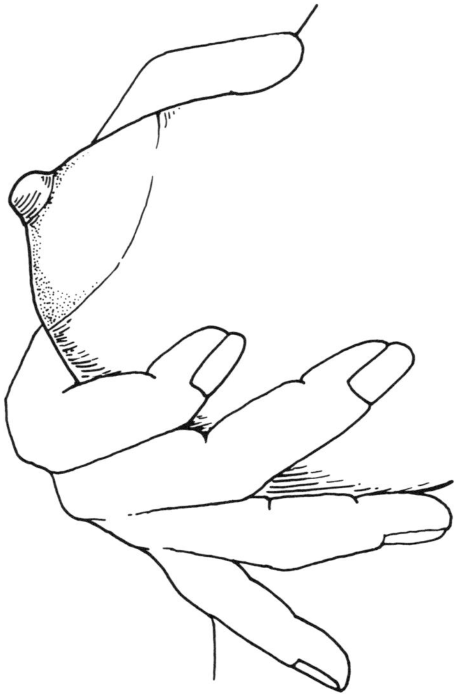

Figure 7-4. The breast should be supported throughout the feeding using the C-cup hold.

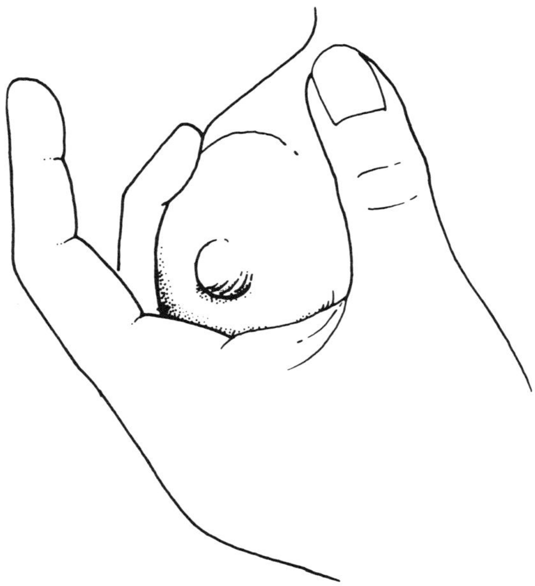

Figure 7-5. For additional support, the index finger can be used to support the infant's chin, or the thumb and index finger can come forward to support the jaw.

Although feeding recommendations are not well-defined, table 7-6 summarizes a suggested guideline for feedings and supplements for prematurely born infants after hospital discharge. Table 7-7 provides recipes for enriched formulas and increasing caloric density of standard infant formulas.

Table 7-6. NICU Discharge Feeding Guidelines for Infants < 37 Weeks' Gestational Age and ≥ 2000 Grams Birthweight*

Birthweight < 1000 g **or** Birthweight ≥ 1000 g **and** discharge weight < 2000 g **or** Serum prealbumin < 10 mg/dl **or** Growth < −2 SD/5th percentile at discharge† **or** Bronchopulmonary dysplasia‡ or osteopenia§	Birthweight ≥ 1000 g **and** Discharge weight > 2000 g **and** Growth ≥ −2 SD or 5th percentile†
Formula-fed 1. 24 kcal/oz premature infant formula w/Fe until 1850 g/4 lb (or at most 3500 g/7 lb 11 oz) 2. 22 kal/oz enriched formula from 1850 g (or 3500 g) until 9 mo to 1 yr corrected age 3. Standard 20 kcal/oz formula may be considered once catch-up growth is completed‖ up to 1 yr corrected age 4. Either formula provides 2 mg/kg/day iron; may need additional iron for a total of 4 mg/kg/day	**Formula-fed** 1. Standard 20 kcal/oz with iron formula or enriched 22 kcal/oz formula up to 1 yr corrected age 2. Supplement with ½ to one dose of multivitamin drops every day if standard formula is used 3. Either formula provides 2 mg/kg/day iron; may need additional iron for a total of 4 mg/kg/day
Breast-fed 1. See figure 7-3. 2. Provide high-protein, high-mineral supplement such as human milk fortifier or enriched formula until nutrient deficiency is corrected; explore alternative feeding techniques (i.e., cup, syringe, etc.) with family to minimize exposure to artificial nipple 3. Supplement with one dose/day of multivitamin drops and iron 2-4 mg/kg/day	**Breast-fed** 1. See figure 7-3. 2. If breast milk supply is insufficient, supplement with standard or enriched formula 3. Supplement with one dose of multivitamin drops every day 4. Supplement with 2-4 mg iron/kg/day

Note: Reassess growth and intake of all infants at two weeks follow-up visit.

*These are general guidelines; discharge instructions must be individualized to accommodate specific needs. Infants > 37 weeks' gestational age or > 2000 g birth weight without chronic disease or condition may be discharged on standard nutrition regimen for normal term infants.

†Growth is evaluated in standard deviations from the mean on the Oregon Growth Chart and in percentile rank on the National Center for Health Statistics (NCHS) charts or the Gairdner/Pearson growth charts; growth parameters that plot below the 25th percentile on the VLBW Infant Health and Development Program (IHDP) growth charts are roughly equivalent to the 5th percentile on the NCHS or Gairdner/Pearson charts or at −2 SD on the Oregon chart.

‡If bronchopulmonary dysplasia is significant at discharge and requires treatment with supplemental oxygen, diuretics and/or steroid therapy, nutritional needs may be altered (see chapter 14 for additional information).

§Osteopenia: serum phosphorus < 4 mg/dl, serum alkaline phosphatase > 600 IU/L, or evidence of bone demineralization on x-ray.

‖Catch-up growth is considered complete when growth parameters achieve expected genetic potential for corrected age.

Vitamin and Mineral Supplements

Supplements are often needed during the first year following premature birth. Considerations include the following:

- A multivitamin is likely to be needed when relatively low volumes (i.e., < 700 ml/day of standard formula or nonfortified human milk meet the caloric needs of the baby (e.g., infants ≤ 3.5 kg).

Table 7-7. Recipes for Mixing Special Formulas for Prematurely Born Infants

Similac NeoCare
Similac NeoCare Powder 3 scoops plus 5 oz water yields 5½ oz of 22 kcal/oz formula
One scoop powder equals 41 kcal

Human Milk Fortifiers
Similac Natural Care. Usually mixed 1:1 with expressed human milk to yield approximately 22 kcal/oz; can also be fed full strength as a supplementary feeding to breast-feeding

Enfamil Human Milk Fortifier. One packet to 25 cc expressed human milk yields a feeding of about 24 kcal/oz; works well as a supplement to breast-feeding when the mother has an adequate supply of pumped milk

Similac NeoCare. Although not originally intended as a human milk fortifier, can be used as such, since it is available as a powder; one scoop to 270 cc (9 oz) expressed human milk yields about 24 kcal/oz

Increased Caloric Density Standard Formula
Concentrated liquid. 13 oz plus 9 oz water yields 24 kcal/oz formula. (A simplified recipe of one 13-oz can plus 1 cup of water yields 24.8 kcal/oz formula)

Powder. 8 scoops plus 12 oz water yields about 13½ oz of 24 kcal/oz formula (When measuring formula powder, 8 loosely packed scoops is approximately equal to ⅔ cup loosely packed or ½ cup firmly packed powder.)

Note: See appendix C for more detailed nutrient composition information.

- Premature infant formulas and enriched infant formula have higher concentrations of vitamins and minerals than standard formulas.
- Adequacy of calcium, phosphorus, and vitamin D is of special concern due to the risk of bone demineralization and osteopenia.
- Iron supplementation should begin no later than 2 months of age at a dose of 2–4 mk/kg.[49] Iron-fortified formulas provide about 2 mg/kg when fed at about 120 kcal/kg. Additional iron can be supplied as ferrous sulfate drops or, when appropriate, in infant cereal.

Solid Food

Introduction of solid foods can usually occur at the corrected age of 4–6 months. Beginning spoon feedings earlier may be appropriate if the infant seems to be catching up developmentally earlier than expected. Conversely, spoon feeding may be delayed if extraordinary neurological impairment is apparent. At least two studies have documented that infants born prematurely are offered significant amounts of solid foods earlier than the above recommendations.[44, 50] Foods usually consumed include cereals, strained fruits, and vegetables. These foods are not good sources of high biological value protein, calcium or zinc—important nutrients during rapid growth. Continued use of an enriched infant formula would ensure better intake of these nutrients.

Summary

Feeding recommendations for prematurely born infants should be based at discharge on birth weight, discharge weight, and nutritional status; should advance through the normal progression using corrected age; and should consider special medical conditions (see table 7-8).

Referral to the Women, Infants and Children Food Supplemental Program (WIC) is appropriate for many families discharged from the Neonatal Intensive Care Unit (NICU). Special arrangements to advance the infant food package based on corrected, rather than chronological, age is usually possible and appropriate. Many infants discharged from the NICU are seen for follow-up by multiple providers: special premature follow-up clinic, visiting nurse, well child care/private pediatrician, surgical/gastroenterology/neurology/ophthalmology/cardiology specialists, occupational and/or physical therapists, WIC, and others. The nutritional care plan should be coordinated, at least

Table 7-8. Nutritional Concerns of Medical Problems Following Prematurity

Clinical Entity	Significant nutritional issues	Suggestions
Bronchopulmonary dysplasia (BPD)	Increased energy needs Decreased fluid tolerance At risk for osteopenia At risk for oral defensiveness and feeding progression delays	Recommend increased caloric density feeding and supplemental vitamins and minerals, as appropriate Offer anticipatory guidance to caregivers
Necrotizing enterocolitis (NEC)	Extended course on TPN in hospital increases risk for cholestasis and bone demineralization At risk for strictures Surgical resection of bowel may result in short bowel syndrome	Follow liver enzymes and x-rays, as appropriate Maintain a high index of suspicion with reports of feeding intolerance Provide enteral intake suitable to digestion/absorption ability; may require a protein hydrolysate formula
Gastroesophageal reflux (GER)	More common in preterm than term infants May result in poor growth, if severe	Recommend semiupright position and/or thickening of formula with ≈ 1 tsp rice cereal/oz formula Investigate medication options if growth rate slows
Neurological impairment/ cerebral palsy (CP)	Inability to progress from liquid to semisolid and solid foods, and slow to develop self-feeding skills At risk for significant growth failure	Provide anticipatory guidance for caregivers Give advice on stable positioning during feeding and on adaptive feeding equipment Work closely with occupational and physical therapists

Reference: Groh-Wargo S, Thompson M, Cox JH, eds. Nutritional care for high-risk newborns. rev. ed. Chicago: Precept Press, 1994.

initially, with the NICU dietitian and/or physician. If complicated care continues for several years, a dietitian should be identified to assist the family in the development of appropriate nutrition goals and specific feeding plans. Resources for both patient families and health professionals are given below. The rewards of good nutritional assessment and planning are the best possible growth and development for these special infants.

References

1. National Center for Health Statistics. Vital statistics of the United States, 1988, vol. 1. Natality. DHHS Pub. No. (PHS) 90-100. Public Health Service. Washington, D.C.: U.S. Government Printing Office, 1990.
2. Maternal and Child Health Bureau, Health Resources and Services Administration, Public Health Service, U.S. Department of Health and Human Services. Child Health USA '94. DHHS Publication No. HRSA-MCH-95-1, July 1995.
3. Hogue CJR, Buehler JW, Strauss LT, et al. Overview of the national infant mortality surveillance (NIMS) project-design, methods, results. Pub Health Rep 102:126, 1987.
4. Halsey CL, Collin MF, Anderson CL. Extremely low birth weight children and their peers: A comparison of preschool performance. Pediatrics 91:807, 1993.
5. Hack M, Merkatz IR, McGrath SK, et al. Catch-up growth in very-low-birth weight infants. Am J Dis Child 138:370, 1984.
6. Ross G, Krauss AN, and Auld AM. Growth achievement in low-birth-weight premature infants: Relations to neurobehavioral outcome at one year. J Pediatr 103:105, 1983.
7. Hack M, Merkatz IR, Gordon D, et al. The prognostic significance of postnatal growth in very-low-birth weight infants. Am J Obstet Gynecol 143:693, 1982.
8. Saigal S, Rosenbaum P, Stoskopf B, et al. Follow-up of infants 500-1,500 gm birth weight delivered to residents of a geographically defined region with perinatal intensive care facilities. J Pediatr 100:606, 1982.
9. Casey PH, Kraemer HC, Bernbaum J, et al. Growth patterns of low birth weight preterm infants: A longitudinal analysis of a large, varied sample. J Pediatr 117:298, 1990.
10. Ernst JA, Bull MJ, Rickard KA, et al. Growth outcome and feeding practices of the very-low-birth weight infant (less than 1500 grams) within the first year of life. J Pediatr 117:S156, 1990.
11. Altigani M, Murphy JF, Newcombe RG, et al. Catch-up growth in preterm infants. Acta Paediatr Scand (suppl) 357:3, 1989.
12. Brandt I. Growth dynamics of low-birth-weight infants with emphasis on the perinatal period. In: Falkner F, Tanner JM, eds. Human growth. vol 2. Postnatal growth. New York: Plenum Press, 1978; 557–617.
13. Casey PH, Kraemer HC, Bernbaum J, et al. Growth status and growth rates of a varied sample of very-low-birth weight, preterm infants: A longitudinal cohort from birth to three years of age. J Pediatr 119:599, 1991.
14. Kitchen WH, Ford GW, Doyle LW. Growth and very low birth weight. Arch Dis Child 64:379, 1989.
15. Kitchen WH, Doyle LW, Ford GW, et al. Very low birth weight and growth to age 8 years. Am J Dis Child 146:40, 1992.
16. Scottish Low-Birth Weight Study Group. The Scottish low birthweight study: I. Survival, growth, neuromotor and sensory impairment. Arch Dis Child 67:675, 1992.
17. Stice J. Routine nutrition care in follow-up. In: Groh-Wargo S, Thompson M, Cox JH, eds. Nutritional care for high-risk newborns. rev. ed. Chicago: Precept Press, 1994.
18. Manser JJ. Growth in the high-risk infant. Clin Perinatol 11:19, 1984.
19. Committee on Nutrition of the Preterm Infant, European Society for Paediatric Gastroenterology and Nutrition. Nutrition and feeding of preterm infants. Acta Paediatr Scand (suppl) 336:1, 1987.
20. Lucas A, King F, Bishop NB. Postdischarge formula consumption in infants born preterm. Arch Dis Child 67:691, 1992.
21. Bhatia J, Rassin DK. Feeding the premature infant after hospital discharge: Growth and biochemical responses. J Pediatr 118:515, 1991.
22. Barros FC, Huttly SRA, Victoria CG, et al. Comparison of the causes and consequences of prematurity and intrauterine growth retardation: A longitudinal study in southern Brazil. Pediatrics 90:238, 1992.
23. Hack M, Breslau N, Weissman B, et al. Effect of very-low-birth weight and subnormal head size on cognitive abilities at school age. N Engl J Med 325:231, 1991.
24. Kramer MS, McLean FH, Oliver M, et al. Body proportionality and head length "sparing" in growth-retarded neonates: A critical reappraisal. Pediatrics 84:717, 1989.
25. Davies P. Size at birth and growth in the first year of life of babies who are overweight and underweight at birth. Proc Nutr Soc 39:25, 1980.
26. Albertsson-Wikland K, Wennergren M, et al. Longitudinal follow-up of growth in children born small for gestational age. Acta Paediatr 82:438, 1993.
27. Vohr BR, Lipsitt LP, and Oh W. Somatic growth of children of diabetic mothers with reference to birth size. J Pediatr 97:196, 1980.
28. Smith DW, Truog W, Rogers JE, et al. Shifting linear growth during infancy: Illustration of genetic factors in growth from fetal life through infancy. J Pediatr 89:225, 1976.
29. Sher PK, Brown SB. A longitudinal study of head growth in pre-term infants. II: Differentiating between 'catch-up' head growth and early infantile hydrocephalus. Dev Med Child Neurol 17:711, 1975.
30. Hamill PVV, Drizd TA, Johnson CL, et al. Physical growth: National Center for Health Statistics Percentiles. Am J Clin Nutr 32:607, 1979.
31. Babson, SG, Benda GI. Growth graphs for the clinical assessment of infants of varying gestational age. J Pediatr 89:814, 1976.
32. Gairdner D, Pearson J. Growth and development record: Preterm—2 years, length/weight/head circumference. Welwyn Garden City, Hertfordshire, England: Castlemead Press, 1988.
33. Baumgartner RN, Roche AF, Himes JH. Incremental growth tables: Supplementary to previously published charts. Am J Clin Nutr 43:711, 1986.
34. Guo S, Roche AF, Fomon SJ, et al. Reference data on gains in weight and length during the first two years of life. J Pediatr 119:355, 1991.

35. Guo S, Roche AF, Moore WM. Reference data for head circumference and 1-month increments from 1 to 12 months of age. J Pediatr 113:490, 1988.
36. Roche A, Himes JH. Incremental growth charts. Am J Clin Nutr 35:629, 1982.
37. Fomon SJ. Infant nutrition. Philadelphia: Saunders, 1973.
38. Morris SE, Klein MD. Pre-feeding skills: A comprehensive resource for feeding development. Tucson: Therapy Skill Builders, 1987.
39. Lawrence RA, Breastfeeding: A guide for the medical profession. 4th ed. St. Louis: Mosby, 1994; 405–72.
40. Kubit JG. Lactation issues. In: Groh-Wargo S, Thompson M, Cox JH, eds. Nutritional care for high-risk newborns. rev. ed. Chicago: Precept Press, 1994.
41. Abrams SA, Schanler RJ, Tsang RC, et al. Bone mineralization in former very low birth weight infants fed either human milk or commercial formula: One-year follow-up observation. J Pediatr 114:1041, 1989.
42. Chan GM. Growth and bone mineral states of discharged very low birth weight infants fed different formulas or human milk. J Pediatr 123:439, 1993.
43. Cox JH. Nutritional concerns at transfer or discharge. In: Groh-Wargo S, Thompson M, Cox JH, eds. Nutritional care for high-risk newborns. rev. ed. Chicago: Precept Press, 1994.
44. Lucas A, Bishop NJ, King FJ, et al. Randomized trial of nutrition for preterm infants after discharge. Arch Dis Child 67:324, 1992.
45. Nako, Y, Fukushima N, Tomomasa T, et al. Hypervitaminosis D after prolonged feeding with a premature formula. Pediatrics 92:862, 1993
46. National Research Council, Food and Nutrition Board. Recommended dietary allowances. 10th ed. Washington, D.C.: National Academy of Sciences, 1989.
47. Friel JK, Andrews WL, Matthew JD, et al. Improved growth of very low birth weight infants. Nutr Res 13:611, 1993.
48. Bishop NJ, King FJ, Lucas A. Increased bone mineral content of preterm infants fed with a nutrient enriched formula after discharge from hospital. Arch Dis Child 68:573, 1993.
49. Groh-Wargo S. Recommended enteral nutrient intake. In: Groh-Wargo S, Thompson M, Cox JH, eds. Nutritional care for high-risk newborns. rev. ed. Chicago: Precept Press, 1994.
50. Ernst J, Bull M, Rickard K, et al. Feeding practices of the very low birth weight infant within the first year. J Am Diet Assoc 82:158, 1983.

Resources for Health Professionals

Groh-Wargo S, Thompson M, Cox JH, eds. Nutritional care for high-risk newborns, rev. ed. Chicago: Precept Press, 1994.
Morris SE, Klein MD. Pre-feeding skills: A comprehensive resource for feeding development. Tucson, Ariz.: Therapy Skill Builders, 1987.
Taeusch HW, Yogman MW, eds. Follow-up management of the high-risk infant. Boston: Little, Brown, 1987.
Ekvall SW. Pediatric nutrition in chronic diseases and development disorders: Prevention, assessment and treatment. New York: Oxford University Press, 1993.
Bernbaum JC, Hoffman-Williamson M, eds. Primary care of the preterm infant. St. Louis: Mosby Year Book, 1991.

Resources for Families of Prematurely Born Infants

Parent Support Organizations

Parents for Prematures
Box 3046
Kirkland, WA 98083-3046
206/283-7466

Parent Care, Inc.
101½ S. Union Street
Alexandria, VA 22314
703/836-4678

Written Information

Harrison H. The premature baby book. New York: St. Martin's Press, 1983.

Breast-Feeding Equipment

Medela, Inc.
P.O. Box 660
4610 Prime Parkway
McHenry, IL 60050
1-800/435-8316

Ameda-Egnell, Inc.
765 Industrial Drive
Cary, IL 60013
1-800/323-8750

Lact-Aid International Inc.
Box 1066
Athens, TN 80206
615/744-9090

Breast-Feeding Pamphlets/Videos

O'Leary M. You can breast-feed your preterm infant (video and pamphlets, 1989). Health Sciences Center for Educational Resources, SB-56, University of Washington, Seattle, WA 98195, 206/545-1186.

Danner S, Cerutti E. Nursing your premature baby (pamphlet, 1990). Childbirth Graphics L&D, Box 20540, Rochester, NY 14602-0540, 716/272-0300.

Breast-feeding your premature baby (pamphlet, 1990). LeLeche League International, Box 1209, Franklin Park, IL 60131, 847/455-7730.

Nutrition Manual for At-Risk Infants and Toddlers
Janice Hovasi Cox, editor

8

OBESITY

Janice Hovasi Cox, MS, RD

Obesity results when energy intake exceeds energy expenditure. This seems to be a relatively simple concept, but childhood obesity is rather arbitrary in specific definition and is complex in nature, etiology, and treatment. This chapter provides general guidelines for the identification of obese infants and children, suggested etiologies, and recommendations for treatment. Because obesity is a complex condition, successful treatment often involves the concerted efforts of all family members, physician, dietitian, psychologist and/or social worker, and exercise physiologist.

Identification

Overweight or obesity in the infant or child is not specifically identified by a weight for age that plots above a specific percentile, but rather by the relationship of weight to length or height. Growth monitoring includes measurement of weight for age, length or height for age, head circumference for age, and weight for length or height, which are then plotted on the National Center for Health Statistics (NCHS) growth charts[1] (see chapter 5). Obesity has been defined as:

- Weight for length or height index that is more than 120–130% of the ideal (50th percentile); that is, a weight for length or height index that is 20–30% *above* ideal (50th percentile), *not* 120–130% *above* ideal[2,3] *and*
- Weight for length or height index greater than the 95th percentile (NCHS) *or*
- Triceps skin fold exceeding the 85th percentile (in children over 1 year old).

Overweight may be identified as:

- Weight for length or height index at least 110% of ideal (50th percentile) or weight for length or height index

10% *above* ideal (50th percentile) *and*
- Weight for length or height between the NCHS 90th and 95th percentiles.[1,4]

It is important to distinguish obesity from normal growth acceleration patterns to avoid overzealous treatment, unnecessary emotional stress for families, and planting the seeds for eating disorders later in life. The growth pattern characteristic of obesity is generally seen as weight gain accelerating first, with weight for length/height gradually exceeding the NCHS 95th percentile (or 130% of average weight for length/height). Accelerated linear growth and increased lean body mass may also accompany obesity, although the weight for length/height ratio by definition remains high.[2,5] Accelerated linear growth is often accompanied by accelerated increases in bone age (although final height is not affected) and increases in fat-free mass that may account for up to 20% of the increase in weight.[2]

Accelerated weight gain associated with obesity must be distinguished from that seen in "catch-up" growth. When parameters of growth at birth are lower (due to maternal or intrauterine influences) than genetic potential, catch-up growth generally occurs during the first 13 to 24 months of age.[4,6] Catch-up growth may also occur after a period of growth lag due to inadequate nutrition associated with illness or adverse environment, with accelerated weight gain and repletion of adipose stores preceding accelerated linear growth, or increases in lean body mass.[7] In catch-up growth, head growth accelerates first, or initially plots at a higher percentile than weight and/or length. Obesity is distinguished from catch-up growth in that head growth does *not* accelerate—or catch up—first or before length; head growth may or may not accelerate later. Figure 3 in chapter 5 gives an example of accelerated weight gain characteristic of obesity. Although often difficult to measure in infants and young children, triceps and subscapular skin folds and upper arm fat area greater than the 95th percentile may help distinguish children with high weight due to increased adiposity from those with increased muscularity.[1,5]

Obesity is associated with several syndromes—Prader-Willi, Down, Turner's, Bardet-Beidl, Alström, Carpenter's, Klinefelter's, Cushing's, and Albright hereditary osteodystrophy—although obesity does not usually become manifest, even in Prader-Willi, until after 2 years of age. Many of these syndromes include other signs and symptoms such as mental retardation, hypogenitalism, short stature, polydactyly, blindness, or deafness.[8] Other diseases or conditions that significantly reduce mobility and physical activity, e.g., myelodysplasia or cerebral palsy, are also associated with obesity. Side effects associated with obesity, such as hypertension or bowing of the legs (Blount disease) are generally not seen until later in childhood or adolescence. In severe obesity, especially in infants/children with enlarged tonsils, sleep apnea may be seen.[2]

Etiology

Reports on the etiology of obesity are numerous and varied. Several concepts seem to recur or generally concur:

- Endocrine disease is not usually considered unless length or height is below normal.[9]
- Greater birth weights are associated with greater weight throughout infancy and early childhood, although there is wide variation in growth patterns during the first year as genetic factors supersede intrauterine effects on growth.[10–14]
- Obesity during infancy does not correlate with adult obesity,[15–18] although macrosomic infants of mothers who had diabetes mellitus during pregnancy may have an increased incidence of obesity later in life.[16]
- Adiposity normally increases during the first year of life, then decreases.[16,20]
- Adiposity then starts to increase again ("adiposity rebound") around ages 6–7 years; earlier and higher "rebound adiposity" (before 5½ years of age) and obesity during later childhood (6–11 years) or adolescence does correlate with obesity during adulthood.[6,16–18]
- Although it has been reported that breast-feeding is associated with lower (but normal) weight-to-length ratios during the first year of life, most studies do not show a prolonged effect of breast-feeding on growth.[21–26]
- Early introduction of solid foods does not correlate with increased incidence of obesity.[15,23,26]
- When an ad libidum diet is presented to infants and young children, size of meal varies greatly while daily intake remains relatively constant (± 10%).[27]
- Hunger and satiety cues are present, but may be misinterpreted and superseded by caregivers.[27]

Less agreement exists about the influence of other factors on obesity: genetic factors (estimates range from 5% to 80%),[28–33] resting metabolic rates (same or lower in obese subjects or subjects born to obese parents),[31–36] energy intake (same or higher in obese subjects),[31, 37] activity levels,[31, 37–39] and environmental influences.[15, 38–40] Varied findings are likely due to (1) lower correlations of infant/toddler obesity with obesity later in life; (2) contributions of various factors toward total energy expenditure (fat-free mass, fat mass, gender, skeletal muscle metabolism, age, growth, and activity); (3) various ways of estimating energy intake and need based on actual weight or estimates of lean body weight; (4) difficulty in measuring energy expenditure in toddlers, (5) unreliability of dietary intake recording, and (6) the presence of confounding variables in any given situation.

Most likely, several genetic factors may predispose a child to obesity, but environmental, personality, and social influences allow this predisposition to become manifest. It is important to note that even small differences in energy intake and expenditure can result in significant weight gains over time. An intake of only 50–100 kcal per day above energy expenditure could bring a toddler's weight-for-length status from the 50th or 75th percentile to above the 95th percentile in just 6–12 months. This also means that even though resting metabolism accounts for the largest part of daily energy expenditure, factors that account for even a small amount of energy may be significant in the development of obesity.

Treatment

Before treatment can be considered, the family's understanding and attitudes about their infant's/child's obesity must be considered. If the family does not desire change, or view change as possible, treatment cannot be successful. If the family seems motivated to make changes toward control of weight gain, a registered dietitian can be helpful in addressing the following:

- Estimate energy needs based on ideal *weight for length or height* using the NCHS percentile charts[1] (appendix F) and the guidelines given in appendix L. Ideal weight for length may be estimated as:
  —25th percentile if muscle mass is low due to primary diagnosis, decreased muscle tone, or low activity levels
  —50th percentile if muscle mass is or should be within normal limits (arm muscle area between 25th and 75th percentiles)[20]
  —75th percentile if muscle mass is increased (arm muscle area equal to or greater than the 75th percentile).[20]
- If weight *maintenance* is recommended during infancy or for mild obesity in childhood; modify intake and activity to maintain weight but continue to support linear growth until weight-for-length percentile ranking is within normal limits (i.e., until the infant/child "grows into" his/her weight).
- If weight *loss* is indicated (if obesity is accompanied by sleep apnea,[2] child is more than 140% of ideal weight, or obesity is interfering with normal development or mobility) and energy intake is lower than the Recommended Dietary Allowance, carefully review recommendations to ensure adequate intake of protein, electrolytes, minerals, and vitamins.
- Estimate energy imbalance by evaluating present weight for length or height status: 1 lb (0.45 kg) of excess weight roughly indicates excess intake of 3,500 kcal. Example: a child who is 5 lb (2.3 kg) overweight and who gained this excess weight over a period of six months (185 days), has consumed roughly 95 excess kcal/day [(3,500 kcal/lb x 5 lb) ÷ 185 days = 95 kcal/day].
- If intake history or records are available and reliable, excess intake may also be calculated by comparing these with estimated needs as above.
- Reduce intake by calculated excess or about 10–20% of usual intake to maintain weight or reduce intake by 200 to 350 kcal/day (or 20–30% of usual intake) to support a gradual weight loss of 1 to 2 lb (0.5–1 kg)/mo if weight loss is medically indicated.
- Help parents identify and appropriately respond to their infant's/child's hunger and satiety cues and cues that may signal other needs.
- Help parents identify their role in providing access to appropriate foods and regulating the timing of meals and snacks; it is the child's responsibility to control how much or if food is eaten.[41]
- Identify food or beverage consumption patterns or behaviors that support excessive weight gain and give parents guidelines to modify or avoid these behaviors. Emphasize *family* (not just the individual child) life-style changes toward:

—Increasing regular physical activity that is fun for the entire family
—Setting limits on sedentary activities (such as television viewing)
—Replacing high-fat foods with lower fat foods
—Replacing high-calorie beverages with lower calorie beverages
—Increasing consumption of foods with more fiber and complex carbohydrates
—Controlling the kinds of foods that are available
—Scheduling three regular meals per day with one to two snacks at peak hunger times
—Separating meals and snacks from other activities
—Using smaller plates and portion sizes
—Storing food out of sight and reach during nonmeal/snack times
—Eating only at the table (not on the run, at the counter, in front of TV, etc)
—Avoiding extreme dietary regimens.

- To maintain lean body mass and support continued linear growth, make sure that there is adequate intake of other nutrients, especially fluid, protein, essential fatty acids, and minerals, particularly if the variety of the diet is limited due to preference, tolerance, disease or disability.
- Protein-sparing modified fasting has been used in older children and adolescents with some success. However, linear growth does decelerate (temporarily), and electrolyte/mineral supplementation is necessary to achieve positive mineral balance. This approach to weight loss is *not* recommended for infants or young children.[15]
- Monitor linear growth and arm muscle area (or prealbumin status if possible for infants and children with altered linear growth patterns associated with their primary disease or condition).
- Help parents devise reward systems for success that are not food centered.

Although several parent education tools are available,[42, 43] nutrition education and/or counseling should be tailored to meet the individual medical, physical, and psychosocial needs of the child and family within the framework of the family's learning styles, abilities, and functional level of literacy and understanding. The child should be included in the educational process whenever possible. For example, foods can be grouped and color coded: (1) high-calorie, low-nutrient content: red (stop—eat in limited quantities); (2) moderate-calorie, moderate-nutrient content: yellow (caution—eat in moderation); (3) lower calorie, high-nutrient content: green (go—eat as desired).

As many family members or caregivers as possible should be included in treatment plans in order to provide consistency and common understanding of concepts and goals. A single caregiver who is not supportive of the program, either through ignorance or volition, can undermine the best plans or attempts at weight control. Family counseling by a qualified social worker or psychologist may be needed in situations in which the child experiences chronic, unresolved marital conflict, overprotection, or overinvolvement of one parent with exclusion of the other.[15] Counseling may also benefit families in which a handicapped child is overfed out of sympathy or compassion by helping family members find ways to comfort, console, or demonstrate their love in ways that are better for the child. Exercise physiologists and physical therapists may be needed to identify safe and appropriate activities for children with physical disabilities.

Those who provide treatment or counseling to families must be aware of the complex nature of obesity and consider the broad scope of influences that affect the obese child. This awareness is the foundation for a comprehensive treatment plan; sensitivity engenders a cooperative spirit and positive self-image for both the child and the parent that augurs well for weight management success.

References

1. Hamill PVV, Drizd TA, Johnson CL, et al. Physical growth: National Center for Health Statistics percentiles. Amer J Clin Nutr 32:607-29, 1979.
2. Dietz WH. Childhood obesity. In: Suskind RM, Lewinter-Suskind, eds. Textbook of pediatric nutrition. New York: Raven Press, 1993.
3. Dietz WH. Nutrition and obesity. In: Grand RJ, Sutphen JL, Dietz WH, eds. Pediatric nutrition: Theory and practice. Boston: Butterworths, 1987.
4. Ashworth A, Millward DJ. Catch-up growth in children. Nutr Rev 44:157–63, 1986.

5. Forbes GB. Lean body mass and fat in obese children. Pediatrics 34:308, 1964.
6. Albertsson-Wikland K, Wennergren G, Wennergren M, et al. Longitudinal follow-up of growth in children born small for gestational age. Acta Pædiatr 82:438–43, 1993.
7. Fomon SJ. Nutrition of normal infants. St. Louis: Mosby, 1993.
8. Wharton RH. Unusual syndromes associated with obesity. Semin Pediatr Gastroenterol Nutr 1:8–12, 1990.
9. Collipp PJ. Obesity in childhood. In: Stunkard AJ, ed. Obesity. Philadelphia: Saunders, 1980; 405–414.
10. Binkin NJ, Yip R, Fleshood L, et al. Birth weight and childhood growth. Pediatrics 82:828–34, 1988.
11. Pomerance HH, Krall JM. The relationship of birth size to the rate of growth in infancy and childhood. Am J Clin Nutr 39:95–99, 1984.
12. Davies DP. Size at birth and growth in the first year of life of babies who are overweight and underweight at birth. Proc Nutr Soc 39:25–33, 1980.
13. Wright CM, Matthews JNS, Waterston A, et al. What is a normal rate of weight gain in infancy? Acta Pædiatr 83:351–56, 1994.
14. Kramer MS, Barr RG, Leduc DG, et al. Infant determinants of childhood weight and adiposity. J Pediatr 107:104–107, 1985.
15. Crocker RW. Childhood obesity. In: Queen PM, Lang CE. Handbook of pediatric nutrition. Gaithersburg, Md.: Aspen, 1993; 560–72.
16. Rolland-Cachera MF, Deheeger M, Bellisle F, et al. Adiposity rebound in children: A simple indicator for predicting obesity. Am J Clin Nutr 39:129–35, 1984.
17. Zack PM, Harlan WR, Leaverton PE, et al. A longitudinal study of body fatness in childhood and adolescence. J Pediatr 95:126–34, 1979.
18. Gasser T, Ziegler P, Seifert B, et al. Prediction of adult skinfold and body mass from infancy through adolescence. Ann Hum Biol 22:217–33, 1995.
19. Vohr BR, Lipsitt LP, Oh W. Somatic growth of children of diabetic mothers with reference to birth size. J Pediatr 97:196–99, 1980.
20. Frisancho AR. Anthropometric standards for the assessment of growth and nutritional status. Ann Arbor, Mich.: University Press, 1990.
21. Dewey KG, Heinig MJ, Nommsen LA, et al. Growth of breast-fed infants from 0–18 months: The DARLING study. Pediatrics 89:1035–41, 1992.
22. Köhler L, Meeuwisse G, Mortensson W. Food intake and growth of infants between six and twenty-six months of age on breast milk, cow's milk formula, or soy formula. Acta Pædiatr Scand 73:40–48, 1984.
23. Jung E, Czajka-Narinf DM. Birthweight doubling and tripling times: An updated look at the effects of birthweight, sex, race, and type of feeding. Am J Clin Nutr 42:182–89, 1985.
24. Saarinen UM, Siimes MA. Role of prolonged breast feeding in infant growth. Acta Pædiatr Scand 68:245–50, 1979.
25. Kramer MS. Do breast-feeding and delayed introduction of solid foods protect against subsequent obesity? J Pediatr 98:883–87, 1981.
26. Wolman PG. Feeding practices in infancy and prevalence of obesity in preschool children. J Am Diet Assoc 84:436–38, 1984.
27. Birch LL, Fisher JA. Appetite and eating behavior in children. Pediatr Clin North Am 42:931–53, 1995.
28. Kimm SY. The role of dietary fiber in the development and treatment of childhood obesity. Pediatrics 96:1010–14, 1995.
29. Stunkard AJ, Sorensen TIA, Hanis C, et al. An adoption study of human obesity. N Engl J Med 314:193–98, 1986.
30. Stunkard AL, Harris JR, Pedersen NL, et al. The body mass index of twins who have been reared apart. N Engl J Med 322:1483–87, 1990.
31. Roberts SB, Savage J, Soward WA, et al. Energy expenditure and intake in infants born to lean and overweight mothers. N Engl J Med 318:461–66, 1988.
32. Griffiths M, Payne PR. Energy expenditure in small children of obese and non-obese parents. Nature 260:698–700, 1976.
33. Davies PS, Wells JC, Fieldhouse CA, et al. Parental body composition and infant energy expenditure. Am J Clin Nutr 616:1026–29, 1995.
34. Epstein LH, Wing RR, Cluss P, et al. Resting metabolic rate in lean and obese children: Relationship to child and parent weight and percent overweight change. Am J Clin Nutr 49:331–36, 1989.
35. Luke A, Roizen NJ, Sutton M, et al. Energy expenditure in children with Down syndrome: Correcting metabolic rate for movement. J Pediatr 125:829–38, 1994.
36. Goran MI, Kaskoun M, Johnson R. Determinants of resting energy expenditure in young children. J Pediatr 125:362–67, 1995.
37. Waxman M, Stunkard AJ. Caloric intake and energy expenditure of obese boys. J Pediatr 96:187–93, 1980.
38. Romanella NE, Wakat DK, et al. Physical activity and attitudes in lean and obese children and their mothers. Int J Obes 15:407–14, 1991.
39. Dietz WH, Gortmaker SL. Do we fatten our children at the television set? Obesity and television viewing in children and adolescents. Pediatrics 75:807–12, 1985.

40. Dietz WH, Gortmaker SL. Factors within the physical environment associated with childhood obesity. Am J Clin Nutr 39:619–24, 1984.
41. Satter E. Child of mine: Feeding with love and good sense. Palo Alto, Calif.: Bull Publishing, 1986.
42. Klein MD, Delaney TA. Feeding and nutrition for the child with special needs: Handouts for parents. Medvescek, CR, ed. Tucson, Ariz.: Therapy Skill Builders, 1994.
43. Aspen Reference Group, Caregiver education guide for children with developmental disabilities. Rockville, Md.: Aspen, 1994.

Nutrition Manual for At-Risk Infants and Toddlers
Janice Hovasi Cox, editor

9

FAILURE TO THRIVE

Ingrida Mara Melbardis, RD

When an infant's or a child's growth and physical development patterns do not meet standard expectations, we may suspect that the infant/child is "failing to thrive." Although there is little consensus about the exact definition of "failure to thrive" (FTT), its prevalence among children in the United States is thought to be as high as 10% in rural outpatient clinics and 3–5% in pediatric patients admitted to teaching hospitals.[1, 3] Using standard growth charts, such as the National Center for Health Statistics (NCHS) charts with reference percentiles (see appendix F), the following criteria are the most commonly used guidelines for identifying infants or children who are failing the thrive:

- Weight for age falls across two major percentiles over a period of three months in infants or six months in children 12 months old or older.[3]
- The rate of gain in weight is less than the -2 SD value during an interval of two months or longer for infants less than 6 months of age or during an interval of three months or longer for infants over 6 months of age, *and* the weight-for-length ratio is less than the 5th percentile.[4]
- Weight for age is less than the 3rd to 5th percentile, or less than 80–85% of the 50th percentile.[2]

Although FTT is ultimately due to inadequate intake, absorption, or metabolism of one or more nutrients, the etiology of FTT may be varied and multifactorial and is often classified into three subgroups: nonorganic (50%), organic (25%), or combined/mixed (25%).[5]

- *Non-organic FTT* (also known as primary FTT) involves psychosocial issues. Stressors in the home environment or characteristics of the parent, infant, or child may inhibit bonding between the infant/child and parent, leading to a poor feeding relationship. Table 9-1 lists common causes of nonorganic FTT.[6–8]

Table 9-1. Nonorganic (Psychosocial) Causes of Failure to Thrive

Caretaker	Inadequate understanding of infant/child feeding or nutritional needs[6] Psychosocial stress Inadequate duration or number of feedings Inattention to or misinterpretation of hunger cues Feeding times not used for positive, loving interaction Neglect/abuse[7, 8] Parental drug abuse Parental depression, feelings of isolation, or mental illness
Infant	Difficult temperament Slow feeder Delayed feeding skills Subtle hunger cues Apathy due to neglect or inadequate stimulation
Environment	Multiple interruptions/distractions during feedings Improper/lack of food or feeding utensils Poor financial situation Lack of adequate clothing or shelter

- *Organic FTT* (also known as secondary FTT) refers to infants/children who are unable to nutritionally compensate for increased nutrient needs and/or impaired intake, absorption, or metabolism of nutrients that is caused by a disease or medical condition. Table 9-2 lists common causes of organic FTT.
- *Combined or mixed FTT* refers to infants/children who have a disease or medical condition that predisposes them to FTT and whose families have compounding psychosocial issues that preclude adequate feeding.

Table 9-2. Organic Causes of Failure to Thrive

Increased metabolic needs*	HIV/AIDS* Cystic fibrosis* Anemia Lead poisoning	Congenital heart disease* Chronic renal insufficiency* Recurrent respiratory infections Bronchopulmonary dysplasia*
Inadequate intake due to oral-motor dysfunction	Cleft palate* Esophageal strictures* Zinc deficiency (dysgeusia) Pyloric stenosis*	Central nervous system dysfunction* Gastroesophagel reflux† Pierre Robin syndrome/micrognathia Dysfunctional feeding skills†
Increased gastrointestinal losses	Cystic fibrosis* Short gut* Malabsorption‡	Chronic nonspecific diarrhea‡ Inflammatory bowel disease Food allergy
Medications/medical therapy	Ritalin Dilantin	Chemotherapy Radiation therapy
Altered metabolic needs	Inborn errors of protein, carbohydrate, or fat metabolism	
Other	Intrauterine viral infections or maternal drug abuse	

*See individual chapters for more detailed discussion of disease states.
†See chapter 4.
‡See chapter 6.

Nutrition Assessment

Careful assessment of growth patterns, medical history, diet, and environment is needed to determine the cause(s) of FTT so that a course of management can optimize the potential for growth and development.

Growth assessment

It is important to distinguish FTT from normal growth deceleration patterns to avoid overzealous medical evaluation and unnecessary emotional stress for families. Growth deceleration during the first one to two years of life may reflect a discrepancy between intrauterine growth and genetic potential. This deceleration is generally symmetrical. Familial short stature and constitutional growth delay do not respond to nutritional manipulations; they are likely to be an expression of normal growth in some families.[9] Infants who experience intrauterine growth retardation may continue to be smaller than their peers, although growth velocity is within normal limits (see chapter 5 for more in-depth descriptions of growth and sample growth charts of infants and young children with various patterns of growth deceleration.)

Assessment of growth should include the following:

- Use of standard methods for measurement of weight, length or height, and head circumference.[4]
- Accurate plotting of growth parameters: "correcting" age for premature birth up to 24–36 months of age (see chapter 7), plotting recumbent length on the NCHS 0–36 months growth charts, and plotting standing height on the NCHS 2–18 years growth charts.
- Serial growth measurement and recording of weight, length, and head circumference from birth to present (or as many data points as possible) to determine whether changes in growth are acute or chronic, symmetrical, or asymmetrical.
- Calculating growth velocity and comparing these to norms (see tables 5-1 through 5-6).
- Although triceps skin fold and arm muscle area are difficult to measure and are of limited value in infants, these measurements may help identify young children with low muscle mass and/or low adiposity.[10]
- When linear growth parameters fall below the normal range, parental size-specific adjustments can be used to further evaluate linear growth.[11]
- History of medical disease or condition that includes diminished growth, such as inborn errors of metabolism, trisomy 21, Turner's syndrome, Russell-Silver's syndrome, etc.

During acute undernutrition, weight-for-length ratios begin to decrease because weight gain is most affected by acute changes in nutrition, while linear growth continues at the expense of weight gain, presumably using body stores of nutrients. Thus, growth deceleration associated with undernutrition is usually asymmetrical. If nutritional needs continue to exceed intake (due to poor intake, increased needs, and/or increased losses) for more than two to four months, linear growth may also begin to decelerate. As linear growth continues to decelerate, or "stunting" occurs with chronic undernutrition, the weight-for-length ratio appears to normalize.[2] Infants and children who have been chronically and severely undernourished may also demonstrate the following signs of protein-energy malnutrition (PEM):[12]

- *Marasmus*, a deficiency primarily of energy-providing foods; a chronic condition of semistarvation; infant/child adjusts to some extent by reduced growth; in advanced stages it is characterized by muscular wasting and absence of subcutaneous fat.
- *Kwashiorkor*, a protein deficiency; hypoalbuminemia, pitting edema, abnormalities of skin and hair, enlarged fatty liver; subcutaneous fat is usually preserved, but muscle wasting is often masked by edema.
- *Marasmic kwashiorkor*, a deficiency of both calories and protein; edema, gross wasting; usually stunted growth.
- Waterlow's classification of the severity of *malnutrition*:[13]

mild malnutrition:	80-90% of expected weight
moderate malnutrition:	70-79% of expected weight
severe malnutrition:	< 70 % of expected weight

Infants or children with moderate to severe malnutrition, marasmus, kwashiorkor, or marasmic kwashiorkor often require hospitalization during the initial rehabilitation to monitor and maintain fluid and electrolyte balance.

Stunting also occurs in psychosocial-deprivation dwarfism. Although inadequate intake may contribute to initial growth lag, energy intake is often at or above normal levels. Chronic stress and psychosocial deprivation are thought to cause changes in energy expenditure and growth response to growth hormone, resulting in delayed linear growth. Weight for length is usually within normal limits. Psychosocial-deprivation dwarfism is characterized by other distinct features such as apathy, withdrawal, depression, or temper tantrums; bizarre behavior, such as pain agnosia or self-mutilation; polyphagia and polydypsia; gorging and vomiting; stealing food or eating garbage or pet food; drinking stagnant water from toilet bowls or fish tanks; and developmental delay.[14]

If assessment of growth reveals deceleration that cannot be explained by genetic history, dietary intake and feeding assessment are indicated to develop a course of management and to provide comprehensive information to others who may be involved in the infant's or child's care.

Dietary Intake and Feeding Assessment

Nutrition and feeding screening tools are given in appendixes A, B, and D. These tools may help identify (1) adequacy of foods offered and accepted—both kind and amount, (2) method of feeding and developmental progression, (3) presence and parental perception of hunger and satiety cues, (4) feeding behaviors that may interfere with adequate nutrition, and (5) clinical findings that may signal altered nutrient needs or unusual losses. Interpretation of nutrition screening is given in chapter 3; interpretation of the feeding screening tool is given in chapter 4.

When growth falls below expected norms, it is important to more closely evaluate the quantity of food consumed in addition to quality and type of food. Beyond nutrition screening, a detailed food frequency and/or a 24-hour dietary intake recall provides a more specific and comprehensive evaluation of typical dietary intake. If intake appears sporadic, or if the parent has difficulty relating a detailed history of usual intake, a three- to seven-day food intake diary may be needed. Energy, protein, mineral, and vitamin intake is then compared to the Recommended Dietary Allowances (RDA) for the specific age of the infant or child. Energy and fluid needs vary with age and size. Appendix L provides recommendations for estimating normal energy needs for infants and toddlers. Appendix K provides recommendations for estimating fluid needs of infants and toddlers.

Observing the infant/child and parent during a feeding can provide useful information about feeding abilities and mealtime interaction between infant/child and parent (see appendix E). Although a feeding may present an opportunity for parent education and behavior modification, it is important to provide suggestions and guidance in a positive, nonjudgmental manner to prevent parental feelings of defensiveness, failure, or lack of confidence. It may be less threatening to ask questions rather than to give directives. For example, if the parent is holding the bottle at such a shallow angle that very little milk is reaching the nipple, asking "How does your baby like the bottle held this way?" while gently repositioning the bottle may be less threatening than stating "Hold the bottle this way." Then explain why the baby might like the bottle held in a more upright position.

Nutrition Treatment/Care Plan

Table 9-3 lists feeding problems in infants and young children that may contribute to FTT. Once identified, some problems can be easily resolved, such as incorrect formula dilution or use of rehydration solutions, water, or juice in place of breast milk or formula. Providing simple instructions and essential utensils for formula preparation and allowing parents to demonstrate correct formula preparation can be done in a positive and supportive manner. Guidelines for use of rehydration solutions, water, and juice can be easily explained. Switching to a formula that is enriched or higher in caloric density may bring marginally adequate intake up to normal. However, many feeding problems contributing to FTT that are not this straightforward may require referrals to other agencies or programs, in-depth assessment of nutrient needs, workable plans to meet those needs, education/counseling, and regular follow-up.

Referrals

Although the cause of faltering growth may be difficult to distinguish during the initial encounter, the medical and social history, anthropometric measurements, and feeding observations help establish the need for referrals to other professionals or agencies. Referral to a physician is needed when the following are identified or suspected: dehy-

Table 9-3. Feeding Problems, Treatment/Care Plans for Infants and Children Who Fail to Thrive

	Feeding problems	Treatment/care plan
Breast-feeding	Insufficient supply	Increase feeding frequency; ensure adequacy of maternal health, diet/hydration; observe feeding—latch-on, let-down, efficient suck/swallow, emptying of breast, satiety cues; avoid maternal use of medications/drugs that may interfere with milk production, alcohol, or smoking; consider referral to lactation consultant; nursing supplementer using a standard-strength infant formula
	Intake inadequate to meet metabolic demands	A calorie-dense formula may be used in a nursing supplementer and given while the infant is nursing at the breast; supplementing the breast-fed infant in this manner will help maintain maternal milk supply and avoid nipple confusion; carbohydrate, fat, vitamin and/or mineral supplements may be given by dropper, teaspoon, or spouted cup when switching from one breast to the other; pumped breast milk may be fortified with infant formula powder or liquid formula concentrate
	Immature or dysfunctional sucking pattern	Referral to feeding specialist
Formula	Inadequate supply	Referral to food supplemental programs (WIC), food stamps, community food "pantries," social service agencies; guidance regarding intake of rehydration solutions, juice or water if prolonged or inappropriate use of these liquids prevents adequate intake of formula
	Intake inadequate to meet metabolic demands	Increase caloric density of the formula by adding less water to formula powder or liquid formula concentrate; increasing formula concentration maintains proportional intake of other nutrients, particularly protein, zinc, iron, calcium, phosphorus, magnesium, and electrolytes; intakes of at least 120–180 ml/kg/day (1.8–2.7 oz/lb/day) can provide adequate intake to support normal or catch-up growth if 1 kcal/ml (30 kcal/oz) formula is used
	Nutrient intake exceeds expected needs, but weight gain remains less than expected	Additional carbohydrate or fat may be added to feedings, provided macronutrient ratios are kept within a balanced range, as given in table 9-4
	Intake not sufficient to meet fluid needs (see appendix L)	Concentration of formula is not indicated; tube-feedings must be considered
Food	Inadequate supply	Referral to food supplemental programs (WIC), food stamps, community food "pantries," social service agencies
	Inadequate variety	Assess adequacy of macro- and micronutrients; review appropriate guidelines for feeding children; consider supplementation with a multivitamin/mineral preparation or therapeutic supplementation of nutrients, if necessary
	Intake inadequate to meet metabolic demands	Supplement diet with nutrient-dense foods such as cheese, cream cheese, margarine, powdered milk, peanut butter, or proprietary supplements such as Pediasure (Ross Laboratories), Kindercal (Mead Johnson), or a variety of breakfast drinks; a variety of chewable multivitamin with mineral supplements are available for children with increased needs for these nutrients—these may be crushed and added to soft or pureed texture foods if necessary; if growth does not improve with oral intake alone, supplemental tube-feeding may need to be considered

Table 9-3. Feeding Problems, Treatment/Care Plans for Infants and Children Who Fail to Thrive (continued)

	Feeding problems	Treatment/care plan
Food (cont.)	Delayed progression to increased food texture	Modify current diet to provide some foods with increased textures, gradually advancing diet as tolerated; refer to a feeding therapist if child is resistant to diet change (oral hypersensitivity, poor oral-motor skills, etc.) (See chapter 4, tables 4-2, 4-7 and 4-8)
	Child refuses to take solids	Provide some thickened liquids, gradually increasing the texture; try offering these foods on a finger, nipple or toy; refer to a feeding therapist (oral hypersensitivity, poor oral-motor skills, etc.)
Behavior/ development	Inefficient feeding (feedings take longer than 30 min for an infant or longer than 45 min for a toddler)	Concentrate formula/provide more nutrient-dense foods; a different nipple style (preemie, orthodontic) may be better tolerated; alter texture of food to require less oral manipulation (see chapter 4)
	Frequent coughing, gagging, choking while eating and drinking	Refer to a feeding specialist for a swallow evaluation
	Lacking age-appropriate feeding skills	Adjust diet consistency/texture to maximize infant's/child's abilities; refer to feeding specialist for further oral-motor skill development
	Poor positioning	Review proper positioning; refer to occupational/physical therapists for adaptive seating equipment, if necessary
	Improper feeding utensils	Review age-appropriate utensils; refer to social service agencies if lack of utensils is due to financial constraints; refer to feeding therapist if adaptive feeding utensils are needed
Elimination	Diarrhea/constipation	See chapter 6
Environment	Multiple interruptions/distractions during feedings	If parent, infant, or child is easily distracted, remove as many distracting variables as possible during feeding times; strong contrasts of color or light, strong odors, television, radio or other loud noises, or the activity of other family members may be distracting and prevent adequate feeding
	Poor interaction of caregiver and infant/child	Help parent identify and learn how to respond to infant's/child's cues of hunger/satiety; encourage interaction between caregiver and infant/child; if parents' needs supersede the infant's or child's need to be fed, refer to psychology, mental health, or social service agency

dration (table 6-2), chronic significant vomiting or diarrhea (tables 6-4 and 6-9), or medical disease/condition (table 9-2). Symptoms of feeding skill delay or dysfunction that may require the intervention of a feeding therapist are given in table 4 of chapter 4. If it is apparent that access to food, clothing, or shelter is inadequate, these needs must be addressed before other expectations can be met. Referral to food supplemental programs, neighborhood "pantries," or social service agencies must be done in a timely manner. Psychosocial dysfunction within the family unit may preclude adequate feeding of one or more of the children, and may require referral to psychology services or mental health or social service agencies.

Estimating and Meeting Nutritional Needs

Whether the cause of FTT is organic or nonorganic, estimating the present intake of nutrients compared to growth is a helpful step. Nutrient needs may be increased in various organic causes of FTT (see table 9-2 and all of section III of this book). If growth is faltering and reported intakes are normal or high, unusual losses through vomiting, diarrhea, or metabolic demands must be considered. If intake is low due to fatigue or immature or dysfunctional feeding skills, concentrated feedings or tube-feedings must be considered. If intake is low due to parental neglect, family dysfunction, or inadequate access to food, individualized care plans must be developed to encompass treatment of the primary psychosocial or economic problem to support successful treatment of the infant or child who is failing to thrive.

Intake may seem adequate when needs are calculated for actual weight, but it may fall below expected needs for ideal weight. Because length/height may be low for age, and body weight may be low for length/height—or may be affected by the presence of edema—calculation of nutrient needs to promote optimal growth is often based on ideal weight for age or ideal weight for length/height or "height-age" rather than actual weight. To estimate energy needs:

- Plot weight for age and length/height for age on the appropriate NCHS growth chart.
- Find the age at which length/height would be at the 50th percentile = height-age.
- Plot weight for length/height.
- Find the ideal body weight (IBW) for length/height:
  —50th percentile weight for length/height if normal activity and muscle mass is expected, or
  —10–25th percentile weight for length/height if activity is limited (e.g., myelomeningocele) or below-normal muscle mass is expected due to inactivity or diagnosis (cerebral palsy, muscular dystrophy).
- Then calculate energy and protein needs using the equations given in table 9-4.

Energy needs may be increased by 20–100% to support adequate catch-up growth.[2, 9] Although initial weight gain is rapid during refeeding, lean body mass may increase more gradually.[4] Some studies have indicated that higher protein intakes takes of up to 15% of total calories may yield improved lean body mass ratios.[15] Infants and children who are severely malnourished may require a more gradual reintroduction of adequate feedings to avoid refeeding syndrome, characterized by diarrhea and a drop in serum phosphorus and potassium. Initial feedings may need to be started as low as 25–50 kcal/day and advanced by 20–25 kcal/kg every one or two days until estimated needs are met[2, 16, 17] (see table 9-4).

Nutrition Treatment/Care Plans

Nutrition treatment/care plans must reflect not only the infant's or child's nutrient needs, but must consider and respect the cultural, socioeconomic, psychological, and physical circumstances of the family. Parents may feel inadequate, incompetent, frustrated or defensive about their offspring's growth regardless of whether growth failure is caused by organic or nonorganic factors. The term *FTT* may be intimidating."Growth problem" or "difficulty gaining weight" may be less threatening terminology. Addressing parents' feelings and perceptions begins a working relationship. Identifying reasonable goals with parents and encouraging them to be actively involved in problem solving improves compliance and ultimate outcome.[6] (Table 9-3 gives suggested treatment/care plans for feeding problems that may cause infants or children to fail to thrive.)

Education

Nutrition education and counseling must meet individual medical, physical, and psychosocial needs of the infant/child and family within the framework of the family's learning styles, abilities, and functional level of liter-

Table 9-4. Estimating Needs for Catch-up Growth

Energy	150–240 kcal/kg/day × actual weight in kg *or* kcal/kg/day for height-age* × IBW† in kg *or* $\frac{\text{kcal/kg/day for weight-age* } \times \text{ ideal weight for age}}{\text{actual weight}}$
Protein	3.1–4.4 g/kg/day × actual weight in kg *or* g/kg/day for height-age (or weight-age) × IBW† in kg *or* $\frac{\text{g/kg/day for weight-age } \times \text{ ideal-weight for age(kg)}}{\text{actual weight (kg)}}$ *or* 8–15% of total energy intake
Carbohydrate	35–60% of total energy intake
Fat	35–50% of total energy intake (at least 4% of total energy intake as essential fatty acids)
Micronutrients	Recommended Dietary Allowances for height-age or actual age, whichever is higher Iron: 1–2 mg/kg/day to meet normal needs 4–6 mg/kg/day in divided doses if iron deficiency anemia is present Zinc: 1.6–9.8 mg/kg/day

*See text and appendix L.

†Ideal weight for length or height (see text).

References: 2–4, 13, 18, 19.

acy and understanding. Basic information may be needed, such as coaching a parent to physically demonstrate formula preparation or providing step-by-step pictured instructions for special dietary recommendations. Other families may make changes more easily if given detailed information or a variety of options from which to choose. Printed education materials for parents that describe increasing formula density, supplementing the breast-fed infant, and increasing the toddler's energy and protein intake are available from several sources. Parents may place more value on educational materials that are individualized in some way to meet their own offspring's specific needs.

Follow-up

During nutritional rehabilitation, the rate of weight gain is usually greater than average for age or height-age. Weight gains of 60 g/day are not unusual until normal weight for length or height has been attained.[4] Improved weight gain generally precedes improved linear growth. The weight-to-length/height ratio may increase above the 50th percentile before improved linear growth occurs. Parents should be advised that their infant/child may start to look "chubby," but that this is normal.[9] When growth potential is attained, appetite decreases to support normal needs for age and size. If parents become concerned about increased weight gain, they should be encouraged to discuss this with their infant's/child's dietitian before changing the feeding regimen. Ultimate linear catch-up growth depends on (1) length of time needed to correct poor weight gain, (2) genetic potential, (3) parental height, (4) intrauterine factors, and (5) birth size.[20–22]

Infants and children who fail to thrive are more likely to have developmental, cognitive, and behavioral difficulties.[22,23] A multidisciplinary team including the parents, pediatrician, social worker, dietitian, and nurse is often needed to effect desired outcomes. Others, such as feeding therapists (occupational therapists, physical therapists, or speech pathologists) and mental health care providers should be consulted as needed. Frequent follow-up is often necessary to refine and adjust care plans when needed and to monitor compliance with dietary and/or psychosocial interventions/recommendations until normal growth parameters are attained.

Appropriate and timely intervention along with frequent follow-up may provide the best success rate for catch-up growth and diminish other long-term effects in infants/children who fail to thrive.[24–28]

References

1. Mitchell W, Gorrell R, Greenberg R. Failure to thrive: A study in a primary care setting. Pediatrics 65:971, 1980.
2. Rathbun J, Peterson K. Nutrition in failure to thrive. In: Grand R, Sutphen J, Dietz W, eds. Pediatric nutrition theory and practice. Boston: Butterworths, 1987; 627.
3. Peterson K. Failure to thrive. In: Queen P, Lang C, eds. Handbook of pediatric nutrition. Gaithersburg: Aspen, 1993; 366.
4. Fomon S, Nelson S. Size and growth. In: Fomon S. Nutrition of normal infants. St. Louis: Mosby, 1993; 36.
5. Gotlin R, Kappy M, Eisenbarth G, Chase HP. Endocrine disorders. In: Hay Jr W, Groothuis J, Hayward A, Levin M, eds. Current pediatric diagnosis and treatment. 12th ed. Norwalk: Appleton & Lange, 1995; 881.
6. McCann J, Stein A, Fairburn C, Dunger D. Eating habits and attitudes of mothers and children with non-organic failure to thrive. Arch Dis Child 70:234, 1994.
7. Taitz LS, King JM, Growth patterns in child abuse. Acta Paediatr 343 (suppl):62, 1988.
8. Peterson K, Washington JS, Rathbun J. Team management of failure to thrive. J Am Diet Assoc 84:810, 1984.
9. Maggioni A, Lifshitz F. Nutritional management of failure to thrive. Pediatr Clin North Am 42: 791, 1995.
10. Frisancho AR. Anthropometric standards for the assessment of growth and nutritional status. Ann Arbor: University of Michigan Press, 1993.
11. Himes JH, Roche AF, Thissen D, Moore WM. Parent-specific adjustments for evaluation of recumbent length and stature of children. Pediatrics 75:304–13, 1985.
12. Lewinter-Suskind L, Suskind D, Murthy KK, et al. The malnourished child. In: Suskind RM, Lewinter-Suskind L, eds. Textbook of pediatric nutrition, 2d ed. New York: Raven Press, 1993; 127–40.
13. Waterlow JC. Classification and definition of protein-calorie malnutrition, Br Med J 3:566, 1972.
14. Vargas A, Tenore A. Nutritional considerations in the development and treatment of psychosocial-deprivation dwarfism. In: Suskind RM, Lewinter-Suskind L, eds. Textbook of pediatric nutrition. 2d ed. New York: Raven Press, 1993; 275–78.
15. Kabir I, Malek M, Rahman M, Khaled M, Mahalanabis D. Changes in body composition of malnourished children after dietary supplementation as measured by bioelectrical impedence. Am J Clin Nutr 59:5, 1994.
16. Bredow M, Jackson A. Community based, effective, low cost approach to the treatment of severe malnutrition in rural Jamaica. Arch Dis Child 71:297, 1994.
17. Fjeld C, Schoeller D, Brown K. Body composition of children recovering from severe protein-energy malnutrition at two rates of catch-up growth. Am J Clin Nutr 50:126, 1989.
18. Jackson AA, Doherty J, de Benoist MH, Hibbert J, Persaud C. The effect of the level of dietary protein, carbohydrate and fat on urea kinetics in young children during rapid catch-up weight gain. Br J Nutr 64:371, 1990.
19. Golden MHN, Golden BE. Effects of zinc supplementation on the dietary intake, rate of weight gain, and energy cost of tissue deposition in children recovering from severe malnutrition. Am J Clin Nutr 30:1545, 1977.
20. Forchielli ML, McColl R, Walker WA, Lo C. Children with congenital heart disease; a nutrition challenge. Nutr Rev 52:348, 1994.
21. Hansen SR, Dorup I. Energy and nutrient intakes in congenital heart disease. Acta Paediatr 82:166, 1993.
22. Fitzhardinge PM, Inwood S. Long-term growth in small-for-date children. Acta Paediatr (suppl) 349P 27, 1989
23. Golden MH. Is complete catch-up growth possible for stunted malnourished children? Eur J Clin Nutr 48(suppl):S58, 1994.
24. Bithoney WG, McJunkin J, Michalek J, Egan H, Snyder J, Munier A. Prospective evaluation of weight gain in both nonorganic and organic failure-to-thrive children: an outpatient trial of a multidisciplinary team intervention strategy. J Dev Behav Pediatr 10:27, 1989.
25. Heikens GT, Schofield WN, Dawson S, Grantham-McGregor S. The Kingston project. I. Growth of malnourished children during rehabilitation in the community, given a high energy supplement. Eur J Clin Nutr, 43:45, 1989.
26. Martorell R, Khan LK, Schroeder DG. Reversibility of stunting: Epidemiological findings in children from developing countries. Eur J Clin Nutr 48 (suppl):S45, 1994.
27. Wahling TM, Georgieff MK. The effects of illness on neonatal metabolism and nutritional management. Clin Perinatol 22:77, 1995.
28. Suwa S. A boy with psycho-social short stature followed up from infancy to adulthood. Acta Paediatrica 37:283, 1995.

Parent Education Materials

Aspen Reference Group, Caregiver education guide for children with developmental disabilities. Rockville, Md.: Aspen, 1996. (1) Promoting weight gain, (2) Snacks to promote weight gain, (3) Sample menu for promoting weight gain, (4) High-calorie food fortifiers.

Klein MD, Delaney TA. Feeding and nutrition for the child with special needs: Handouts for parents. Medvescek CR, ed. Tucson: Therapy Skill Builders, 1994. (1) High calorie formulas. (2) Increasing formula concentrations, (3) Choosing the right nipple, (4) Helping your child transition from liquids to strained foods, (5) Helping your child transition from strained foods to soft, lumpy foods, (6) What to do about failure to thrive, (7) Calorie boosters: Tips for tanking up, (8) Calorie boosters that pack a punch, (9) Calorie boosters: Fueling with food group variety, (10) Calorie boosters: Mealtime makeovers.

Nutrition Manual for At-Risk Infants and Toddlers
Janice Hovasi Cox, editor

10

NEUROLOGICAL COMPROMISE

Sally Bonnema, MA, RD

Infancy and early childhood marks a period of tremendous growth and development for which nutrition and the ability to feed are cornerstones. Neurological compromise often has an impact on the nutrition status and feeding abilities of the infant or child. This impact may become more apparent with time as growth, development, and the acquisition of new feeding skills evolve or fail to evolve along established norms (see chapter 4). Just as sound nutrition practices are basic to growth and development, appropriate diet modification or supplementation for the special needs infant/child improves nutritional status and enhances growth and functioning abilities.[1]

Infants and children described in this chapter differ by diagnosis, yet share many of the same characteristics or conditions that increase their nutritional risk. Collectively, the literature has addressed this population as children with developmental disabilities. As defined in the Developmental Disabilities Assistance and Bill of Rights Act of 1990 (Public Law 101–496), the term *developmental disability* in infants or children under 5 years of age refers to substantial motor or cognitive delays or specific congenital or acquired conditions that are associated with a high probability of delay if services are not provided.[2] The incidence of developmental delay for children in the United States has been estimated at 3%, with up to 90% of these children exhibiting at least one nutrition-related concern.[3-5]

Although some motor or cognitive delays may be due to a single etiology, many infants and children demonstrate more than one disabling condition. For example, a child with cerebral palsy caused by anoxia may also have seizures.[5] Many of these disabilities are complex in nature, affecting both motor and cognitive development. Motor disabilities range from mild, with minimal or no impairment of function, to impairment so severe that movement is dominated by decerebrate posturing and primitive reflexes. Oral-motor skills and feeding abilities may also be affected. Neurologically compromising medical diagnoses and conditions that may affect nutrition are listed in table 10-1.

Although nutritional requirements for special needs infants and children mirror the nutrient needs of their normal cohorts, their needs may be influenced by their condition and/or its treatment. General nutrition problems associated with specific conditions that are associated with developmental disabilities are listed in table 10-2. The

Table 10-1. Medical Diagnoses/Conditions with Neurologic and Nutrition Implications

Genetic
- Chromosomal abnormalities:
  - fragile X
  - trisomy 13
  - trisomy 18
  - trisomy 21 (Down syndrome)
- Neurometabolic disorders (including inborn errors of protein, carbohydrate, or fat metabolism)
- Neuromuscular dystrophies (including adrenoleukodystrophy)
- Spina bifida

Congenital
- Drug exposure
- Fetal alcohol syndrome
- Hydrocephalus
- Hypothyroidism (untreated)
- Intrauterine growth retardation
- Intrauterine hypoxia
- Intrauterine infections:
  - cytomegalovirus
  - herpes simplex virus
  - syphilis
- Small for gestational age
- Uncontrolled maternal neurometabolic disorder during pregnancy

Perinatal or birth trauma
- Asphyxia
- Intraventricular hemorrhage
- Kernicterus
- Meconium aspiration
- Prolonged hypoglycemia or acidosis
- Sepsis

Acquired conditions
- Cerebral palsy (spastic, hypotonic, ataxic, athetoid)
- Epilepsy (seizure disorders)
- Trauma:
  - Abuse/neglect ("shaken baby" syndrome, battering, etc.)
  - Accidents (closed head injuries, falls, near-drowning, asphyxia, poisoning, etc.)

Adapted with permission from Nevin-Folino NL. Neurological impairment. In: Groh-Wargo S, Thompson M, Cox JH, eds. Nutritional care for high-risk newborns. rev. ed. Chicago: Precept Press, 1994.

severity of nutritional problems encountered varies widely based on age, body composition, energy expenditure, altered growth rates, medications, physical impairment, environment, functioning ability, and the capacity for training.[5-8]

Nutrition Assessment

Growth

Various medical conditions that affect neurological function in infants and toddlers may also affect growth, as shown in table 10-2. Chromosomal disorders, syndromes of unknown etiology, maternal infections such as rubella and cytomegalic virus, fetal alcohol syndrome, or intrauterine cocaine exposure may cause prenatal onset of growth delay.[9] Infants who are proportionally small for gestational age and do not show signs of catch-up growth during the first year of life, particularly in head circumference, are more likely to exhibit developmental delay and

Table 10-2. Frequently Reported Nutrition-Related Problems in Infants with Neurologic Impairment

Condition	Growth delay	Altered energy needs	Altered nutrient needs	Feeding problems	Constipation or diarrhea	Other
Cerebral palsy	+	+	+	+	+	Poor appetite, altered muscle tone
Seizures		±	+	±	+	Drug/nutrient interactions
Birth asphyxia	+	+		+	+	
Drug exposure or FAS*	+	+		+	+	Poor appetite
Sepsis		+		+		
Neurometabolic disease	±	+	+	+		May need specialized formula or supplements
Chromosomal abnormalities	+	+	±	+	+	
Spina bifida	+	+	+	+	+	
Prader-Willi syndrome	+	+		+	+	

Adapted with permission from Nevin-Folino NL. Neurological impairment. In: Groh-Wargo S, Thompson M, Cox JH, eds. Nutritional care for high-risk newborns. rev. ed. Chicago: Precept Press, 1994.

\+ indicates problem usually present
± indicates problem may be present
* FAS = Fetal alcohol syndrome

are likely to remain small for age throughout childhood.[10] Postnatal growth delay may be characteristic of some metabolic diseases, chromosomal anomalies, quadriplegic cerebral palsy, psychosocial deprivation, and syndromes such as Rett, Turner's or Down. [11]

Although postnatal growth delay in neurologically compromised infants and children may be associated with poor nutritional status, several nonnutritional factors may be involved. Diminished growth of bone and muscle may occur in infants and toddlers who are unable to ambulate or bear full body weight on their legs.[7, 8, 12] This may be due to decreased production and release of growth factors at the bone site. Normally, production and release of these factors are stimulated by the mechanical stress associated with movement and weight bearing.[8] Delayed bone age may accompany delayed linear growth. [11]

Serial height/length, weight, and head circumference measures should be plotted on standard growth charts such as the National Center for Health Statistics (NCHS) charts given in appendix F or growth charts that have been developed for specific diagnoses such as quadriplegic cerebral palsy, Turner's, Williams, Down, and Prader-Willi syndromes (see figures 10-1 through 10-5). The rate of weight gain and linear growth may be calculated and compared to norms for age or height-age to help identify ongoing growth delay or catch-up growth, as discussed in chapter 5.

Measuring growth in infants and children with developmental delay is often challenging. The presence of limb contractures, scoliosis, abnormal postures, supportive or corrective bracings or casts, and the inability to cooperate can decrease the accuracy of weight and linear measurements.[13-15] Standard techniques for measuring weight and length/height should be used whenever possible.[16] If practical, weight should be measured without supportive or corrective devices. If this is not practical, weight changes over time can be compared to norms, as suggested in chapter 5. Although these devices can be weighed at one visit, then subtracted from subsequent measurements of weight, the devices may be changed frequently to accommodate growth and developmental progress.

Due to physical disabilities, alternative measures for height and length have been developed to assess growth. A reliable picture of growth can be obtained when measurements are taken periodically using a consistent method and standard technique.[15] Alternative length/height measures include the following list (these measurements are reproducible and may be compared with published norms as suitable approximations of linear growth):[15-19]

- Crown-rump length for infants and children up to 2 years of age and sitting height for children 2 years and above. Because the legs grow more rapidly during childhood than the trunk, the ratio of crown-rump or sitting height to total length or height is not constant, but is highest during infancy and gradually decreases during childhood.[19]

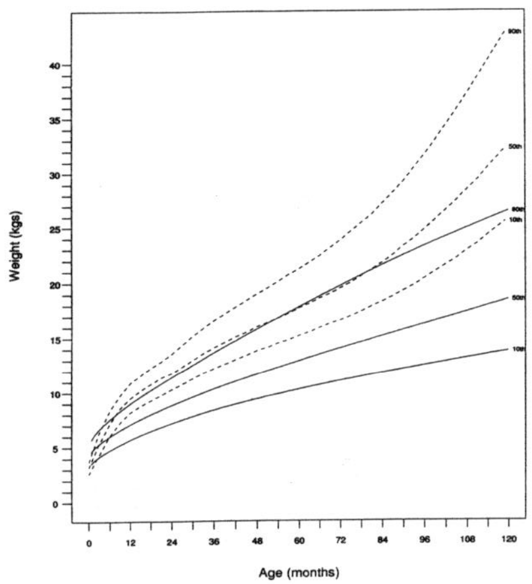

FIG 2. Weight for age for girls aged 0 to 120 months. The solid line represents girls with quadriplegic cerebral palsy and the dotted line represents the National Center for Health Statistics standard curve for 10th, 50th, and 90th percentiles.

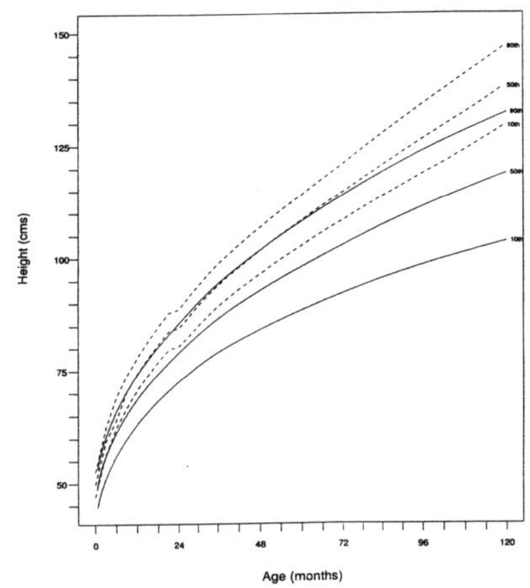

FIG 3. Length for age for girls aged 0 to 120 months. The solid line represents girls with quadriplegic cerebral palsy and the dotted line represents the National Center for Health Statistics standard curve for 10th, 50th, and 90th percentiles.

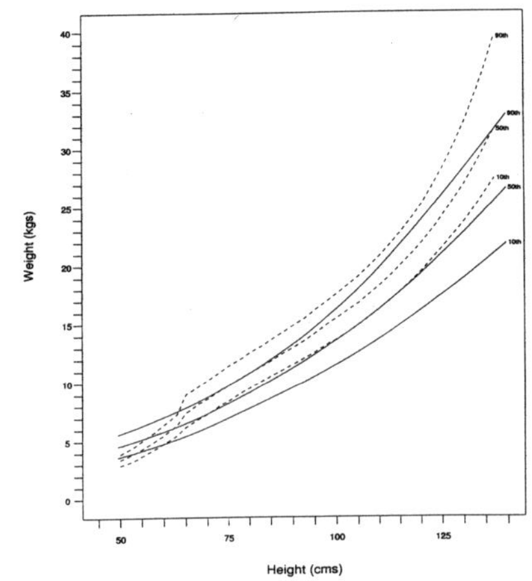

FIG 4. Weight for length for girls aged 0 to 120 months. The solid line represents girls with quadriplegic cerebral palsy and the dotted line represents the National Center for Health Statistics standard curve for 10th, 50th, and 90th percentiles.

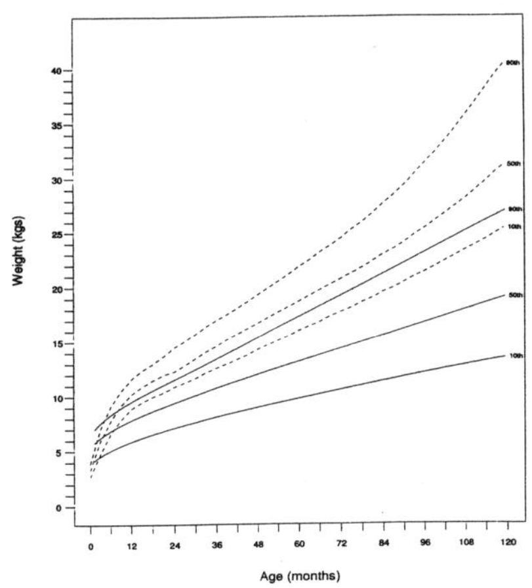

FIG 5. Weight for age for boys aged 0 to 120 months. The solid line represents boys with quadriplegic cerebral palsy and the dotted line represents the National Center for Health Statistics standard curve for 10th, 50th, and 90th percentiles.

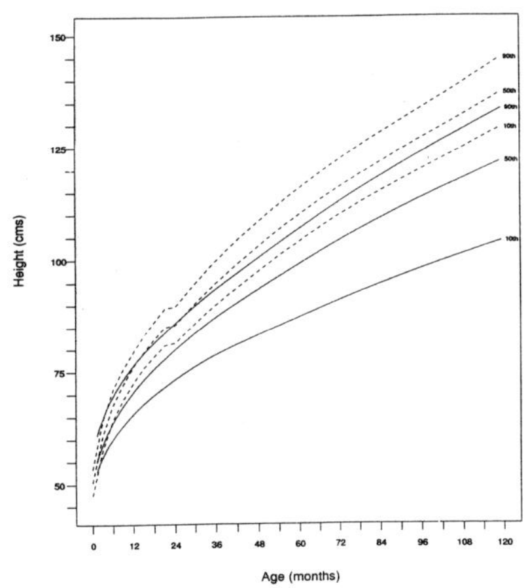

FIG 6. Length for age for boys aged 0 to 120 months. The solid line represents boys with quadriplegic cerebral palsy and the dotted line represents the National Center for Health Statistics standard curve for 10th, 50th, and 90th percentiles.

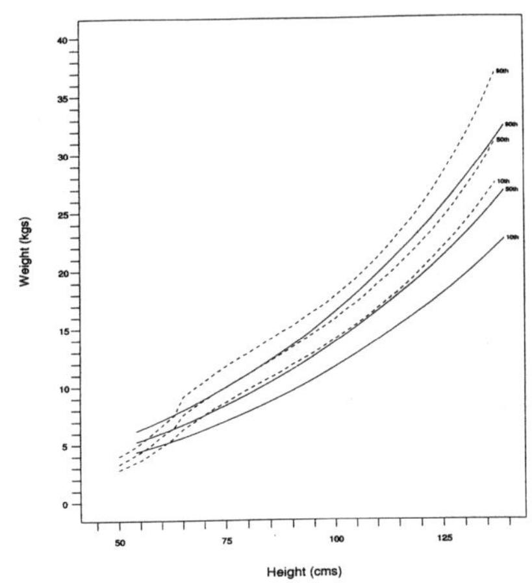

FIG 7. Weight for length for boys aged 0 to 120 months. The solid line represents boys with quadriplegic cerebral palsy and the dotted line represents the National Center for Health Statistics standard curve for 10th, 50th, and 90th percentiles.

Figure 10-1. Growth graphs for infants and children with quadriplegic cerebral palsy. (Krick J, Murphy-Miller P, Zeger S, Wright E. Pattern of growth in children with cerebral palsy. J Am Diet Assoc 96:680–85, 1996. © American Dietetic Association)

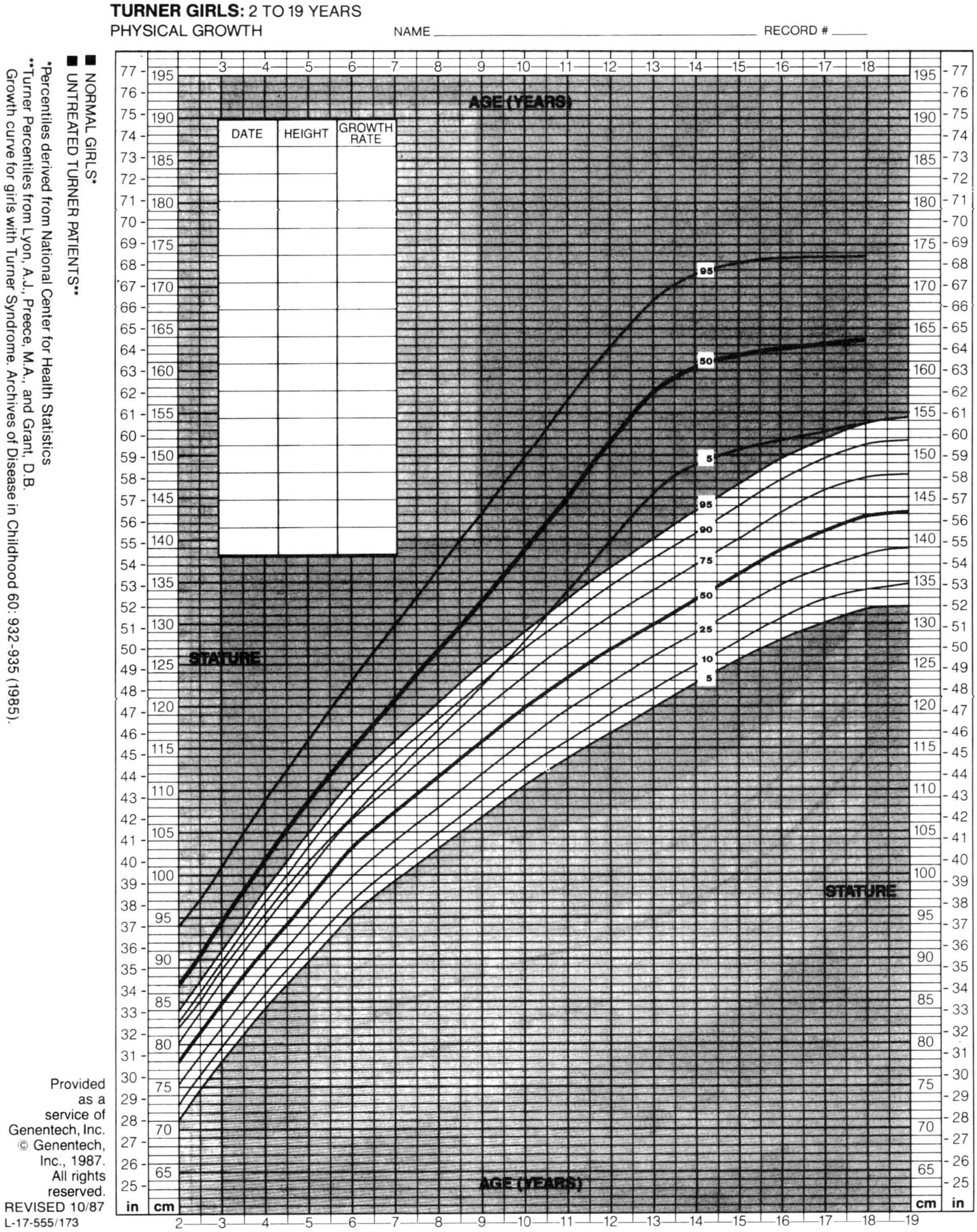

Figure 10-2. Growth graphs for girls with Turner syndrome. (Reprinted with permission. © Genentech, Inc. 1987.)

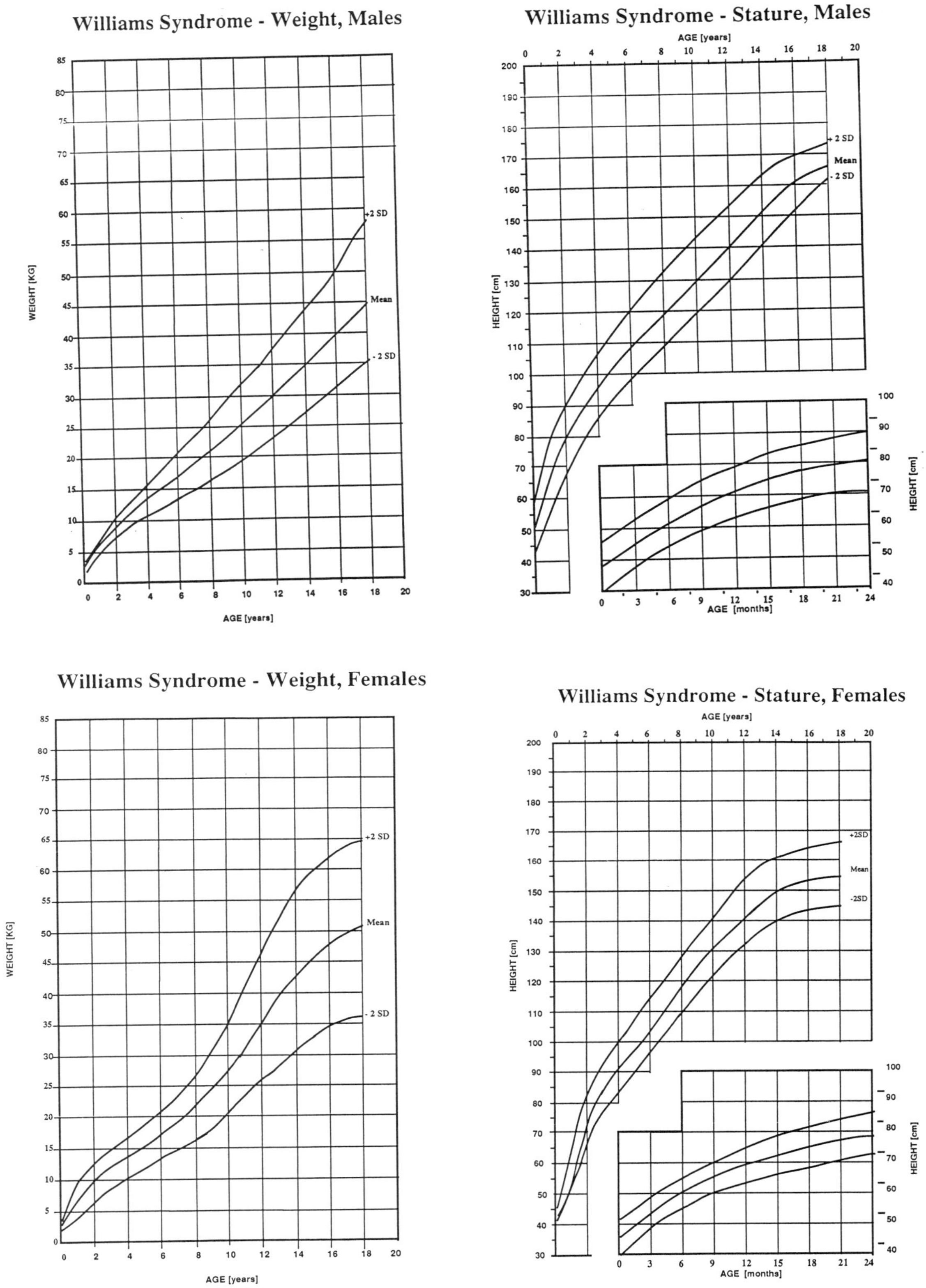

Figure 10-3. Growth graphs for children with Williams syndrome. (Reprinted with permission from Morris CA, Demsey MS, Leonard CL, et al. height and weight of males and females with Williams syndrome. Williams Syndrome Association National Newsletter, summer 1991, pp 29–30.)

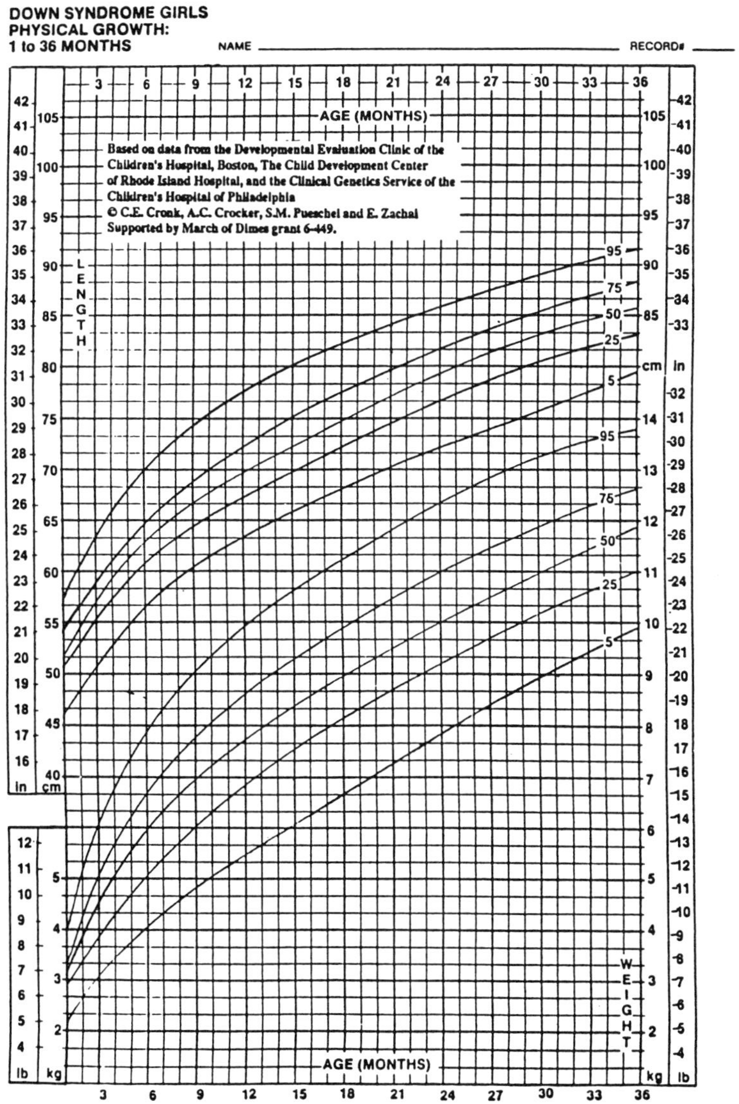

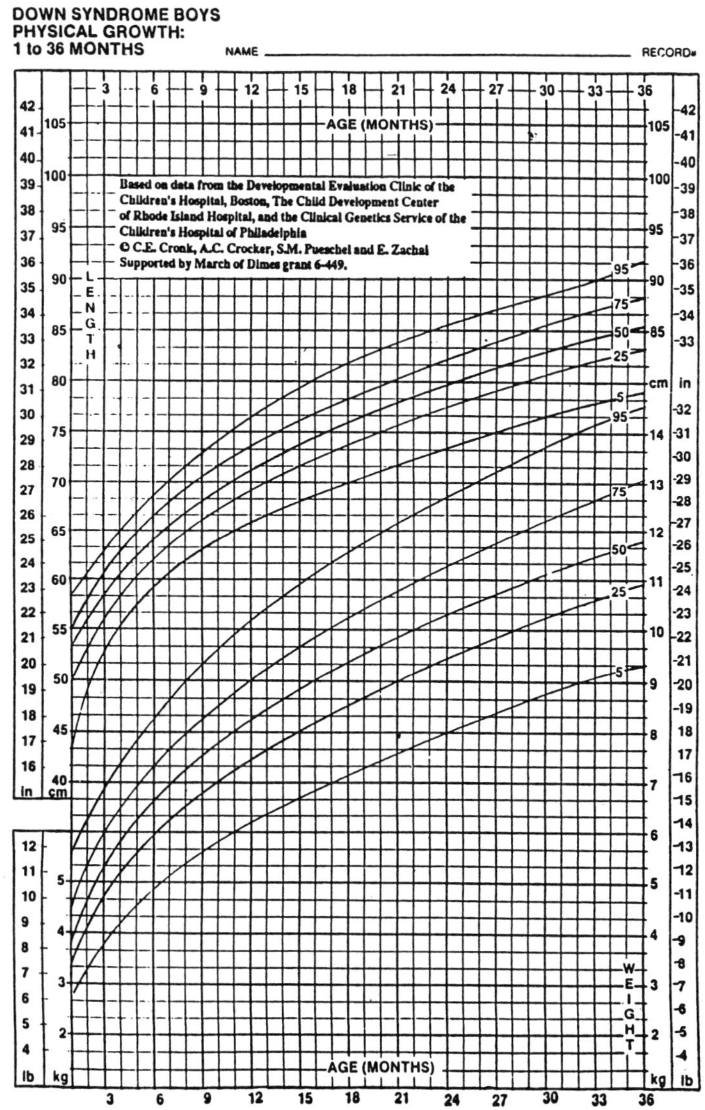

Figure 10-4. Growth graphs for infants and children with Down syndrome. (Cronk C, Crocker AC, Pueschel SM, et al. Growth charts for chidlren with Down syndrome. Reproduced by permission of Pediatrics 81:102–10, © 1988.)

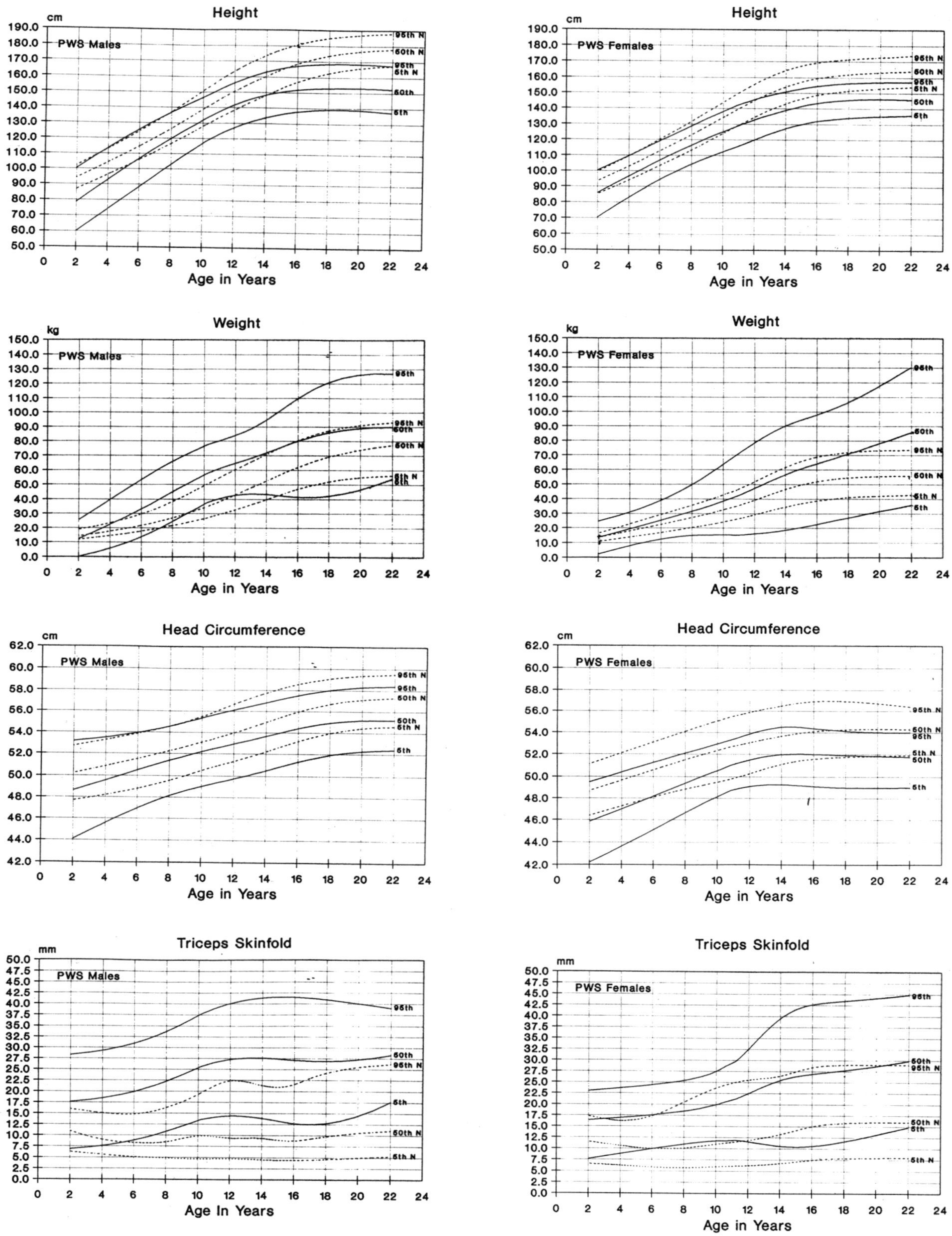

Figure 10-5. Growth graphs for children with Prader-Willi syndrome. (From Butler MG, Meany FJ. Standards for selected anthropometric measurements in Prader-Willi syndrome. Reproduced by permission of Pediatrics 88:853–58 © 1991.)

- For children 3 years and over, segmental body measures such as arm span, upper arm length, or tibial length may be used to assess linear growth.[3, 12, 15-26]
- Arm span correlates well with stature in normal children 3 years of age and older[21, 27] and has routinely been used as an alternative for length or height in children with myelomeningocele.[23] Accurate measurement of arm span requires two trained observers and a calibrated anthropometer, measuring the distance between the tips of the middle fingers when arms are fully extended at shoulder height.[3]
- Single total arm length, measured from the acromion process (the bony projection of the scapula that forms the point of the shoulder) to the styloid process (protuberance at the distal end of the lateral surface of the supinated forearm), may be determined by a single trained observer and may be better tolerated by the child.[28] A ratio of stature to total arm length may then be applied to obtain estimated stature, which can then be plotted on standard growth charts to determine percentile rank.[13, 22]
- Upper arm length is obtained by measuring the distance between the acromion process (as above) and the olecranon (elbow) in the midline on the posterior aspect of the right upper arm. Measurements obtained may then be compared to published norms.[21, 22]
- Tibial length is the distance between the medial tibial epicondyle (the bulging prominence at the proximal end of the tibia) and the medial malleolus (the rounded projection at the distal end of the tibia that forms prominence on the inner surface of the ankle). It is most accurately measured using an anthropometer, although flexible steel tapes can also be used. Tibial length may be plotted on special standardized charts,[15, 28] or stature may be estimated by the following equation and plotted on standard growth charts:

$$\text{estimated stature (in cm)} = [3.26 \times \text{tibial length in cm}] + 30.8 \text{ cm}$$

Even after reliable measures of weight and stature are obtained, interpreting the plotted data and determining ideal weight for length or height may be difficult. Weight for length or height may plot below or above established norms. Neurologically impaired infants and children often have feeding problems. If access to nutrition is inadequate, weight for length or height may be low. If stunting (decreased linear growth) occurs due to chronic or severe undernutrition and sustained inadequate weight gain, weight for length or height may appear to normalize.

Because their muscle mass may be relatively low, some infants and toddlers may appear obese even though weight plots within the norm for age and length or height. Muscle tissue contains a relatively high proportion of intracellular fluid, thus is heavier than adipose tissue. If muscle tissue is underdeveloped due to genetic predisposition or lack of normal physical use and exercise, ideal weight for length or height may be at the 5th to 25th percentile, or lower than normally expected. Weight for length or height at or above the 50th percentile may represent excess adiposity, which may further impair developmental progress if muscle tissue is hypotonic or underdeveloped.

Measurements of mid-arm circumference and triceps skin fold may be useful in assessing adiposity and identifying normal or limited muscle mass in children over 1 year of age.[16, 29] Caution must be used in estimating total body fatness from one skin fold measurement, especially in nonambulatory children. Total body fatness may be overestimated in some children, as fat folds have been shown to increase over paralyzed limbs.[24, 29]

Altered Energy Needs

The standard method of estimating energy needs using the Recommended Dietary Allowances (RDA) is often inappropriate for infants and children with neurological compromise.[26, 28, 30, 31] Children with conditions such as Down or Prader-Willi syndrome or myelomeningocele may exhibit decreased growth, diminished muscle mass, hypotonia, or increased adiposity; also, they may have lower energy and/or other nutrient requirements when compared with normal children of the same age.[26, 30, 31] Physical impairments that reduce activity, particularly ambulation, as often seen in children with spastic cerebral palsy, hypotonia, or myelomeningocele, may further reduce energy requirements and complicate maintenance of ideal body weight.[7, 32, 33] Children with hyperactivity, hypertonia (increased muscle tone), spastic or athetoid (fluctuating high- and low-tone) muscle activity, or increased involuntary movements that accompany frequent uncontrolled seizure activity may have significantly increased energy needs.[3, 33-35] Energy expenditure needed to perform an activity that approaches the child's physical limitations maybe higher than normal.[26]

Such medications as central nervous system stimulants can result in appetite suppression and decreased growth. Corticosteroids can blunt growth, accelerate appetite, and enhance muscle tissue catabolism, causing increased adiposity or obesity.[31] Tranquilizers or sedatives may reduce activity and energy needs, whereas amphetamines used to control hyperactivity have been related to suppression of weight gain and linear growth.[5] Various medications may also affect appetite, intake, and elimination.[36]

Altered Nutrient Needs

Medications used to treat developmental or behavioral problems and seizure disorders among infants and children may alter the absorption, metabolism, and/or excretion of several nutrients. Anticonvulsant, antireflux, muscle relaxant, stimulant, and laxative medications may be used in this population. Drug/nutrient interactions for these and other medications are given in appendix J.

Neurometabolic disease may involve errors in metabolism of various nutrients: carbohydrate, protein/amino acids, fats/fatty acids, minerals, vitamins, or other micronutrients. Some diseases require rigorous adherence to feeding schedules, some require meticulous avoidance of the offending nutrient, and others require a measured balance of nutrient administration within a narrow margin between safe and adequate.

Neonatal screening is available in many states for phenylketonuria (PKU), galactosemia, and maple syrup urine disease (MSUD), only 3 of more than 50 known neurometabolic disorders. Most of these disorders appear during infancy accompanied by such symptoms as failure to thrive, vomiting, diarrhea, lethargy, altered muscle tone, seizures, respiratory distress, jaundice, hepatomegaly, and/or other abnormal clinical features.

Due to the complicated nature of diagnosis and treatment, infants and toddlers with suspected neurometabolic disease are seen and managed at designated centers in each state. These centers provide physicians and registered dietitians who have specific training and experience in treating neurometabolic diseases. Specific laboratory testing must also be readily available.

Feeding Problems

Feeding problems in children with neurological compromise may be identified through use of such screening tools as those listed in appendixes A, B, D, and E. Infants and children with neurologic impairment may be delayed in developing normal feeding skills. Oral-motor dysfunction, abnormal muscle tone, posture (extension more prominent than flexion), and behavioral or psychosocial problems can result in reduced nutrient intake that may have a negative impact on growth and nutritional status. Feeding skill problems commonly associated with neurological compromise are listed in table 10-3.

Physical impairments may contribute to feeding difficulty and extend the amount of time needed to complete a meal. Fatigue may contribute to reduced intake and increased frustration on the part of the child and the caregiver. Sensory processes in the neurologically impaired infant and child may vary significantly from normal. These children may have strong adverse reactions to sensory input, or may require increased stimulation to evoke a desired response.[37] Oral hypersensitivity may cause a strong gag reflex at a slight touch of the tongue, whereas oral hyposensitivity may require a large bolus of food to initiate a swallow.[28] Chronic vomiting may be caused by a hyperactive gag reflex, gastroesophageal reflux (GER), or rumination—the chronic regurgitation of ingested food (which may or may not be reswallowed) that frequently results in chronic undernutrition.[28, 39] If recurrent pain or aspiration is associated with vomiting, food avoidance behaviors may occur.

Infants and toddlers depend on others for their care, including food selection and preparation, and rely on others to interpret and appropriately respond to their hunger and satiety cues. Yet, their neurological condition may limit their ability to communicate these cues, respond appropriately to their caregiver, or progress in feeding skills in a normal way. Children with neurological compromise may be cognitively ready to self-feed but may lack adequate motor control and development. Each of these factors may limit the variety or amount of foods and beverages consumed[36] (see chapter 4).

Each of these complications may also delay the acquisition of new feeding skills or the normal progression to foods with greater texture. It is important to keep in mind that the developmentally disabled child requires time and repeated opportunities to develop normal or adaptive feeding skills. For some children, feeding difficulties may be severe enough to prevent adequate intake; in these cases, alternate methods of nutrition support should be considered.

Constipation/Diarrhea

Decreased physical activity and hypertonic or hypotonic abdominal muscle tone may contribute to delayed gastric emptying, slow peristalsis, and constipation. Impaired oral function that limits fluid and/or fiber intake and frequent vomiting that contributes to poor hydration each can contribute to hard and infrequent stools. Chronic use of anticonvulsant or tranquilizing medications commonly produces the side effect of constipation (see appendix J).

Table 10-3. Feeding Skill Problems Commonly Associated with Neurological Compromise

Feeding skill	Description of problem
Sucking	Sucking may be poorly initiated, arrhythmical, weak, unsustained, or inefficient, resulting in poor intake or prolonged feeding times
Swallowing	*Oral phase.* If facial or oral muscles are weak or hypotonic, or if lips retract or tongue thrust is prominent, organizing and moving a liquid or semisolid bolus to the back of the mouth may be difficult and may cause choking or difficulty in swallowing the bolus. Food may collect in the cheeks if it cannot be moved to the center and back of the mouth for swallowing
	Pharyngeal phase. If the swallow is delayed or incomplete, food or liquids may pool in the sinuses present in the pharynx, increasing risk of aspiration into the lungs
	Esophageal phase. Decreased motility of the esophagus or gastroesophageal reflux may further increase the risk for aspiration of food into the lungs when the pharyngeal phase of swallowing is slow or ineffective. A hyperactive gag reflex may cause vomiting of any food that has been swallowed
Biting	A phasic bite may prevent the ability to bite harder or thicker foods, while a tonic bite reflex does not allow a normal release of food. The jaw may remain clenched for long periods of time, preventing further feeding
Chewing	Chewing requires adequate perception of food and its position in the mouth, adequate lip closure to keep food in the mouth, cheek and tongue control to transfer food to the teeth for chewing and back to the center and the back of the mouth for swallowing. Dental problems such as poor oral hygiene and dentition, enamel hypoplasia, bruxism, malocclusion, dental caries, and gum hyperplasia may affect intake
Self-feeding	Eye-hand, hand-to-mouth, pincer grasp, combined shoulder, elbow and wrist coordination each contributes to successful self-feeding. When feeding skills are either delayed or dysfunctional, constant assistance may be needed during feedings well beyond infancy. Parents may feel discouraged or overwhelmed by feedings that are difficult, stressful, or prolonged

References: 25, 26, 36, 37.

Nutrition Treatment

Nutrition intervention is designed and implemented to increase quality of health, limit episodes of illness, and reduce medical costs[40] by achieving the following:

- Delay or prevent further neurological damage or disability in neurometabolic disease (inborn errors of metabolism).[41]
- Provide adequate nutrition to maximize linear growth potential.
- Determine ideal weight for length or height, allowing for differences in muscle mass, mobility and ambulation.
- Provide adequate nutrition to support ideal weight-for-length status, preventing underweight or overweight status from further compromising developmental progress.
- Maintain optimal nutrition status in spite of medications or other treatments that may alter nutrient needs.
- Maintain optimal nutrition status in spite of altered feeding methods (such as tube-feeding), feeding problems, or delayed development of feeding skills.
- Provide support and guidance for the selection of foods and nutrient supplements to maximize oral nutrition or facilitate progression of feeding skills.
- Provide parents with adequate information to meet their infant's/child's nutrition needs and limit or prevent nutrition problems.

Estimating Energy Needs

Energy intake should promote adequate growth and prevent extremes of underweight or overweight. Energy needs are often determined using body weight or body surface area, assuming that weight, muscle mass, and activity levels are within the normal range for age and length or height. Because the growth of neurologically compromised infants and children may be well above or below established norms, estimates of energy needs are usually based on height, ideal weight for length or height, estimated basal energy needs, and estimated activity levels.

Ideal weight for length or height is normally considered to be at or close to the 50th percentile on the NCHS growth charts. If muscle development is below normal, ideal weight for length or height may be less the 50th percentile (see table 10-4). Estimated basal energy needs are given in tables 10-5 and 10-6. Factors that allow for estimated energy needs for tone, activity and growth are given in table 10-7. Several methods for estimating the energy needs of neurologically compromised infants and children have been proposed and are given in figures 10-6 through 10-8. Because there is such wide variation in energy needs and so little research has been reported regarding energy needs in this population, frequent monitoring of growth and nutritional intake provides the most accurate estimation of energy needs.

Estimating Other Nutrient Needs

Nutritional care for infants and children with neurometabolic disease is complex and may involve dietary intake alterations of protein, various amino acids, monosaccharides, disaccharides, long-chain or medium-chain fatty acids, carnitine, vitamins, and minerals. Management of neurometabolic disease is described in detail elsewhere.[42, 43]

Protein. Neurologically impaired infants and children probably require normally recommended amounts of protein. Children with delayed or dysfunctional feeding skills may find it difficult to consume adequate amounts of high-protein foods. It may also be more difficult for the child with low energy needs to consume adequate amounts of protein while limiting energy intake.[30, 33] If growth is significantly delayed, the recommended intake of protein may be based on the RDA for ideal weight for length or height and height-age rather than age or actual weight.[44, 45]

Carbohydrate and fat. Carbohydrate is the primary source of energy, and as with standard pediatric recommendations, it is suggested that at least 50% of energy needs be met by carbohydrate, with no more than 10% as sucrose.[30] Carbohydrate can be increased or decreased as needed to adjust energy intake. Fat increases palatability and satiety and also supplies essential fatty acids. Fat is uniquely calorie dense and should represent approximately 30-35% of total energy intake. Fat may be increased or decreased to adjust intake of energy to meet estimated needs.[30]

Table 10-4. Estimating Ideal Body Weight Based on Estimated Muscle Mass

Weight for length or height percentile (NCHS)*	Mid-arm muscle area†
50th percentile	Normal muscle mass (arm muscle area >10th percentile)
25th to 50th percentile	Decreased muscle mass (arm muscle area 5th–10th percentile)
5th to 10th percentile	Low muscle mass (arm muscle area < 5th percentile)

Note: Muscle mass is estimated using measurements of upper mid-arm circumference and triceps fat fold and the method for determining mid-arm muscle area for children given in appendix N.

*See appendix F.

†Reference: 16.

Table 10-5. Basal Metabolic Rates for Children Based on Body Surface Area

kcal x square meter body surface area* x 24 hours = daily basal energy expenditure†

Age (yr)	1	2	3
Boys (kcal/m²/hr)	53.0	52.4	51.3
Girls (kcal/m²/hr)	53.0	52.4	51.3

*Body surface area may be determined using a nomogram, measured weight and length or height (appendix M).

†Estimated basal energy needs must then be multiplied by a factor to accommodate estimated activity levels and growth given in table 10-7. See figure 10-6.

From Fleish A. Le metabolisme basal standard et sa determination au moyen du "Metabolcalculator." Helv Med Acta 81:23–44, 1951.

Fluid. Many infants and children with developmental delay may not be able to ask for a drink or respond to thirst. Because thin liquids are the most difficult food to control orally and swallow, many children with oral-motor difficulties may not be able to close their lips or swallow thin liquids efficiently. And because these infants and children are at increased risk for dehydration and constipation, dietary manipulation may be required to meet their fluid needs. Thickeners or liquids in thicker forms may be helpful in maintaining adequate hydration and fluid intake. (For estimating fluid needs, see appendix K.)

Vitamins and minerals. Vitamin and mineral requirements are based on the RDA for height age or ideal body weight, unless utilization and/or metabolism is compromised by medications (see appendix J for drug/nutrient interactions). Serum calcium, phosphorus, and alkaline phosphatase may be measured annually to assess vitamin D status if an anticonvulsant that affects vitamin D status is used chronically.[46, 47] Alkaline phosphatase levels may be elevated during growth and with hepatic dysfunction.[47, 48] If hypocalcemia, hypophosphatemia, and elevated alkaline phosphatase are present, radiographic follow-up or bone densitometry may be indicated to detect bone demineralization. If demineralization is detected, 600 to 800 IU of vitamin D is often recommended, with 1 to 1.5 times the

Table 10-6. Basal Metabolic Rates for Infants and Children Based on Weight

kcal/hr (for weight and age) x 24 hr = daily basal energy expenditure*

Age 1 wk to 10 mo		Age 11 to 36 mo		
Weight (kg)	kcal/hour M/F	Weight (kg)	kcal/hour M	kcal/hour F
3.5	8.4	9.0	22.0	21.2
4.0	9.5	9.5	22.8	22.0
4.5	10.5	10.0	23.6	22.8
5.0	11.6	10.5	24.4	23.6
5.5	12.7	11.0	25.2	24.4
6.0	13.8	11.5	26.0	25.2
6.5	14.9	12.0	26.8	26.0
7.0	16.0	12.5	27.6	26.9
7.5	17.1	13.0	28.4	27.7
8.0	18.2	13.5	29.2	28.5
8.5	19.3	14.0	30.0	29.3
9.0	20.4	14.5	30.8	30.1
9.5	21.4	15.0	31.6	30.9
10.0	22.5	15.5	32.4	31.7
10.5	23.6	16.0	33.3	32.6
11.0	24.7	16.5	34.0	33.4

*Estimated basal energy needs must then be multiplied by a factor to accommodate estimated activity levels and growth given in table 10-7. See figure 10-6.

Adapted with permission from Altman PL, Dittmer DS, eds. Metabolism. Bethesda, Md.: Federation of American Societies for Experimental Biology, © 1968.

RDA for calcium and phosphorus.[49] Measurement of serum calcium levels may be necessary to prevent hypercalcemia even when clinical rickets are present.[49]

The mean corpuscular volume (MCV) of red blood cells in infants and children on diphenylhydantoin therapy may be monitored to identify megaloblastic anemia as a sign of folic acid deficiency.[46] If evident, treatment with folic acid 1 to 1.5 times the RDA is generally adequate.[49] Valproic acid may alter carnitine status. If carnitine abnormality is suspected, treating with 50-100 mg/kg/day is usually sufficient, although smaller doses may be needed if nausea and diarrhea become a problem. [46]

Management of Feeding Problems

Delayed or dysfunctional oral skills. Management of abnormal oral-motor skills is best addressed by a qualified professional such as a speech pathologist, occupational therapist, or physical therapist who is trained and has experience feeding infants and children. Criteria for referral to a feeding therapist are given in table 4 of chapter 4. Feeding programs may be developed that require use of adaptive equipment and alteration of food texture. Liquids and thin pureed foods may require thickening with commercial products (see appendix C). Foods with varied or harder textures may require blending for better tolerance.

Dental problems. For prevention of dental caries and for good dental hygiene, limiting intake of simple carbohydrates and use of a fluoride supplement are encouraged. Bruxism and malocclusion are common and may require adjusting the texture of foods to soft or puree. Referral for orthodontic evaluation may be indicated.

Constipation and diarrhea. For resolving constipation, encourage adequate fluid consumption (see appendix K). If possible, increase intake of high-fiber foods such as wheat bran, whole wheat cereals and bread, cooked or raw vegetables, legumes, and fruit with skins and small seeds. If high-fiber foods are used, for each 4-oz serving, provide an additional 4-oz of fluids. For the child who receives tube-feedings, fiber may aid in stimulating gastrointestinal motility and help the stool retain more moisture. If abdominal muscle tone is higher or lower than normal, massage techniques may enhance gastric motility.

Table 10-7. Factors for Accommodating Energy Needs for Altered Muscle Tone, Activity, and Growth

Estimated basal energy needs must be multiplied by a factor to accommodate altered tone levels:

hypotonia	0.9
hypertonia	1.1

Estimated basal energy needs must be multiplied by a factor to accommodate altered activity levels:

confined to bed	1.15
confined to wheelchair	1.2
crawling	1.25
ambulatory	1.3
athetoid cerebral palsy	1.5–2.0
normal activity	1.7–2.0

Energy needs for growth (5 kcal/g of weight gain) must be added to estimate total daily energy needs:

normal growth	30–150 kcal/day
catch-up growth	150–300 kcal/day

From Krick J, Murphy PE, Markham JFB, et al. A proposed formula for calculating energy needs of children with cerebral palsy. Develop Med Child Neural 34:481–87, 1992.

Down syndrome	16.1 kcal/cm: male 1-3 yr 14.3 kcal/cm: female 1-3 yr
Prader-Willi syndrome	10-11 kcal/cm: maintenance 8-9 kcal/cm: weight loss
Myelomeningocele	7 kcal/cm: weight loss

Figure 10-6. Energy needs of selected populations of children with developmental disabilities. (Adapted with permission from Rokusek C, Heindicles E. Nutrition and feeding for the developmentally disabled. South Dakota University Affiliated Program, Interdisciplinary Center for Disabilities, © 1985.)

Tube-Feeding

For a number of developmentally delayed or neurologically impaired infants and children, the coordination of suck/swallow or mastication/swallow in a safe and timely fashion exceeds their physical and/or cognitive abilities. Decreased ability to consume adequate nutrition on a chronic basis hinders weight gain, thus affecting growth and prompting consideration of alternate feeding methods for supplemental or total nutrition. Alternative feeding methods may also be warranted by the presence of gastroesophageal reflux, choking or gagging on liquids or solid foods, or other factors that may increase the risk of aspiration and upper respiratory infections. If the digestive and absorptive functions of the gastrointestinal tract are intact, enteral feeding is the preferred method of nutrition support.

Specifically, enteral feeding may be indicated when (1) oral intake meets <80% of energy needs or <100% of *minimal* fluid needs, (2) total oral feeding time >4–6 hours/day, (3) weight loss or no weight gain >3 months, (4) weight for length or height <5th percentile, and (5) triceps skin fold or mid-arm muscle area <5th percentile.

The most commonly used routes to provide enteral nutrition are nasogastric, nasoduodenal, nasojejunal, gastrostomy, and jejunostomy. The most appropriate route is determined by the length of time enteral feedings are needed, the potential to orally feed, the degree of aspiration risk based on medical condition(s), past medical history, and individual history of feeding experiences. The general benefits of tube-feedings include increased weight gain and linear growth, muscle mass, subcutaneous adipose stores, and improved nutritional status. The types of enteral

Estimating Energy Needs (Neurological Compromise)

1. Determine height-age by finding the age at which the infant's or child's length or height would plot at the 50th percentile using the National Center for Health Statistics growth charts (appendix F).
2. Determine ideal weight for length or height by using the 5th to 50th percentile weight for length or height from the NCHS growth charts, depending on estimated muscle mass (table 10-7).
3. Using height-age and ideal weight for length, find recommended total estimated energy needs in table 10-4 or 10-5, or appendix L.
4. Adjust for decreased or increased level of activity if necessary.

Example: An 18-month-old girl has quadriplegic cerebral palsy, a mid-arm muscle area at the 5th percentile, and:

length:	29 in. (73.7 cm)	< 5th percentile for age
weight:	16 lb. 1 oz (7.3 kg)	< 5th percentile for age

1. Height-age = Length would plot at 50th percentile if she were 11½ mo old
2. Ideal weight for length with low muscle mass = 5–10th percentile = 8.1–8.4 kg
3. Total estimated energy needs for height age from appendix L:

   98 to 105 kcal/kg/day

4. Activity level is significantly lower than normal; normal activity accounts for 20 kcal/kg/day; subtract (albeit somewhat arbitrarily) 10 kcal/kg/day for inactivity:

   88 to 95 kcal/kg/day × 8.1 to 8.4 kg = 713 to 798 kcal/day

This level of energy intake should support catch-up growth or a weight that is normal for length.

Note: Monitoring growth in follow-up: Energy intake can be adjusted if initial estimate of energy needs does not support desired growth outcome.

Figure 10-7. Estimating total energy needs of infants and children with neurological compromise using the RDA (Recommended Dietary Allowances). See appendix L.

feeding routes in infants and children, their specific indications, benefits, and potential complications are listed in table 10-8.

Tube-feeding may be a temporary source of nutrition, improving nutritional status and growth until the infant or child is able to be nourished adequately by mouth. If they are tolerated at all, oral feedings should be encouraged to (1) prevent further loss of feeding skills; (2) promote the normal progression of eating, from liquids to variety of solid food textures; (3) support a positive feeding environment and parental bonding; and (4) build toward eventual independent feeding. To assist the infant/child in meeting these goals, a safe, well-structured feeding program that normalizes eating skills/behaviors and treats maladaptive compensatory behaviors before they become firmly engrained is a sound approach for helping to support functional eating.[50, 51] A qualified feeding therapist can provide a plan of therapy to enhance or develop normal feeding skills.

Hunger and satiety cues may not be as clear when tube-feedings are used. The registered dietitian can help parents identify subtle feeding cues and provide guidance regarding the volume of feeding needed to support optimal growth and development. Increases in feeding volumes are required frequently during infancy (every 1–2 weeks) and young childhood (every 1–2 months) to meet changing needs during rapid growth. As feeding skills progress, the registered dietitian can provide guidance for selecting foods and tapering tube-feedings or modifying tube-feeding schedules to enhance hunger-induced motivation for eating while preventing nutritional compromise.

Formula selection. Selection of the appropriate formula is based on the infant or child's medical and nutritional status, nutrient requirements, age or height-age, gastrointestinal function, and feeding route. Additional consideration is given to the individual feeding history and tolerance, parents' preference, and formula specifics such as caloric density, osmolality, renal solute load, nutrient composition, availability, ease of preparation, and cost.[50, 51]

For infants, breast milk or a commercial infant formula best meets their nutritional needs. For children over 1 year of age, a variety of pediatric formulas are available (see appendix C). Concentrated infant formulas, homemade blenderized formulas, or a number of adult formulas may be modified to meet specific nutritional requirements.

Estimating Energy Needs (Cerebral Palsy)

Basal metabolic rate (BMR) may be calculated based on body surface area or weight. Total daily energy needs may be estimated by multiplying BMR times factors that accommodate muscle tone and activity (given in table 10-7), adding estimated energy needs for growth as follows:

Total Energy Needs (kcal/day) = [BMR × tone factor × activity factor] + growth*

Example: An 18-month-old girl with quadriplegic cerebral palsy is 29 in. long (73.7 cm) and 16 lb. 1 oz (7.3 kg) (considerably underweight for both age and length) and is generally hypertonic, but confined to a wheelchair.

A. Using body surface area, age, sex: BMR (kcal/day) = BSA × kcal/m²/hr × 24 hr

BSA = body surface area (See appendix M for body surface area nomogram.)
kcal/m²/hr for age and sex are given in table 10-5.

1. Body surface area (appendix M) is 0.39 m².
2. Basal metabolic rate (table 10-5) is 52.4 kcal/m²/hr

$0.39\ m^2 \times 52.4\ kcal/m^2/hr \times 24\ hr = 496$ kcal/day basal energy needs

3. Tone factor is: 1.1
   Activity factor is: 1.2
   Normal weight gain: 6 g/day or 6 × 5 = 30 kcal/day
   Catch-up growth: 30 g/day or 30 × 5 = 150 kcal/day

[490 kcal/day × 1.1 × 1.2] + 30 to 150 kcal/day = 677 to 797 kcal/day

B. Using age, sex, and general category of body weight:
BMR (kcal/day) = kcal/kg/hr (for weight category, age and sex) x 24 hr

1. Energy in kcal/kg/hr for age and sex are given in table 10-6. BMR factor for this example is 17.1 kcal/hr:

17.1 kcal/hr × 24 hr = 410 kcal/day

2. Tone factor is: 1.1
   Activity factor is: 1.2
   Normal growth: 6 g/day or 6 × 5 = 30 kcal/day
   Catch-up growth: 30 g/day or 30 × 5 = 150 kcal/day

[410 kcal/day × 1.1 x 1.2] + 30 to 150 kcal/day = 572 to 692 kcal/day

*Krick J, Murphy PE, Markham JFB, et al. A proposed formula for calculating energy needs of children with cerebral palsy. Develop Med Child Neurol 34:481–87, 1992.

Figure 10-8. Estimating total energy needs of infants and children with cerebral palsy using basal energy needs.

Formula delivery. The method of formula delivery depends on location of the tube, the infant's or child's tolerance, and the family/caretaker's schedule. Intermittent bolus feedings, delivered to the stomach by gravity over 15 to 30 minutes, may be given every two to four hours. Bolus feedings are often the best for physically active children or for children preparing for transition to oral feedings. The feeding regimen can be planned to accommodate a family's busy schedule. Continuous drip method delivers nutrients at a constant rate over a specific period of time. This method of feeding is often beneficial for those who have GER or who are at risk for aspiration. Continuous feeding is most commonly used for those with transpyloric or nocturnal feedings. Enteral feeding pumps may be used to control the rate of formula delivery, but must be able to deliver small amounts of formula and to advance the rate of feeding by small increments. Lightweight, portable pumps allow for greater mobility. The initiation and advancement of tube-feedings is dependent upon the infant's or child's gastrointestinal structure and function. General considerations are provided in table 10-8.[50]

Table 10-8. Types of Enteral Feeding Routes in Infants and Children, Their Indications, Benefits, and Potential Complications

Route	When to use	Benefits	Potential complications
Naso/orogastric	No blockage, stricture, or area of tissue erosion between nose or mouth and stomach Short-term use (days, weeks) Supplemental or nocturnal feedings needed Larger osmolality and volume well tolerated	Tube insertion does not require surgery Uses normal digestive processes Allows flexible feeding schedule Gastric acid provides bacteriocidal effect	Infant/child can remove tube more easily Nasal, esophageal, or tracheal irritation Presence of tube may interfere with oral feedings Increased risk of aspiration due to reflux or incorrect placement of feeding tube Compromised pulmonary function due to aspiration Risk of airway obstruction Diarrhea or dumping syndrome
Transpyloric feedings (nasoduodenal or nasojejunal)	No blockage, stricture, or area of tissue erosion between nose or mouth and duodenum or jejunum When increased risk of aspiration is present due to inadequate gag reflex, delayed gastric emptying, frequent vomiting, or severe gastroesophageal reflux	Either may help prevent aspiration Nasojejunal tubes may be less likely to migrate or dislodge	Gastric reflux may still be possible with duodenal feedings; nasoduodenal tubes may migrate or dislodge, increasing risk of reflux and aspiration Potential for intestinal perforation with stiff or large-bore tubes Diarrhea or dumping syndrome
Gastrostomy or jejunostomy tube	Blockage, stricture, or area of tissue erosion between nose or mouth and duodenum or jejunum present When increased risk of aspiration is present due to inadequate gag reflex, delayed gastric emptying, frequent vomiting, or severe gastroesophageal reflux Incompetent lower esophageal sphincter Long-term feeding (>6 wk) Surgical tolerance expected	Percutaneous endoscopic (PEG or PEJ) placement does not usually require anesthesia Bypasses mouth, stomach and pyloric sphincter, reducing interference with oral feedings when at least some oral feedings are possible Reduces gastroesophageal reflux and vomiting Gastrostomy tube can be converted to transpyloric feeding	PEG or PEJ not indicated in infants or children with multisystem organ failure; surgical placement requires anesthesia Surgical or infectious complications Feedings may be more difficult to establish Tube occlusion or migration

Note: See text for general indications, benefits and complications of enteral feedings.

Ketogenic Diet

The ketogenic diet, designed to establish and maintain ketosis, was developed for children with intractable, myoclonic, and atonic epileptic seizures that are nonresponsive to anticonvulsant medications. This diet seems to be most effective in children under the age of 10 years,[45,52] but it is not generally recommended for children under the age of 2 because maintaining ketoacidosis in this age group is often difficult. Although the complete mechanism is still uncertain, in sustained ketosis or accumulation of ketone bodies, the ketone bodies are believed to behave as inhibitory neurotransmitters, heightening the seizure threshold and producing an anticonvulsant effect.

The diet is very high in fat and severely restricted in carbohydrate. A ratio of 4:1 or 3:1 in fat energy to carbohydrate plus protein energy is generally recommended. Protein intake is quite limited, but should meet the RDA for age. Fluid intake is limited to maintain minimal hydration. The conventional high-fat ketogenic diet using long-chain triglycerides is inadequate in B-complex vitamins, iron, calcium, and vitamins C and D. Although ketosis is maintained using less fat when medium-chain triglycerides (MCT) replace some of the fat in the diet, both diets must be supplemented with vitamins, iron, and calcium. All supplements and medications, including vitamins, minerals, analgesics, and antibiotics must be given in forms that are sugar-free. Use of this diet has been limited by its expense and technicality, the high compliance required, and the lack of palatability.

References

1. Stalling VA, Charney EB, Davies JC, Cronk CE. Nutrition related growth failure of children with quadriplegic cerebral palsy. Dev Med Child Neurol 35:997,1993.
2. McFadden DL, Burke EP. Developmental disabilities and the new paradigm: Directions for the 1990's. Ment Retard 29(1):iii, 1991.
3. Pipes PL, Glass RP. Nutrition and feeding of children with developmental delay and related problems. In: Pipes PL, ed. Nutrition in infancy and childhood, 4th ed. St. Louis: Times Mirror/Mosby, 1989; 361.
4. Palmer S, Eckvall S. Pediatric nutrition in developmental disorders. Springfield, Ill.: Thomas, 1978.
5. Palmer S, Horn S. Feeding problems in children. In: Palmer RD, Ekvall S, eds. Pediatric nutrition in developmental disorders. Springfield, Ill.: Thomas, 1978; 107.
6. Suskind RM, Nutritional support of the developmentally disabled child. In: Suskind RM, ed. Textbook of pediatric nutrition, 2d ed. New York: Raven Press, 1993; 485.
7. Position of the American Dietetic Association: Nutrition in comprehensive program planning for persons with developmental disabilities (technical support paper). J Am Diet Assoc 87:1068, 1987.
8. Krick J, Murphy-Miller P, Zeger S, et al. Pattern of growth in children with cerebral palsy. J Am Diet Assoc 96:680–85, 1996.
9. Crane JP, Kopta M. Comparative newborn anthropometrics data in symmetric vs asymmetric intrauterine growth retardation. Am J Obstet Gynecol 138:518, 1990.
10. Hack M, Breslau N, Weissman B, et al. Effect of very low birth weight and subnormal head size on cognitive abilities at school age. N Engl J Med 325:231, 1991.
11. Holm VA. Growth in children with developmental disabilities. Nutrition focus for children with special health care needs. 9(2): 1–5, 1994.
12. Position of the American Dietetic Association: Nutrition in comprehensive program planning for persons with developmental disabilities. J Am Diet Assoc 92:614, 1992.
13. Stevenson RD. Use of segmental measures to estimate stature in children with cerebral palsy. Arch Pediatr Adolesc Med 149: 658, 1985.
14. Tobis JS, Saturen P, Larios G, Posniak AO. Study of growth patterns in cerebral palsy. Arch Phys Med Rehabil 42:475, 1961.
15. Spender QW, Cronk CE, Charney EB, Stallings VA. Assessment of linear growth of children in cerebral palsy: Use of alternative measures to height or length. Dev Med Child Neurol 31:206, 1989.
16. Frisancho AR. Anthropometric standard for the assessment of growth and nutritional status. Ann Arbor: University of Michigan Press, 1990.
17. Davies JC, Antonucci DL, Charney EB, Stallings VA. Use of upper arm length and percent body fat for nutritional assessment of children with cerebral palsy. Dev Med Child Neurol 31(suppl):39, 1989.
18. Feucht S. Assessment of growth. Nutr Focus 4(6):1–5, 1989.
19. Lohman T, Roche AF, et al. Anthropometric standardization reference manual. Champaign, Ill.: Human Kinetics Books, 1988.

20. Engstrom FM, Roche AF, Mukherjer D. Differences between arm-span and stature in white children. J Adolesc Health Care 2:19, 1981.
21. Belt D, Ekvall S, Cook C, Oppenheimer S, Wessel J. Linear growth measurement: A comprehension of single arm length and arm span. Dev Med Child Neural 28:319, 1986.
22. Snider R, Schneider C, Owing CL, Reynolds HM, Golomb DH, Schork, MA. Anthropometry of infants, children and youths to age 18 for product safety design. Bethesda, Md.: Consumer Product Safety Commissions (report no. UM-HSRI-77–17), 1977.
23. Zorab PA, Prine FJ, Harrison A. Estimation of height from tibia length. Lancet 1:195, 1963.
24. Lee MMC. Thickening of the subcutaneous tissues in paralyzed limbs in chronic hemiplegia. Hum Biol 31:187, 1959.
25. Twin Cities Dietetic Association. Children with special health care needs. In: Manual of pediatric nutrition. St. Paul: Twin Cities Diet Assoc, 1990; 459.
26. Bandini L, Patterson B, Ekvall S. Cerebral palsy. In: Ekvall SW, ed. Pediatric nutrition in chronic disease and developmental disorders: Prevention, assessment and treatment, New York: Oxford University Press, 1993; 93.
27. Engelbach W. Endocrine medicine. vol. 1. Springfield, Ill.: Thomas, 1932.
28. Stevenson RD. Feeding and nutrition in children with developmental disabilities. Pediatr Ann 24:255, 1995.
29. Frisancho AR. New norms of upper limb fat and muscle areas for assessment of nutritional status. Am J Clin Nutr 34:2540, 1981.
30. Cloud HH. Developmental disabilities. In: Queen PM, Lang CE, eds. Handbook of pediatric nutrition. Gaithersberg, Md.: Aspen, 1993; 401.
31. Nelson JK, Moxness KE, Jensen MD, Gastineau CF. Other nutritional considerations in developmental delay. In: Mayo Clinic diet manual, a handbook of nutrition practices. 7th ed. St. Louis: Mosby, 1994; 453.
32. Green EM, McIntosh EN. Food and nutrition skills of mentally retarded adults assessment and needs. J Am Diet Assoc 85:611, 1985.
33. Hahn TJ, Hahn BH. Osteopenia in patients with rheumatic disease. In: Principles of diagnosis and therapy: Semin Arthritis Rheum 6:165, 1976.
34. Dietz WH. Nutrition requirements and feeding of the handicapped child. In: Grand RJ, Sutphen JL, Dietz WH, eds. Pediatric nutrition theory and practice. Stoneham, Mass.: Butterworth, 1987; 387.
35. Wodarski LA. Nutrition intervention in developmental disabilities: An interdisciplinary approach. J Am Diet Assoc 85:218, 1985.
36. Cloud, HH. Feeding problems of the child with special health care needs. In: Ekvall SW, ed. Pediatric nutrition in chronic disease prevention, assessment and treatment. New York: Oxford University Press,1993; 203.
37. Morris SE, Klein MD. Pre-feeding skills. Tucson: Therapy Skill Builders, 1987.
38. Heine R, Reddihough DS, Catto-Smith AG. Gastro-esophageal reflux and feeding problems after gastrostomy in children with severe neurological impairment. Dev Med Child Neuro 37:320, 1995.
39. Rast J, Elline-Allen JA, Johnston JM. Dietary management of rumination: Four case studies. Am J Clin Nutr 42:95, 1985.
40. Mandelbaum BR, Tolo VT, McAfee PC, Burest P. Nutritional deficiencies after staged anterior and posterior spinal reconstructive surgery. Clin Orthop 234:5, 1988.
41. Nevin-Folino NL. Neurological impairment. In: Groh-Wargo S, Thompson M, Cox JH, eds. Nutritional care for high-risk newborns. rev. ed. Chicago: Precept Press,1994; 350.
42. Acosta PB. Nutrition support protocols. Columbus, Ohio: Ross Laboratories, 1989.
43. Acosta PB. Nutrition support of inborn errors of metabolism. In: Queen PM, Lang CE, eds. Handbook of pediatric nutrition. Gaithersburg, Md.: Aspen, 1993; 315–65.
44. Kram K. Dietary assessment criteria, reliability and depth. In: Smith M, ed. Guides for the assessment of the mentally retarded and the developmentally disabled. Proceedings of the 3rd National Nutrition Workshop for Nutritionalists of University-Affiliated Facilities, 1974.
45. The Chicago Dietetic Association and the South Side Suburban Dietetic Association. Manual of clinical dietetics. Chicago: American Dietetic Association, 1988; 151.
46. Wodarski LA. An interdisciplinary nutrition assessment and intervention protocol for children with disabilities. J Am Diet Assoc 90: 1563, 1990.
47. Latner, AL. Clinical biochemistry. Philadelphia: Saunders, 1975.
48. Babbit LR. Nutrition concerns for children with seizure disorders. Nutrition focus for children with special health care needs 9(4): 1–5, 1994.
49. Brizer L. Drug-nutrient interactions concerns for children with special health care needs. Nutrition focus for children with special health care needs 7(6): 1–5, 1992.
50. Lingard CD. Enteral nutrition. In: Queen PM, Lang CE, eds. Handbook of pediatric nutrition. Gaithersburg, Md.: Aspen, 1993; 249–78.
51. Nardella MT. Practical tips on tube feedings for children. Nutr Focus 10(2):1–8, 1995.
52. Pryor H, Thelander H. Growth deviations in handicapped. Clin Pediatr 6:501, 1967.

Parent Education Materials

See chapter 4 for recommendations regarding feeding progression.

Nutritional care for the child with developmental disabilities. United Cerebral Palsy, Attn: Tina Shaddix, RD, 24330 11th Avenue North, Birmingham, AL 35223. Phone: (205) 251-0165.
Brochures providing relevant nutrition information for those involved in the care and treatment of the developmentally disabled child are listed below. Each brochure addresses a major concern and provides dietary measures to alleviate the problem identified. (1) Meal planning for the childhood years, (2) Promoting weight gain, (3) Management of constipation, (4) Weight control for the overweight child, (5) Oral-motor development and feeding techniques.

Klein, MD, Delaney, TA. Feeding and nutrition for the child with special needs. Tucson: Therapy Skill Builders, 1994.

Section 2: Breast and bottle feeding: Formula concentrations (increasing and decreasing), formula preparation, positioning for helping baby suck, nipple selections, feeding progressions

Section 3: Introducing foods from a spoon: Thickening foods and drinks, transitioning from liquids to strained foods and soft, lumpy foods, oral hypersensitivity management, gagging management, appropriate spoon selection

Section 6: Oral-motor treatment strategies: Chewing management; cheek, jaw, tongue, swallow education and management; preparation for feeding, managing oral hypersensitivity

Section 7: Nutrition treatment strategies: Anemia, constipation, fluid facts, massage techniques for constipation, tube feeding complications, diarrhea management, long term diarrhea, drug/nutrient interactions, food sensitivities, cow's milk allergy, lactose intolerance, management of the overweight and underweight child, calorie cutters and calorie boosters

Section 8: Conditions affecting feeding and nutrition: BPD, cardiac, cerebral palsy/muscle tone, cleft lip and palate, Down syndrome, GER, meningomyelocele, Prader-Willi syndrome, prematurity, Rett syndrome, rickets, seizure disorder

Section 9: Tube feedings: Types of tube feedings; feeding tips; positioning for tube feedings; tube feedings and growth; formula choices; medications through the tube; tube feeding complications: nausea, vomiting, skin irritation, constipation; GER; transitioning to oral feedings; transitioning tube feeding to school

Wolf L, Glass R. Feeding and swallowing disorders in infancy: Assessment and management. Tucson: Therapy Skill Builders, 1992.

Evans Morris S, Dunn Klein M. Pre-feeding skills: A comprehensive resource for feeding development. Tucson: Therapy Skill Builders, 1987.

DiLima, S, Niemeyer S. Caregiver education guide for children with developmental disabilities. Aspen Reference Group. Gaithersberg, Md.: Aspen, 1996.

Chapter 6, on nutrition and feeding, includes the following camera-ready handouts:
Mealtime goals and guidelines, iron deficiency anemia, weight control, risk factors for obesity, snacks for weight control, promoting weight gain, snacks to promote weight gain, high-calorie food fortifiers, nutritional management of constipation, increasing fiber, increasing fluid intake, oral-motor development and feeding skills, enhancing oral-motor skills, guidelines for the progression of food texture, introducing liquids from a cup, oral treatment techniques, feeding treatment techniques, swallowing problems, tube feeding: nasogastric and gastrostomy tubes, nutrition for your gastrostomy fed child

Nutrition Manual for At-Risk Infants and Toddlers
Janice Hovasi Cox, editor

11

SPINA BIFIDA (MYELOMENINGOCELE)

Nancy L. Nevin-Folino, MEd, CS, RD, LD, and Gloria Pina, RN, CPNP

Spina bifida is a defect in the spinal canal caused by abnormal fetal development during the first trimester of pregnancy. Defects range in severity from nonapparent and asymptomatic (spina bifida occulta) to protrusion of both the spinal cord and its covering through the spinal column (myelomeningocele). Other terms used to describe spinal canal defects include myelodysplasia, myeloschisis, and neural tube defects. The frequency and severity of health-related problems associated with myelomeningocele depend, in part, on where the lesion is located. Lesions occurring higher on the spinal column are often associated with greater problems.[1] Nutrition concerns associated with spina bifida are listed in table 11-1.

Growth Assessment

Routine measurement of growth is needed for infants and children with myelomeningocele so that deviations from the norm can be identified and addressed promptly. Because several methods may be used to measure growth, consistency is paramount for meaningful and valid growth evaluation. Weight, length, weight-for-length and head circumference measurements are most commonly used for infants and toddlers. Triceps skin folds may be used with older children, but are often not helpful in younger children due to wide variability.

Length

Recumbent length should be measured and plotted on the National Center for Health Statistics (NCHS) percentiles, birth to 36 months (appendix F) and compared to previous measurements, observing trends and deviations from previous growth pattern.

Measurement may be difficult if deformities of the lower extremities or scoliosis are present. Arm span may be

Table 11-1. Nutrition Concerns Associated with Spina Bifida

Problems associated with growth:
- Deformities of the lower extremities
- Scoliosis
- Short stature
- Underweight
- Obesity

Problems associated with lack of sensation in the lower extremities
- Lack of ambulation
- Spontaneous bone fractures
- Obesity
- Trophic ulcers

Problems associated with bowel and bladder control
- Bowel incontinence
- Constipation
- Bladder incontinence
- Frequent bladder or urinary tract infections

Problems associated with feeding
- Hydrocephalus/mental retardation/learning problems
- Arnold Chiari malformation
- Underweight
- Obesity
- Drug/nutrient interactions

used in children over 3 years of age and is described elsewhere.[2] If there is a difference between length measured using right and left lower extremities, the longer measurement is usually used. Although lower lesions (sacral vertebrae) are not as strongly associated with decreased stature, children with mid-lesions (lumbar 3–5) or high lesions (lumbar 2 and above) may have significantly decreased stature (below the 3rd percentile), particularly if these lesions are associated with decreased ambulation.[3] Deviations in linear growth may be caused by neuroendocrine or skeletal abnormalities,[4] but are often not evident until the second to sixth year.[5] Treatment with growth hormone has been shown to significantly improve the growth rate and length of children with neural tube defects, but has only been studied in children 4 years of age or older.[4]

Weight

Weight should be measured and plotted on the NCHS percentiles, birth to 36 months (appendix F) and compared to previous measurements, observing trends and deviations from previous growth pattern. A chair scale or bed scale may be needed to weigh nonambulatory children or children who cannot sit independently. Weight should be measured without special equipment such as braces, shoes, and the like.

Weight gain generally follows normal parameters until 3 to 4 years of age.[2,5] Diminished weight gain during infancy may occur if feeding skills are delayed or altered with more severe forms of the Arnold-Chiari malformation. Excessive weight is common, particularly in nonambulatory children, due to a lower basal metabolic rate that accompanies lower muscle mass, lower activity levels, and increased intake.

Weight for Length

At 2 to 6 years of age, weight gain may continue at a normal or accelerated rate, while linear growth may continue at a normal or decelerated rate. The result is often obesity. Obesity may be more apparent on visual examination than weight or weight for length plotted on percentile charts. Muscle tissue is heavier per unit of volume than adipose tissue. If muscle tissue is reduced and adipose tissue comprises a greater proportion of total body weight, weight and weight for length may plot within normal limits, even though the child clearly appears obese.[2,6]

Excessive fat stores may be more apparent on the trunk, while the legs may actually appear thin.[6] Increased

Clinical Assessment of the Infant/Toddler with Spina Bifida

Infant/Child's Name ______________________ DOB ____________ Chart No. ____________

Bowel Information:

Usual stool frequency:	1/day _____	2+/day _____	3–4/week _____	other ________			
Time of day: _____ am/pm	Relationship to meals:	before	after	no relationship			
Consistency/color:	yellow/green	brown	seedy	soft/mushy	liquid	hard/marble	
Abdominal cramping:	Yes	No	Frequency:	occasionally	daily	more frequently	
Presence of blood:	Yes	No	Frequency:	occasionally	daily	more frequently	
Presence of mucous:	Yes	No	Frequency:	occasionally	daily	more frequently	

Method:

Enema	Frequency:	____________	Type:	____________
Suppository	Frequency:	____________	Type:	____________
Laxative	Frequency:	____________	Type:	____________
Physical activity	Frequency:	____________	Type:	____________
Digital Stimulation	Frequency:	________	Manual evacuation/Frequency:	________

Child participation: ________________________________

Toileting:

Urge sensation: Present Absent/Unreliable Sits on toilet: Assisted Unassisted

Resistance/reluctance: Yes No Strains/pushes: Yes No

Length of time: ________

Soiling ("Accidents" if Toilet Trained):

Frequency:	Occasionally	Daily	More Frequently		
Protective garments:	Yes	No	Type ______________		
Indicates when soiled:	Yes	No			
Participation in cleaning:	Dependent	Shows interest	Assists	Needs reminding	Independent

Bladder Information:

Frequency of urination: ______________ Method: ______________

Frequency of infection: ______________ Medications: ______________

Nutrition:

Fluid intake: ________________________________

Fiber intake: ________________________________

Skin breakdown/pressure sores: Yes No Spontaneous fractures: Yes No

Interviewer's Signature ______________________ Date ____________

Figure 11-1. Information-gathering form for clinical assessment of child with spina bifida.

adiposity may cause increased difficulties with ambulation or trophic ulcers and may further compromise nutritional status.[6]

Head Circumference

Head circumference follows normal growth curves unless hydrocephaly is present. If a ventriculoperitoneal shunt is placed, head circumference may decrease initially, then increase at normal or decelerated rates, reflecting brain growth (see chapter 5).

Clinical Assessment

Standard screening tools used to identify clinical signs and symptoms of nutrition problems may be used (appendixes A and B), focusing on fluid intake, bowel and bladder function, and medications. Detailed information such as that given in figure 11-1 may be needed to further define clinical problems. Neurogenic bowel and bladder occurs frequently in infants and children with neural tube defects, causing constipation and frequent urinary tract infections.

Medications frequently prescribed for infants and toddlers with neural tube defects include anticholinergic drugs for bladder control, antibiotics for frequent urinary tract infections, laxatives or stool softeners, and anticonvulsants for control of seizures. (See appendix J for a description of drug/nutrient–related concerns.)

Carrying, moving, and repositioning infants and young children become more difficult as they get older. Skin breakdown may occur if the ability to change position and sensation are decreased. Untreated, pressure sores can be a source of infection for both skin and bone tissue. Spontaneous bone fractures may occur in children with neural tube defects. Although fractures and osteopenia are more likely to be associated with limited mobility and lack of weight-bearing exercise, the diet should provide adequate intake of vitamins C and D, calcium, phosphorus, and protein.[2,7]

Feeding Assessment

Feeding problems may be present early in infancy if the neural tube defect is complicated by "bulbar palsy" associated with Arnold-Chiari brain malformation. Decreased head and neck control and varying degrees of laryngopharyngeal paralysis may impair the effectiveness or efficiency of sucking and swallowing. A nutrition assessment should include questions that identify feeding problems such as difficulty sucking or swallowing, frequent episodes of coughing or choking during feedings, or difficulty breathing during feedings (see appendixes A and B). If feeding problems are suspected, referral for in-depth assessment by a feeding specialist may be warranted (see chapter 4).

Although obesity does not usually become evident until 3 to 4 years of age, prevention is the best course of action. Reduced levels of activity in infants and children with high-level neural tube lesions may significantly decrease energy expenditure. Basal metabolic rates may also be lower in older children with myelodysplasia due to decreased muscle mass in lower extremities.[10] Intake history should focus on hunger and satiety cues and the parents' ability to interpret and appropriately respond to these cues. If weight or weight for length is greater than the 65th percentile, or if the infant or child appears obese, a detailed account of daily energy intake should be obtained and evaluated by a qualified dietitian.

Nutrition Care Plan

Goals and treatment plans for nutrition-related problems of infants and toddlers with spina bifida are given in table 11-2. Although growth and energy needs may not vary significantly from the norm until 2 to 4 years of age, if the rate of weight gain is greater than the 50th percentile (see table 11-3), or weight for length is at or above the 65th percentile, energy needs and intake should be addressed promptly. Normal activity levels account for 15% of energy needs in infants, 20–25% in toddlers.[8,9] If the infant/toddler does not have voluntary movement in the lower extremities, energy needs may be at least 10–25% less than normal. Energy needs may be estimated as follows:

- Use 75%–100% of RDA energy intake to meet normal weight goals:

Ages 6 months–1 year	85–110 kcal/kg*/day
Ages 1–3 years	75–100 kcal/kg*/day
Ages 4–6 years	70–90 kcal/kg*/day

*kg of ideal or goal weight for length

- If excessive weight gain occurs, use the infant/child as his or her own control, reducing energy intake by 10% and monitoring growth and intake every six months.

Table 11-2. Nutrition Treatment Plan for Infants and Toddlers with Spina Bifida

Nutrition problem	Goal	Treatment plan
Underweight	Weight for length ≥5th percentile but ≤65th percentile	• Feeding assessment and referral to feeding therapist if needed • Frequent feeding schedule every 3 to 4 hours for infants • Frequent feeding schedule 3 meals and 3 snacks/day for toddlers • Nutrient-dense feeding (e.g., higher calorie dense formulas that can easily be diluted or eliminated when normal weight is achieved • Tube feeding if oral intake is ≥10% below expected needs in spite of above measures; nasogastric tube feeding may be used if expected tube feeding duration is <6 weeks; a gastrostomy tube may be considered if tube feeding is required >6 weeks • Accurate assessment of intake to ensure nutrition adequacy
Obesity	Weight for length ≤75th percentile[11] Rate of weight gain at 75–100% of 50th percentile growth rate (see table 11-3)	• Prevention through appropriate interpretation and response to hunger and satiety cues starting in infancy • Frequent evaluation of growth: ≤1 month, 1–6 months, 6–12 months, every 6–12 months thereafter[11] • Accurate assessment of intake; accurate assessment of energy needs (see text); education of parents toward meeting these needs • Providing lower calorie, nutrient-dense foods to maintain adequate intake of other nutrient needs when limiting energy intake; may need vitamin/mineral or protein supplement • Activity/exercise plan • Psychological evaluation/counseling if needed for depression or noncompliance
Constipation	Predictable and full evacuation of soft formed stools	• Adequate fluid intake (see chapter 6) • Adequate fiber intake for older infant and toddler • Exercise and/or massage • Rectal stimulation—medical or physical
Urinary tract infections	Eliminate or reduce frequency of urinary tract infections	• Adequate fluid intake (see chapter 6) • Vitamin C supplement may be prescribed to acidify urine (pH <6) • Cranberry or blueberry juice (contains E. coli adhesion inhibitor)[12]
Trophic ulcers	Prevention of tissue breakdown Rapid healing to prevent nutrient loss	• Meet RDA for all nutrients, especially protein and zinc, even when energy intake is reduced in management of overweight or obesity
Spontaneous fractures	Optimize bone density	• Meet RDA for calcium, phosphorus, protein, vitamins C and D

Table 11-3. Goals for Weight Gain for Infants and Toddlers with Spina Bifida

Goal for weight gain is 75–100% normal expected growth rate[13, 14]			
Age	Weight gain in g/day	Weight gain in oz/wk	Weight gain in lb/6 mo
0–3 mo	23–30	5–7	—
4–6 mo	16–21	4–5	—
7–9 mo	10–13	2–3	—
10–12 mo	8–10	2	—
12–18 mo	5–7	—	2.25–3
18–24 mo	4.5–7	—	2–2.25
2–5 yr	4–5.5	—	1.7–2.25

- For children and infants 4 months of age and older, use 9-11 kcal/cm of length for weight maintenance.[3]
- When using various calculations for estimating basal or resting energy needs for nonambulatory children, use a factor of 1.2 to 1.4 instead of 1.8 to 2.0.[9, 10]

Summary

Infants and toddlers experience their lives first in their homes and with their families. The treatment and management of spina bifida brings these infants and children in frequent contact with medical, community, and educational services. Nutrition is a strong component of the treatment and management of infants and children with spina bifida. Essential to the prevention and management of nutrition problems that occur specific to this condition are frequent nutrition monitoring by a qualified dietitian; effective communication among medical, community, and educational services and the family; and early education and intervention, along with ongoing support.

References

1. Spina bifida. In: Manual of pediatric nutrition. St. Paul: Twin Cities District Dietetic Association, 1990.
2. Dustrude A, Prince A. Provision of optimal nutrition care in myelomeningocele. Top Clin Nutr 5:34–47, 1990.
3. Ekvall SW. Myelomeningocele. In: Ekvall SW, ed. Pediatric nutrition in chronic diseases and developmental disorders. New York: Oxford University Press, 1993; 109.
4. Rotenstein D, Reigel DH. Growth hormone treatment of children with neural tube defects: Results from 6 months to 6 years. J Pediatr 128:184–89, 1996. (Note: 6 months to 6 years represents the duration of treatment, not age of subjects.)
5. Ekvall SM. Myelomeningocele: Nutrition implications. Top Clin Nutr 3:41–54, 1988.
6. Brizee L. Nutritional concerns associated with spina bifida. Nutrition News 3:1–4, 1988.
7. Management of common nutrition/feeding problems for myelomeningocele. In: Goodall pediatric nutrition reference. Columbus, Ohio: Ohio Department of Health, Division of Family and Community Health Services, 1995.
8. Lowry GH. Growth and development in children, 6th ed. Chicago: Year Book Publishers, 1973.
9. National Academy of Sciences. Recommended dietary allowances, 10th ed. Washington, D.C.: National Academy Press, 1989.
10. Bandini LG, Schoeller DA, Fukagawa, et al. Body composition and energy expenditure in adolescents with cerebral palsy or myelodysplasia. Pediatr Res 29:70–77, 1991.
11. American Dietetic Association Dietitian and Pediatric Practice Quality Assurance Committee. Wooldridge NH, Spinozzi N, Isaacs JS, et al., eds. Quality assurance criteria for pediatric nutrition conditions. Chicago: The Association, 1988.
12. Ofek I, Goldhar J, Zafriri D, et al. Anti-escherichia coli adhesin activity of cranberry and blueberry juices. N Engl J Med 324:1599, 1991.
13. Guo S, Rocke AF, Fomon SJ, et al. Reference data on gains in weight and length during the first two years of life. J Pediatr 119:355, 1991.
14. Baumgartner RN, Roche A, Himes JH. Incremental growth tables: Supplement to previously published charts. Am J Clin Nutr 43:711–22, 1986.

Educational Materials

Educational materials for families that address problems with the nutritional aspects of feeding, underweight, obesity, constipation, and urinary tract infections are available from several sources:

Spina Bifida Association of America
1700 Rockville Pike
Rockville MD 20852
tel. 1-800-621-3141

Dietary Management of the Child with Spina Bifida
Sparks Center
University of Alabama at Birmingham
P.O. Box 313, University Station
Birmingham, AL 35294

Niemeyer S, ed. Caregiver education guide for children with developmental disabilities. Gaithersburg, Md.: Aspen Publishers, 1994. Promoting weight control, promoting weight gain, managing constipation, managing urinary tract infections through diet, tube feedings: nasogastric tubes and gastrostomy tubes, and nutrition for your gastrostomy-fed child.

Klein MD, Delaney TA. Feeding and nutrition for the child with special needs: Handouts for parents. Medvescek, CR, ed. Tucson: Therapy Skill Builders, 1994.

Nevin-Folino N. Nutrition education handouts. Children's Medical Center, One Children's Plaza, Dayton, Ohio 45404. Nutrition guide for babies with spina bifida 0–6 months of age, 6 months to 1 year, 1 year to 5 years; and sample very low calorie meal plan for a child with spina bifida, age 2 to 5 years.

Nutrition management of spina bifida. Nutrition focus for children with special health care needs. 11(3): 1–7, 1996.

Nutrition Manual for At-Risk Infants and Toddlers
Janice Hovasi Cox, editor

12

CONGENITAL HEART DISEASE

Janice Hovasi Cox, MS, RD

Many infants and young children with congenital heart disease (CHD) demonstrate normal growth and development and are able to consume adequate amounts of breast milk, formula, milk, and/or foods to meet their nutrient needs. Cardiovascular anomalies associated with growth or nutritional problems include those that significantly affect hemodynamics, i.e., those with which cardiac output is significantly decreased and/or circulation of adequately oxygenated blood is decreased, causing tissues to be generally hypoxic. Most commonly, these problems include ventricular or atrioventricular septal defects, transposition of the great arteries, tetralogy of Fallot, coarctation of the aorta, hypoplastic left ventricle, and patent ductus arteriosus.[1–3] Growth and nutritional status may be minimally affected if corrective surgery is accomplished during the neonatal period. Problems with growth and nutrition may occur if surgery is palliative or must be delayed.[2] A description of these and other cardiac anomalies that affect growth and nutritional status is given in table 12-1.

Nutrition Assessment

Growth Assessment

The reported incidence of growth failure varies with age, identification criteria, and the specific cardiovascular anomaly. As many as 70–80% of infants and children with cyanotic CHD and 45% of infants and children with acyanotic CHD complicated by congestive heart failure (CHF) may plot below the 16th percentile for weight.[2,4] From 40 to 60% and 18%, respectively, may plot below the 3rd percentile for both height and weight. Weight is usually more affected than length or height. Weight for length is low, especially in infants 6 to 12 months of age.[5] Length or height is more often affected in infants and children with cyanotic CHD.[6,7] Stunting (low weight and length or height) is more common in infants and children under 2 years of age.[8]

Although growth acceleration is seen in most infants and children after surgery, catch-up growth is most

Table 12-1. Common Congential Cardiac Defects

Defect	Description	Symptoms/ treatment	Growth implications
Patent ductus arteriosis	Failure of contraction of ductus arteriosis that connects the PA and aorta	Heart murmur/fluid restriction, pharmacological closure, ligation or division	Weight negatively affected prior to surgery. Growth acceleration following surgery
Ventricular septal defect (VSD)	Communication between ventricles allowing blood flow between them	Congestive heart failure/pulmonary artery banding	Large VSD associated with severe growth failure
Transposition of the great arteries (TGA)	Two parallel and separate circulatory systems exist, one pulmonary and one systemic	Cardiomegaly, cyanosis/Blalock-Hanlon shunt, Mustard procedure	Growth retardation in a third to a half of patients
Pulmonary stenosis	Obstruction to right ventricular outflow	Asymptomatic until late childhood/ valvectomy	Normal growth unless lesion is severe
Aortic stenosis	Obstruction to left ventricular outflow	Severe state diagnosed at birth as cardiac failure and shock/ valvotomy	Growth failure noted in 16% of patients
Tricuspid atresia	Absent atrioventricular connection failure	Slightly increased heart size/Glenn shunt	40% of children have marked weight and height growth retardation
Atrial septal defect (ASD)	Communication between 2 atria persists after birth	Asymptomatic or mild respiratory symptoms/direct closure of defect, patch graft	Normal growth unless lesion is severe; then weight gain is poor
Coarctation of the aorta	Narrowing of aorta beyond left subclavian artery	Elevated upper extremity blood pressure, congestive failure/medical management, resection of narrowed section at 3–10 yr. Blalock-Taussig or Waterston shunt	Growth normal with simple defect
Tetrology of Fallot	Right ventricular outflow obstruction, VSD	Cyanosis, dyspnea/ modified Blalock-Taussig shunt	Moderate growth failure, primarily in weight
Hypoplastic left heart syndrome	Absence or severe hypoplasia of some or all left-sided heart structures	Respiratory distress, pallor, congestive failure/Norwood's procedures, cardiac transplantation, or nontreatment (controversial)	Unknown; early morality (before recent surgical procedures) precluded observations of growth

Used with permission. Greecher CP. Congenital heart disease. In: Groh-Wargo S, Thompson M, and Cox JH, eds. Nutritional care for high-risk newborns. rev. ed. Chicago: Precept Press, 1994.

significant when reparative (vs. palliative) surgery is done early. Weight, length, and head circumference have been shown to reach estimated genetic potential within 6 to 12 months when reparative surgery is performed before 7 months of age.[9] Continued growth delay after surgery may be due to genetic or intrauterine factors, residual cardiac compromise, or the effects of early nutritional compromise.[2] Growth subsequent to heart transplant may be diminished due to large doses of corticosteroids needed to avoid transplant rejection.[10]

Growth is monitored frequently, because early detection of a compromise in growth allows timely nutrition intervention, better preparing the infant for surgery and postoperative recovery, supporting normal growth and development, and facilitating the normal progression of feeding skills.[1, 10] Referral to a registered dietitian may be warranted when growth assessment reveals[1]:

- Weight for age or weight for length or height at or below the 5th percentile on the National Center for Health Statistics growth chart (appendix F) or weight ≤90% of estimated ideal body weight for length or height
- Weight gain deceleration (see chapter 5 for normal ranges of daily or weekly weight gain by age)
- Significant decline in percentile rank, crossing at least two major growth channels for weight, length, or head circumference
- Triceps skin fold at or below the 5th percentile (children over a year old).

Table 12-2 lists factors that may contribute to growth failure in infants and children with CHD. Once adequate growth is established through nutrition intervention, average daily weight gain can be monitored every one to two weeks in the young infant or monthly in the older infant or toddler (see chapter 5).

Dietary Intake Assessment

Although growth delay is associated with several factors in infants and children with CHD, inadequate nutrient intake is often the most significant. Reported energy intake of infants and young children may average only 80–90% of normal recommendations.[11–13] Intakes of iron, zinc, calcium, or vitamins D, E, C, B_1 or B_6 may also fall below normal recommendations.[14] Energy needs may be higher than normal due to increased work of breathing, frequent infections and/or fever.[5, 8, 10, 11, 14, 15] Decreased absorption may occur due to relative gastrointestinal tissue hypoxia or edema.[10, 16] Hepatomegaly compressing the stomach may reduce gastric capacity, and CHF may cause gut dysmotility or hypoxia. These factors may then cause delayed gastric emptying and premature satiety or frequent vomiting associated with gastroesophageal reflux.[10, 11, 16] Energy intakes of 125 to 175 kcal/kg/day may be needed to support normal or catch-up growth.[11, 12, 17]

Table 12-2. Factors That May Contribute to Growth Retardation in Infants and Young Children with Congenital Heart Disease

Insufficient nutrient intake due to poor appetite, fatigue during feedings, abdominal discomfort associated with gastrointestinal tract hypomotility due to tissue hypoxia
Decreased nutrient absorption
Increased energy needs due to increased work of breathing
Tissue hypoxia
Acidosis
Congenital heart disease as part of a recognizable syndrome associated with intrauterine or postnatal growth retardation
Recurrent respiratory infections
Frequent hospitalizations
Adverse psychosocial conditions
Gastroesophageal reflux
Cardiomyopathies caused by carnitine, thiamin, or selenium deficiencies

A feeding history can reveal problems with inadequate volume of intake, inability to coordinate suck, swallow, and breathing; breathing difficulty associated with feedings; fatigue or tiring with feedings; early satiety; delayed progression of feeding skills; and frequent episodes of vomiting or diarrhea (see appendixes A and B). Parents' perception and reportage of feeding problems are excellent indicators for low growth outcome and low voluntary food intake.[8] If growth is significantly delayed, evaluation of a three-day food intake record may be needed to specifically identify intake of fluid, energy, electrolytes, iron, calcium, and vitamins and to develop feasible nutrition interventions.

Laboratory Assessment

The most common laboratory indexes for nutrition assessment include serum sodium and potassium; urine osmolality or specific gravity; and serum albumin, prealbumin, hemoglobin, and hematocrit. CHF, restrictions in dietary fluid or sodium, and use of diuretics may alter fluid and electrolyte balance.[2] Serum levels of sodium and potassium help to identify changes in intake needs. Fluid intake may need to be increased if urine osmolality is greater than 400–600 mOsm/L or specific gravity is greater than 1.010–1.014, particularly during stress periods when growth plateaus or catabolism of lean tissues occurs.[10, 17] Decreased serum albumin or prealbumin helps to identify malnutrition as in other infants and children, although changes in fluid balance may make these values more difficult to interpret.

If energy intake has been maximized and growth continues to lag, a three-day fecal fat test may be used to identify fat malabsorption. Fat intake must be quantified to validate test results. Test instructions often advise an intake of at least 100 g of fat per day. Because this is not feasible for infants and young children, dietary fat intake of 3 g/kg/day or 30% of total energy intake is usually recommended.[18] Medium-chain triglycerides (MCT) may not be detected if the Van de Kamer laboratory method is used. Replacement of MCT in the diet with long-chain triglycerides may be necessary, or an alternative method of fecal fat analysis may be used.[19, 20] Malabsorption of fat is generally defined as stool fat losses >15% of dietary fat intake in infants under 6 months of age and >7% thereafter.[21]

Polycythemia frequently occurs in response to chronic hypoxemia. This complicates interpretation of laboratory indexes normally used to identify anemia. Serum iron levels may be needed to identify deficiency, as hematocrit levels may be falsely elevated. Ferritin levels may be falsely elevated if infection is present. If an infant or young child is at increased risk for polycythemia, iron deficiency anemia is considered when hematocrit levels are <40–45% and serum iron levels are below normal. Hematocrit levels ≥60–70% may be exacerbated by iron toxicity and may be associated with impaired perfusion and increased risk of cerebrovascular accidents.[17, 22]

Nutrition Treatment

The nutritional requirements of infants and toddlers with significantly altered cardiac function associated with CHD are given in table 12-3 (infants and toddlers with minor cardiac irregularities are not included).

Fluid and Electrolyte Intake

Management of fluid and electrolyte intake requires concerted input from the physician, parents, feeding therapist, and dietitian. Cardiac output, presence of CHF or edema, use of diuretics or fluid restriction, serum sodium and potassium values, feeding skills and tolerance, and renal solute load must be considered. Although fluids are often restricted to control pulmonary edema and CHF, fluid losses may be increased due to fever, diuretic therapy, and/or tachypnea.[23] Fluid intake may be limited by the infant's ability to feed orally.

Fluid tolerance must be determined before further feeding recommendations can be made. If oral fluid or energy intake is not adequate to support normal hydration and growth, tube feedings may be considered. If energy needs exceed fluid tolerance using standard breast milk, infant formulas, or milk, concentrated feedings or feeding supplements may be considered. Electrolyte supplements may be required during diuretic therapy.

Human Milk and Formula

Tachypnea or increased fatigability may make nipple-feeding from breast or bottle more difficult for the infant with CHD. When breast-feeding, it is often helpful to initiate the let-down reflex before placing the infant at the breast. If the infant tires before the breast is fully emptied, the hind milk, which is rich in fat, may be inadequately

Table 12-3. Nutrient Needs of Infants and Toddlers with Significantly Altered Cardiac Function Associated with Congenital Heart Disease*

Nutrient	Amount	Comments
Fluid	135–180 ml/kg/day or ↑ as tolerated 95–150 ml/kg/day (congestive heart failure)	Limited during periods when congestive heart failure is present, or during illness when pulmonary edema and reduced cardiac output may be present; more liberal during convalescence; may require diuretics; oral intake may be limited due to fatigue or high respiratory rate; tube feedings may be indicated if oral fluid intake is inadequate
Energy	150–180 kcal/kg/day (infants) 120–150 kcal/kg/day (toddlers) RDA for ideal weight for length or height, age corrected for prematurity and/or height age may also be used, at least as a starting point 8–10% of total calories as protein 35–65% as carbohydrate 35–50% as fat (4% essential fatty acids)	Increased resting energy expenditure, increased work of breathing, incomplete absorption of fats and catch-up growth may all contribute to increased needs
Protein	2.2–4.0 gm/kg/day (infants) RDA for ideal weight for length or height, age corrected for prematurity and/or height-age (toddlers)	8–10% of total energy intake; higher end of range needed if gastrointestinal losses are suspected; catch-up growth or chronic corticosteroid use after heart transplant may also increase needs
Electrolytes	2.5–4 mEq Na/kg/day 2.0–5.0 mEq K/kg/day	Depending upon cardiac output and effect of diuretics; potassium excretion ↑ with corticosteroids, chlorothiazide and furosemide; sodium needs may be greater if sodium losses exceed fluid losses with diuretic use
Minerals	2–4 mg iron/kg/day (infants) 72–150 mg calcium/kg/day (infants) 1.0–1.5 mg zinc/kg/day (infants) RDA for age, corrected for prematurity and/or height age (toddlers)	Avoid excess iron, particularly with polycythemia that accompanies chronic tissue hypoxia due to risk of impaired perfusion and cerebrovascular accident; calcium, phosphorus, magnesium, and/or zinc excretion may be enhanced with diuretic use or corticosteroid use after heart transplant
Vitamins	RDA for age, corrected for prematurity and/or height-age (infants, toddlers)	Ensure normal vitamin D and mineral intake, as calcium excretion may be increased by diuretic use or corticosteroid use after heart transplant; infants may have decreased exposure to sunlight

*Infants and toddlers with minor cardiac anomalies or arrhythmias, or after reparative surgery (and subsequent catch-up growth) are not included in this chart. Their needs should match the normal Recommended Dietary Allowances.[20]

References: 1, 2, 10, 12, 17, 18, 19

taken. Hind milk that remains after nursing may be pumped and given by dropper, spoon, spouted cup, or nursing supplementer.[24]

Because infants and toddlers with CHD often consume less than the normal Recommended Dietary Allowances (RDA)[25] for energy, intake should be gradually increased by 10–20 kcal/kg/day until a normal or catch-up growth rate is achieved. Ideal weight for length or height must be considered in identifying energy needs in order to allow for increased metabolic needs and catch-up growth.[15] Initial attempts to increase energy intake of infants should include concentration of standard infant formulas alone or in conjunction with breast-feeding (using a nursing supplemental feeding system). Concentrating standard infant formulas increases the intake of all nutrients proportionally and ensures more adequate intake of protein, vitamins, and minerals. This also decreases free water intake and increases the osmolality and the renal solute load. Careful follow-up may be needed when using formula concentrations above 30 kcal/oz (1 kcal/ml), as these may be associated with increased risk of osmotic diarrhea; dehydration may occur more rapidly, particularly in the presence of increased extrarenal fluid losses caused by such conditions as fever, tachypnea, or diaphoresis. (Recipes for concentrating infant formula up to 30 kcal/oz are given in appendix C.)

Nutritionally complete products containing 30 kcal/oz are available in flavored, ready-to-use form for toddlers. These products are not generally recommended for use with infants because they provide a higher renal solute load than infant formulas concentrated to 30 kcal/oz. However, concentrating infant formula increases osmolality, whereas proprietary 30 kcal/oz products are usually isotonic (see appendix C).

If nutrient intake meets the RDA using up to 30 kcal/oz formula but growth continues to lag, energy intake may be further increased using additional carbohydrate or fat. Glucose polymers are easily digested and do not significantly increase the renal solute load or the osmolality of the feeding. Medium-chain triglyceride (MCT) oil or vegetable oils do not increase the renal solute load or the osmolality of the feeding, but may require vigorous mixing to maintain an adequate emulsion and prevent separation. Although the addition of fat can delay gastric emptying, overall intake of energy is significantly increased when fat is added.[11, 26] Although high-calorie formulas are associated with an increase in metabolic rate and oxygen consumption, the increases are transient and probably not clinically significant, inasmuch as high-calorie formulas improve weight gain and overall nutritional status.[11, 12]

When carbohydrate or fat is added to standard-formula products, an appropriate ratio of protein to energy should be maintained, providing *at least* 6–8% (although many studies suggest 8–10%) of total energy intake from protein.[10, 11, 17] The nutrient content of spoon-feedings and other foods must also be considered for toddlers and infants over 4 to 6 months of age. Current carbohydrate and fat products available are listed in appendix C. Sample high-calorie formulas and their nutritional analyses are given in table 12-4.

Solid Food/Beikost/Table Foods

Solid foods may be started around 4 to 6 months of age, as recommended by the American Academy of Pediatrics.[27] Since pureed solid foods form a more cohesive bolus than liquids when swallowed, they may be more easily tolerated by infants who are often tachypneic. Although these foods may be a good source of energy and vitamins A and C, they are often not a good source of protein, minerals, or other nutrients. If a variety of foods are chosen, such as cereal, fruit-flavored yogurt, pudding, white or sweet potato, and ice cream, solid foods can be used to enhance intake energy, protein, vitamins, and minerals. Waiting beyond 6 to 8 months to initiate spoon-feedings may delay oral skill development.[28]

Tube-Feeding

When voluntary nutritional intake has been maximized by increasing the nutrient density of breast milk, formula, and foods but growth continues to lag, tube-feedings may be considered. Continuous feeding may be tolerated better than bolus feeding if reflux or delayed gastric emptying is present. Nocturnal tube-feedings may sufficiently supplement voluntary oral feedings during the day. Continuous tube-feeding may be required in severely undernourished infants or toddlers to effect significant weight gain.[12, 29, 30]

Using supplementary tube-feedings carries several advantages and disadvantages. Advantages include (1) increased overall intake of nutrition and improved weight gain and nutritional status,[5, 11, 12, 29, 30] (2) decreased stress for parents and infants or toddlers surrounding feedings that are difficult or excessively time consuming, and (3) increased energy reserves and time for play or other activities that enhance development.

Disadvantages include nasal irritation, increased gastroesophageal reflux, vomiting, and/or risk of aspiration with constant indwelling nasogastric feeding tube.[5] Parents require instruction in inserting feeding tubes and maintaining their patency, cleanliness, and function. Placement of gastrostomy feeding tubes for long-term use, fundoplication in treatment of gastroesophageal reflux, or pylorotomy to enhance gastric emptying require surgery that is not without risk.

Frequent follow-up is needed to adjust feedings in response to growth and changes in oral food intake. Young infants may need weekly adjustments in feeding volume, whereas older infants and toddlers may need monthly adjustments. A feeding therapist may be needed to enhance oral feeding skills so that the infant/child may be gradually weaned from tube-feedings. As feeding skills progress, a dietitian can provide guidance for selecting foods and tapering tube-feedings or modifying tube-feeding schedules to enhance hunger-induced motivation for eating while preventing nutritional compromise.

Table 12-4. Sample High-Calorie Formulas for Infants or Toddlers with Congenital Heart Disease

Formula 1	Breast-feeding 90 kcal/kg/day with 30 kcal/kg/day (or 5ml/kg/feeding) supplement of 30 kcal/oz standard infant formula. Given with nursing supplementer, medicine dropper, or spouted cup. Provides normal amount of kcal in lower volume
Formula 2	Standard infant formula concentrated to 30 kcal/oz given at 150 ml/kg/day
Formula 3	Standard infant formula concentrated to 27 kcal/oz plus 3 tbsp of Polycose added per 19 oz (or 3½ tbsp added per 22 oz) given at 150 ml/kg/day
Formula 4	Pediasure, Ross Laboratories, Columbus, Ohio
Formula 5	Standard infant formula concentrated to 30 kcal/oz plus 3 tbsp of Polycose and 2½ tsp of vegetable oil added per 17 oz (or 3½ tbsp of Polycose and 1 tbsp of vegetable oil added per 22 oz) given at 135 ml/kg/day. Provides the highest kcal at lowest volume of intake

Nutrients	No. 1	No. 2	No. 3	No. 4	No. 5
Energy (kcal)	121	152	154	159	170
Volume (ml)	164	150	150	150	135
Water (g)	143	127	125	125	113
Protein (g)	2.1	3.4	3.0	4.5	3.0
Fat (g)	6.8	8.2	7.6	7.5	9.1
Carbohydrate (g)	12.9	16.3	18.5	16.5	19.1
Protein (% total kcal)	6.8	8.9	7.8	12.0	7.0
Fat (% total kcal)	50.8	48.3	44.5	44.0	48.0
Carbohydrate (% total kcal)	42.5	42.8	48.0	44.0	45.0
Calcium (mg)	60	114	95	146	103
Phosphorus (mg)	37	88	64	120	78
Magnesium (mg)	6.4	9.1	10.6	29	8.1
Iron (mg)	0.58	2.7	2.6	2.1	2.4
Zinc (mg)	0.39	1.1	1.06		1.0
Sodium (mg)	32	42	42	58	43
Potassium (mg)	102	164	147	173	146
Chloride (mg)	76	100	95	150	100
Vitamin A (IU)	389	456	422	381	404
Vitamin D (IU)	21	91	84	75	81
Vitamin E (IU)	1.4	4.6	4.2	3.4	4.0
Vitamin K (mcg)	2.7	12.2	11.7	5.6	10.8
Thiamin (vitamin B_1) (mcg)	59	152	106	400	135
Riboflavin (vitamin B_2) (mcg)	92	228	212	313	202
Pyridoxine (vitamin B_6) (mcg)	46	91	84	388	81
Cyanocobalamin (vitamin B_{12}) (mcg)	0.14	0.38	0.31	0.88	0.34
Niacin (mg)	0.5	1.6	1.7	2.5	1.4
Folic acid (mcg)	11.2	22.8	21.2	55	20.2
Ascorbic acid (vitamin C) (mg)	8.2	13.7	11.0	15	12.1
Renal solute load (mOsm)	14.5	22.4	20.4	31.8	22.4
Osmolality (mOsm/L)	326	485	492	325	547

Nutrient analysis by NEDNOVA Nutrition Optimizer, Ross Products Division of Abbott Laboratories, Columbus, Ohio

References

1. Greecher C. Congenital heart disease: A nutrition challenge. Nutr Focus 5(1):1–6, 1990.
2. Rosenthal A. Nutritional considerations in the prognosis and treatment of children with congenital heart disease. In: Suskind RM, Lewinter-Suskind L. Textbook of pediatric nutrition. New York: Raven Press, 1993; 383–91.
3. Haworth SG, Bull C. Physiology of congenital heart disease. Arch Dis Child 68:707–11, 1993.
4. Mehrizi A, Drash A. Growth disturbance in congenital heart disease. J Pediatr 61:418–29, 1962.

5. Norris MKG, Hill CS. Nutritional issues in infants and children with congenital heart disease. Crit Care Nurs Clin North Am 6(1):153–63, 1994.
6. Cameron JW, Rosenthal A, Olson AD. Malnutrition in hospitalized children with congenital heart disease. Arch Pediatr Adolesc Med 149:1098–1102, 1995.
7. Salzer, Jr H, Wimmer M, Heil M, et al. Growth and nutritional intake of infants with congenital heart disease. Pediatr Cardiol 10:17–23, 1989.
8. Thommessen M, Heiberg A, Kase BF. Feeding problems in children with congenital heart disease: The impact on energy intake and growth outcome. Eur J Clin Nutr 46:457–64, 1992.
9. Weintraub RG, Menahem S. Early surgical closure of a large ventricular septal defect: Influence on long-term growth. J Am Coll Cardiol 18:552–58, 1991.
10. Forchielli ML, McColl R, Walker WA, et al. Children with congenital heart disease: A nutrition challenge. Nutr Rev 52:348–53, 1994.
11. Yahav J, Avigad S, Frand M, et al. Assessment of intestinal and cardiorespiratory function in children with congenital heart disease on high-caloric formulas. J Pediatr Gastroenterol Nutr 4:778–85, 1985.
12. Unger R, DeKleermaeker M, Gidding SS, et al. Calories count: Improved weight gain with dietary intervention in congenital heart disease. Am J Dis Child 146:1078–84, 1992.
13. Mitchell IM, Davies PS, Day JM, et al. Energy expenditure in children with congenital heart disease, before and after cardiac surgery. J Thorac Cardiovasc Surg 107:74–80, 1994.
14. Hansen SR, Dorup I. Energy and nutrient intakes in congenital heart disease. Acta Pædiatr 82:166–72, 1993.
15. Menon G and Poskitt EME. Why does congenital heart disease cause failure to thrive? Arch Dis Child 60:1134–39, 1985.
16. Sondheimer JM, Hamilton JR. Intestinal function in infants with severe congenital heart disease. J Pediatr 92:572-78, 1987.
17. Rickard K, Brady MS, Gresham EL. Nutritional management of the chronically ill child. Pediatr Clin North Am 24:157–74, 1977.
18. Kopelman H. Pancreatic function testing. In: Wyllie R, Hyams JD, eds. Pediatric gastrointestinal disease. Philadelphia: Saunders, 1993.
19. Jeejeebhoy KN, Ahmed S, Kozak G. Determination of fecal fats containing both medium and long chain triglycerides and fatty acids. Clin Biochem 3:157, 1970.
20. Van de Kamer JK, tenBokkel Huinink H, Weyers HA. Rapid method for the determination of fat in feces. J Biol Chem 177:347, 1949.
21. Fomon SJ, Zeigler ER, Thomas LN, et al. Excretion of fat by normal full-term infants fed various milks and formulas. Am J Clin Nutr 23:1299, 1970.
22. West DW, Scheel JN, Stover R, et al. Iron deficiency in children with cyanotic congenital heart disease. J Pediatr 117:266, 1990.
23. Greecher C. Congenital heart disease. In: Groh-Wargo S, Thompson M, Cox JH, eds. Nutritional care of high-risk newborns. rev. ed. Chicago: Precept Press, 1994; 266–75.
24. Valentine CJ, Hurst NM, Schanler RJ. Hindmilk improves weight gain in low-birth-weight infants fed human milk. J Pediatr Gastroenterol Nutr 18:474–77, 1994.
25. National Research Council Food and Nutrition Board. Recommended dietary allowances. 10th ed. Washington D.C.: National Academy of Sciences, 1989.
26. Cavell B. Gastric emptying in infants with congenital heart disease. Acta Pediatr Scand 70:517, 1981.
27. American Academy of Pediatrics, Committee on Nutrition. On the feeding of supplemental foods to infants. Pediatrics 65: 1178–81, 1980.
28. Coyner AB, Zelle RS. Habilitative approaches to facilitate more adaptive oral patterns related to eating and expressive language. In: Developmentally disabled infants and toddlers: Assessment and intervention. Philadelphia: Davis, 1983; 443.
29. Vanderhoof JA. Continuous enteral feedings: An important adjunct to the management of complex congenital heart disease. Am J Dis Child 136:825–27, 1982.
30. Schwarz S, Gewitz M, See C, et al. Enteral nutrition in infants with congenital heart disease and growth failure. Pediatrics 86:368–73, 1990.

Parent Education Materials

Klein MD, Delaney TA. Feeding and nutrition for the child with special needs: Handouts for parents. Medvescek, CR, ed. Tucson, Ariz.: Therapy Skill Builders, 1994. (1) Nutrition and feeding for the child with congenital heart disease.

Aspen Reference Group, Caregiver education guide for children with developmental disabilities. Rockville, Md.: Aspen Publications, 1994. (1) Enhancing oral-motor skills, (2) Nutrition for your gastrostomy-fed child, (3) Guidelines for the progression of food textures, (4) Oral treatment techniques, (5) Feeding treatment techniques.

Nutrition Manual for At-Risk Infants and Toddlers
Janice Hovasi Cox, editor

13

CYSTIC FIBROSIS

Lori Yelton, MS, RD

Cystic fibrosis (CF) is an autosomal recessive inherited disease seen most often in the Caucasian population. It can affect the respiratory, gastrointestinal, hepatobiliary, and pancreatic systems by a defect in the chloride transport system in the cells. This defect results in a production of thick mucous secretions, especially in the pancreas and lungs, which block the ducts that release the pancreatic enzymes for proper digestion and produce a good environment for infections in the lungs.

Clinical symptoms of CF may include meconium ileus at birth, rectal prolapse, recurrent lung infections, steatorrhea, azotorrhea, unusually foul-smelling stools, excessive flatulence, poor weight gain in spite of a ravenous appetite, and gastroesophageal reflux or vomiting associated with coughing. Delayed growth, loss of adipose tissue, and muscle wasting may occur as clinical signs of malnutrition. Edema, anemia, and hypoalbuminemia may also occur.[1] Steatorrhea may cause increased loss of bile salts and bile acids, trace minerals, fat, and fat-soluble vitamins.[2] About 85% of CF patients eventually experience malabsorption and nutritional compromise.[3] Most CF patients develop initial symptoms of the disease within the first two years of life.[4]

Early diagnosis of CF is vital in order to avoid possible nutrition deficiencies and poor growth. Research has established a clear link between malnutrition and decreased lung function.[5] Advances in understanding the disease, newer antibiotics and therapeutic medicines, as well as improved nutrition and respiratory therapies in the past two decades have increased the median lifespan of the CF patient to nearly 30 years.[6]

Nutritional Assessment

Table 13-1 summarizes the nutrition assessment recommendations of the Cystic Fibrosis Foundation (CFF) Consensus Report.[2]

Table 13-1. Nutritional Status Assessment

Parameter	Minimum Frequency	Indication
Anthropometric measurement		
Weight	Every 3 mo	Routine care
Height (length ≤ 2 yr)	Every 3 mo	Routine care
Head circumference	Every 3 mo until age 2 yr	Routine care
Mid-arm circumference	Every 3 mo	Routine care
Triceps skin fold thickness	Every 3 mo	Routine care
Nutritional assessment		
Dietary intake. *This assessment usually consists of a 24-hour recall with assessment of dietary intake by a registered dietitian*	Yearly	Routine care, at diagnosis
3-day fat balance. *Includes diet records to determine energy intake as well as fat intake to determine net fat absorption*	As indicated	Weight loss, growth failure, clinical deterioration, at diagnosis
Anticipatory dietary guidance	Yearly	Routine care, at diagnosis
Laboratory studies		
CBC. *If there is any evidence of iron deficiency, iron status must be measured (i.e., serum iron, iron binding capacity and ferritin)*	Yearly	Routine care, at diagnosis
Serum or plasma retinol	Yearly	Routine care, at diagnosis
Serum or plasma—tocopherol	Yearly	Routine care, at diagnosis
Albumin	As indicated	Weight loss, growth failure, clinical deterioration, at diagnosis
Electrolytes and acid-base status	As indicated	Prolonged fever, summer heat, infancy, breast-feeding, at diagnosis

Reprinted with permission from the Cystic Fibrosis Foundation.[2]

Anthropometric Measurements

- Measure and plot weight, length, head circumference, and weight for length using standard measurement techniques and the National Center for Health Statistics growth charts (appendix F).
- From 0 to 2 years of age, monitor growth weekly or biweekly until normal growth is established, then reassess every two to three months.
- Optimal weight is a range of 90 to 100% of ideal weight for length or height. Underweight is 85 to 89%, mild malnutrition is 80 to 85%, moderate malnutrition is 75 to 79%, and severe malnutrition is < 75% of ideal weight for length or height.
- A decline in linear growth may signal malnutrition and the need for nutrition intervention. Normal expected linear growth for a specific infant or child may be estimated using mid-parental height.[7]
- After 1 year of age, triceps and subscapular skin folds, upper mid-arm circumference, and upper mid-arm muscle area may be compared to standardized norms for age and gender to identify changes in fat stores and lean body mass.[8]

- Energy requirements for the infant and toddler may vary in patients with CF due to differing ability to consume liquids and solids, degree of malabsorption, current health status, activity, age, and gender (see section below on energy and protein requirements).

Dietary Intake Assessment

During the first two years of life, thorough assessment of dietary intake may be needed frequently until normal growth is established. Thereafter, assessment should be performed at least annually. The most convenient method of dietary intake assessment may be a 24-hour recall. When there is evidence of weight loss, gastrointestinal complaints, or a significant change in stools, a more detailed assessment from records of actual food intake may be needed. Dietary intake is most often specifically evaluated for energy, protein, fat, essential fatty acid, and fat-soluble vitamin intake. In addition to food intake, use of nutritional supplements, vitamins, pancreatic enzyme replacements, symptoms of malabsorption, and fecal fat test results should be monitored.

Clinical Assessment

Malabsorption is most accurately assessed by a three-day fecal fat test to determine the percent of absorption. Fat intake must be quantified to validate test results. Test instructions often advise an intake of at least 100 g of fat/day. Because this is not feasible for infants and young children, dietary fat intake of 3 g/kg/day or 30% of total energy intake is usually recommended.[9] Medium-chain triglycerides (MCT) may not be detected if the Van de Kamer laboratory method is used. Replacement of MCT in the diet with long-chain triglycerides may be necessary, or an alternative method of fecal fat analysis may be used.[10, 11] Malabsorption of fat is generally defined as stool fat losses >15% of dietary fat intake in infants under 6 months of age and >7% thereafter.[12] Without pancreatic enzyme replacement, absorption may be 10–80% of intake.[12] Even with enzyme replacement therapy, some CF patients still have a significant amount of malabsorption. It is important to monitor growth and adjust energy intake recommendations closely. Overt clinical signs of essential fatty acid deficiency have been reported in infants with cystic fibrosis and pancreatic insufficiency, but such symptoms are rare beyond infancy even though biochemical evidence is common.[1, 13]

Pancreatic enzyme replacements consist of lipase, protease, and amylase, dispensed as a bulk powder or as enterically coated microspheres or microtablets contained within a gelatin capsule. Enterically coated enzymes are preserved from breakdown and deactivation in stomach acid, maintaining their potency until they reach the small intestine, where they aid in the digestion of dietary fats, proteins, and starches. Enzymes that are not enterically coated may cause breakdown of mouth and stomach tissues, but may be used for tube-feedings, because the enterically coated microspheres do not pass through standard tubing. Enterically coated microspheres do not dissolve in liquids, nor do they pass through the holes in standard nipples used for bottle-feeding. Infants and toddlers who cannot yet swallow the whole pancreatic enzyme capsule need to have the microspheres removed from the gelatin capsule and mixed with a small amount of strained food such as applesauce, which is then given by spoon. The capsules containing enterically coated enzymes should not be crushed nor chewed because this may destroy the enteric coating, decreasing the enzymes' effectiveness and possibly causing mouth and stomach ulcers. When the microspheres are mixed with strained food (e.g., applesauce), which is often acidic, they should be given immediately and not be stored in the food, as this causes some breakdown of the enteric coating.

Approximately 85% of CF patients have pancreatic insufficiency.[3] The amount of pancreatic enzymes prescribed by the physician is individualized for each patient, depending upon individual weight, diet, nutrient needs, degree of malabsorption present, intestinal pH, and individual gastrointestinal tract anatomy. A guideline for initiation of therapy is 2000–4000 IU of lipase per 120 ml feeding, or, in general, 500 IU lipase/kg.[14] Enzymes are then adjusted according to growth, stool appearance, volume, and consistency. The CFF does not recommend >2000 IU, lipase/kg body weight without specific investigation of malabsorption. Dosages >6000 IU lipase/kg per meal have been associated with colonic strictures.[14, 15] For optimal management of pancreatic enzyme replacement, it is important that patients (1) take the prescribed amounts of pancreatic enzymes at each meal or snack, (2) do not alter enzyme doses without consulting their physician, and (3) take the prescribed pancreatic enzyme and not a generic brand. Because pancreatic enzymes differ in the amounts of lipase, amylase, and protease, the prescribed pancreatic enzyme replacement should reflect the individual's diet. Enzyme dosages range from 4000 to 20,000 IU lipase per capsule. Constipation in CF is often associated with inadequate doses of pancreatic enzyme replacement rather than with excessive dosages.[1, 16]

Laboratory Assessment

Table 13-1 provides the minimum frequency of laboratory assessment in accordance to the CFF Consensus Conference recommendations.[2, 5]

Biochemical measurements of albumin, prealbumin, electrolytes, CBC, serum retinol, and alpha-tocopherol should be determined at diagnosis and at any time there are signs of clinical deterioration. Hypoalbuminemia and hypoproteinemia are usually accurate indicators of malnutrition during infancy.[13] In toddlers, serum albumin and total protein become less reliable indicators of nutritional status because they are affected by many factors such as acute infection and hydration status. Serum prealbumin may be a better indicator of protein stores and nutrition status. Hydration, electrolytes, and acid/base status are often monitored more frequently during the summer months, especially if the infant is breast-fed, has profuse diarrhea, or prolonged fever.[3] Many CF centers use other diagnostic tests to assess exocrine pancreatic function, duodenal aspiration, or fecal fat studies.[17]

Treatment/Nutrition Recommendations

Human Milk and Formula

The CFF Consensus Report indicates that some infants with CF sustain normal growth on human milk when receiving pancreatic enzyme supplementation, even though protein deficiency has been reported.[2] Bile salt–activated lipase present in human milk may enhance fat absorption, and the isomeric configuration of the fatty acids in human milk may support better fat and mineral absorption.[18] If an infant is fed human milk exclusively, serum levels of sodium, albumin, and linoleic acid should be monitored periodically to prevent hyponatremia, hypoproteinemia,[19] and linoleic acid deficiency.[18, 20] Soy protein formulas are not usually recommended for infants with CF based on earlier research indicating the development of hypoalbuminemia and hypoproteinemia in infants with CF fed soy-based formulas.[21]

A cow's milk–based infant formula or protein hydrolysate formula is often the best choice for either supplementation of breast-feeding or total feeding. These formulas provide high-quality protein, and the hydrolysate formulas require less digestion for adequate absorption of macronutrients. In a recent survey, 69% of responding dietitians recommended protein hydrolysate formulas for infants with CF.[22] Protein hydrolysate formulas may be especially beneficial if an infant had a meconium ileus or is diagnosed with failure to thrive. The CFF recommends that all infants with CF receive human milk and/or infant formula for at least the first 12 months and up to 24 months of age.[2]

If an infant is unable to take adequate volumes of human milk or infant formula to sustain a normal growth pattern, supplements may be given in a variety of ways. Powdered or liquid concentrate formulas may be added to human milk or mixed in higher concentrations, usually up to 30 kcal/oz (1 kcal/ml) and given as supplements or as the entire source of nutrition (see appendix C). Supplements of fat or carbohydrate may be given to enhance energy intake, although care should be taken to maintain an appropriate balance of macronutrients: protein 7–18%, carbohydrate 40–50%, and fat 30–54% of total energy intake.[23]

Beikost/Spoon-Feedings/Table Foods

Complementary foods should be introduced in accordance with the American Academy of Pediatrics guidelines, usually around 4 to 6 months of age. Enzyme replacements do not contain disaccharidases and are not given with juices or most fruits. Disaccharidases are present in the small intestine in adequate amounts. Vegetables, cereals, and fruits that contain tapioca or other starches require the amylase present in supplemental enzyme preparations. Meats, mixed foods, and many table foods contain protein, fat, and starches that require enzyme replacement for adequate digestion and absorption of these macronutrients.

As the infant becomes a toddler, certain food preferences may be expressed. The diet should be monitored closely during these years for energy and nutrient adequacy, dietary patterns, and behaviors. Because mealtimes during these ages are often of prolonged duration, replacement enzyme doses may divided and given at the beginning and midway through the meal to improve effectiveness.

A more aggressive means of nutrition support is recommended for patients whose weight-for-height ratio is <85% of ideal.[2] Tube-feedings or parenteral nutrition may be started in order to prevent or decrease malnutrition.[24]

Of the dietitians surveyed who work in CF clinics, 86% recommend tube-feeding or parenteral nutrition support in the malnourished infant as a means of promoting growth.[22]

Energy and Protein Requirements

Energy requirements for the infant and toddler may vary in the CF patient population. Their ability to consume liquids and solids, degree of malabsorption or pancreatic insufficiency, current health status, activity, age, and gender all need to be taken into consideration when calculating caloric requirements. There is evidence that CF infants have a 25–26% higher energy expenditure than matched normal healthy infant controls.[25, 26] The estimated energy needs for an infant or toddler with CF may range from 100% of the Recommended Daily Allowances (RDA) for age and gender if malabsorption is not present or under good control, to 150% of the RDA for those with malabsorption, frequent infections, or other stress factors.[3, 27–29] One study suggests that there may be a constitutional disorder of energy metabolism and that early and specific nutrition therapy should be started during infancy, even before respiratory compromise and/or other stress factors become evident.[26]

The CFF recommendations are based on the World Health Organization's equations for calculation of basal metabolic rate (BMR), to which are added factors for estimated activity levels, lung function, and fat absorption.[29, 30] Calculation of estimated energy needs is explained in figure 13-1. When weight for length or height is low, ideal weight may be used in these calculations to allow adequate energy for catch-up growth. These calculations are used to establish initial nutrition recommendations or therapy. Frequent follow-up is often necessary to further adjust intake and/or enzyme doses to achieve adequate growth and nutrition status.

Calculating Energy Needs for Infants and Toddlers with Cystic Fibrosis

Step 1. Basal metabolism rate (BMR) for infants/children 0–3 years of age (WHO)*

	Female		Male
BMR =	(61.0 kcal × weight in kg) – 51 kcal	or	(60.9 kcal × weight in kg) – 54 kcal

Weight in kg = actual weight or ideal weight for length or height if weight status is low

Step 2. Estimate activity (AC) and disease co-efficients (DC)

Activity:	confined to bed = 1.3	sedentary = 1.5	active = 1.7 – 2.0
Disease:	normal = 0	moderate = 0.3 – 0.5	

Lung function may be measured by Forced Expiratory Volume (FEV):
≥80% of predicted value represents essentially normal lung function
40–79% of predicted value represents moderate lung disease

Step 3. Calculate daily energy expenditure (DEE)

$$DEE = BMR \times (AC + DC)$$

Step 4. Calculate total daily energy requirement (DER)

$$DER = DEE \times (0.93 \div \%\ \text{fat absorption})$$

If a stool fat collection is not available to determine the fractional fat absorption, an approximate value of 0.85 (or 85% fat absorption) may be used to calculate total daily energy requirements

Sample Calculation

An active 18-month-old boy who weighs 11 kg (50th percentile weight for length) has moderate lung disease (FEV 75% of predicted value) and is found to absorb 90% of ingested fat. His total daily energy requirement may be calculated as follows:

BMR = (60.9 kcal/kg × 11 kg) – 54 kcal = 616 kcal
DEE = 616 kcal (1.7 AC + 0.3 DC) = 616 kcal × 2 = 1232 kcal
DER = 1232 kcal × (0.93 ÷ 0.90) = 1232 kcal × 1.03 = 1269 kcal total/day

*WHO – World Health Organization[30]

Figure 13-1. In calculating estimated energy needs, if weight for length or height is low, ideal weight may be used to allow adequate energy for catch-up growth. (Adapted with permission from the Cystic Fibrosis Foundation.)

As with calorie needs, protein needs vary in the CF population. Protein needs are increased with malabsorption and during infection. Without pancreatic enzyme replacement, protein losses may range from 10 to 50% of dietary intake.[31] Even with pancreatic enzyme replacement therapy, stool protein losses may be as much as 18% of dietary intake.[31] Infants are at higher risk for protein deficiency due to their needs during the first year. Because of the lower protein content of human milk, breast-fed infants with CF should be monitored.

With increased clinical severity, protein needs may increase to 200% of the RDA for age and gender.[29, 32] Dietary protein should contribute 7–18% of the total energy intake of infants. As foods are introduced into the diet, the biological value of the protein consumed may vary. Dietary protein should contribute 15–20% of total energy intake in young children, and foods with protein of high biological value should be encouraged.[33]

In the past, dietary fat intake was restricted due to steathorrea. With improved pancreatic enzymes and the recognition of fat as a significant source of energy, a diet high in fat, or 40–50% of the total energy intake, is now recommended.[28, 34]

Vitamin and Mineral Recommendations

Fat-soluble vitamins A, D, E, and K may be malabsorped in patients with pancreatic insufficiency. Supplementation is generally recommended (see table 13-2). With the advent of enteric-coated pancreatic enzymes, absorption of fat-soluble vitamins has improved to the degree that water-miscible forms are no longer routinely given.

Earlier reports documented conjectival xerosis and increased intracranial pressure in infants and night blindness in older patients with CF due to vitamin A deficiency.[1] Although pancreatic enzyme replacement therapy and vitamin supplementation has improved vitamin status, and clinical signs of vitamin A deficiency are not usually seen, low serum levels of vitamin A are often detected. Reduced synthesis of retinol-binding protein or zinc deficiency may be contributing factors in addition to reduced vitamin A absorption.[35] In addition to retinol, the

Table 13-2. Recommended Nutrient Supplementation for Infants and Young Children with Cystic Fibrosis

Age	Infant	1–4 yr
Calories	100–120% RDA* with pancreatic sufficiency; up to 150% of RDA for pancreatic insufficiency, low weight or increased clinical severity[21, 26]	
Protein	15–20% of total calories and up to 200% RDA* with increased clinical severity[13, 28–30]	
Fat	40–50% of total calories[4, 28]	
Multivitamins with A and D	1 dose of liquid multivitamin with iron	1 dose of liquid multivitamin or standard children's multivitamin with 5000 IU vitamin A, 400 IU vitamin D
Vitamin E	0–6 mo: 25 IU/day 6–12 mo: 50 IU/day	100 IU/day
Vitamin K	2.5 mg/wk or 2.5 mg twice per week if on antibiotic therapy	5.0 mg 2×/wk when on antibiotics or if cholestatic liver disease is present
Sodium	2–4 mEq/kg/day or 1/8 or 1/4 tsp of table salt/day for breast-fed or formula-fed babies, especially during summer months[2]	Ad libidum access to salty foods

*RDA - Recommended Dietary Allowances[29]

carotenoids, particularly beta carotene, may be needed in increased amounts in patients with CF for their role as antioxidants. Serum levels of beta carotene are low in children with CF. Although relatively high doses of beta carotene may be needed to achieve normal serum levels in some patients, definitive studies of dose response, efficacy, and toxicity have yet to be completed; therefore, specific dose recommendations have not been proposed.[36]

Laboratory evidence of vitamin E deficiency has been observed at diagnosis of CF in nearly 40% of 7-week-old infants.[1] Although serum levels of vitamins A and D may normalize during the first year of life when pancreatic enzymes and vitamin supplementation within the usual range are provided, vitamin E supplements of 100 mg/day may be required to avert biochemical evidence of deficiency.[37, 38]

Overt vitamin D deficiency is rare in CF patients. This may be due to the ample sources available, including fortified formulas and milk, vitamin and pancreatic enzyme supplementation, and adequate exposure to direct sunlight.[1]

Vitamin K deficiency is also rare, but has been described in newly diagnosed infants. Vitamin K supplementation is recommended throughout the first year,[2] especially if gut flora are not yet mature.[3] Because antibiotics may decrease intestinal microflora production of vitamin K, supplementation is recommended during treatment with these agents.[2, 3]

Except for vitamin B_{12}, there is no evidence of water-soluble vitamin deficiencies in CF. In patients with pancreatic insufficiency, B_{12} is absorbed and metabolized when adequate pancreatic enzymes are used. In patients with meconium ileus who have undergone resection of the terminal ileum, oral or intramuscular B_{12} supplementation may be required. Serum levels of B_{12} are used to identify deficiency state.[4]

Sodium supplementation may be needed for infants who are breast-fed[2] or formula-fed,[3] and for all infants during the hot summer months.[2] Table 13-2 gives dosage recommendations for infants and children up to 4 years of age.

Although fat and bile salt absorption may affect mineral and trace mineral status, clinical evidence of deficiencies of these nutrients has not been widely reported. Decreased cortical thickness of long bones,[39] hypomagnesemia and fatigue during aminoglycoside antibiotic therapy,[40] low zinc levels and growth retardation,[41] and iron deficiency anemia[42] have been reported. However, adequate pancreatic enzyme replacement therapy and normal dietary intakes of vitamins, minerals, and trace metals appear to meet nutritional needs without additional supplementation.[43] Fluoride supplementation may be needed as for normal infants and children if they live in areas where water sources of fluoride are limited or absent.

References

1. Lacaille F, Schmiltz J. Cystic fibrosis. Semin Pediatr Gastroenterol Nutr 4(2):1–15, 1993.
2. Ramsey BW, Farrell PM, Pencharz P, Cystic Fibrosis Consensus Committee. Nutrition assessment and management of cystic fibrosis: A consensus report. Am J Clin Nutr 55:108–16, 1992.
3. Wooldridge NH. Pulmonary diseases. In: Queen PM, Lang CE, eds. Handbook of pediatric nutrition. Gaithersburg, Md.: Aspen, 1993; 422–40.
4. Lloyd-Still JD. Textbook of cystic fibrosis. Bristol, England: John Wright, 1983.
5. Cystic Fibrosis Foundation Consensus Conference. Nutrition assessment and management in cystic fibrosis. Concensus Report. vol. 1, sect. V, April 1990.
6. Creveling S, Light M, Gardner P, Greene L. Cystic fibrosis, nutrition and the health care team. Building block for life 18(3): 1–7, 14–15, 1994. (Published by the Pediatric Nutrition Practice Group of American Dietetic Association.)
7. Himes JH, Roche AF, Thissen D, Moore WM. Parent specific adjustments for evaluation of recumbent length and stature in children. Pediatrics 75:304–13, 1985.
8. Frisancho AR. Anthropometric standards for the assessment of growth and nutritional status. Ann Arbor, Mich.: University Press, 1990.
9. Kopelman H. Pancreatic function testing. In: Wyllie R, Hyams JD, eds. Pediatric gastrointestinal disease. Philadelphia: Saunders, 1993.
10. Jeejeebhoy KN, Ahmed S, Kozak G. Determination of fecal fats containing both medium and long chain triglycerides and fatty acids. Clin Biochem 3:157, 1970.
11. Van de Kamer JK, tenBokkel Huinink H, Weyers HA. Rapid method for the determination of fat in feces. J Biol Chem 177:347, 1949.
12. Fomon SJ, Zeigler ER, Thomas LN, et al. Excretion of fat by normal full-term infants fed various milks and formulas. Am J Clin Nutr 23:1299, 1970.

13. Forstner G, Durie G. Nutrition in cystic fibrosis. In: Grand R, Sutphen JL, Dietz WH, eds. Pediatric nutrition: Theory and practice. Stoneham, Mass.: Butterworth, 1987.
14. Cystic Fibrosis Foundation Consensus Conference. Use of pancreatic enzyme supplements for patients with cystic fibrosis in the context of fibrosing colonopathy: Consensus Report. vol. 6, sect. I, March 1995.
15. Freiman JP, FitzSimmons SC. Colonic strictures in patients with cystic fibrosis: Results of a survey of 114 cystic fibrosis care centers in the United States. J Pediatr Gastroenterol Nutr 22:153–56, 1996.
16. Shalon BS, Adelson JD. Cystic fibrosis gastrointestinal complications and gene therapy. Pediatr Gastroenterol 1, 43:1, 1996.
17. Woodbridge NH. Nutrition management of cystic fibrosis: Nutr Focus 9:6, 1994.
18. Britman J, Hamosh M, Wood D, Freed L, Hamosh P. Lipid composition of milk from mothers with cystic fibrosis. Pediatrics 80: 927–31, 1987.
19. Fleisher DS, DiGeorge AM, Barness LA, Cornfield D. Hypoproteinemia and edema in infants with cystic fibrosis of the pancreas. J Pediatr 64:341–48, 1964.
20. Luder E, Meyer K, Torres G, Bonfonte R. Recommendations for breast feeding in cystic fibrosis centers. Am J Dis Child 144:1153–55, 1990.
21. Abman S, Aaurso F, Bowman M. Persistent morbidity and mortality of protein-calorie malnutrition in infants with cystic fibrosis. J Pediatr Gastroenterol Nutr. 15:3 393–95, 1986.
22. Cowing Cannella P, Bowser EK, Guyer LK, Borum PR. Feeding practices and nutrition recommendations for infants with cystic fibrosis. J Am Diet Assoc 93:292–300, 1993.
23. American Academy of Pediatrics Committee on Nutrition. Commentary on breastfeeding and infant formulas, including proposed standards for formulas. Pediatrics 57:278, 1976.
24. Gerson W, Swan P, Walker A. Nutrition support in cystic fibrosis. Nutr Rev 45:353–60, 1987.
25. Shepherd RW, Holt TL, Vasquez L, Coward WA, Prentice A. Increased energy expenditure in young children with cystic fibrosis. Lancet 1:1300–3, 1988.
26. Girade JP, Tounian P, Sardet A, et al. Resting energy expenditure in infants with cystic fibrosis. J Pediatr Gastroenterol Nutr 18:214–18, 1994.
27. Foster SW, Farrell PM. Enhancing nutrition in cystic fibrosis with comprehensive therapies. J Pediatr Gastroenterol Nutr 22:3, 1996 (edit).
28. Green ME, Buchanan E, Weaver ET, et al. Nutritional management of the infant with cystic fibrosis. Arch Dis Child 72:452–6, 1995.
29. National Research Council Food & Nutrition Board. Recommended dietary allowances, 10th ed. Washington D.C.: National Academy of Sciences, 1989.
30. World Health Organization. Energy and protein requirements. WHO Technical Report Service, series 724, 1985.
31. Gaskin NJ. Cystic fibrosis: Nutritional problems and their management. Semin Pediatr Gastroenterol Nutr 18:214–18, 1994.
32. Michel SH, Mueller DH. Practical approaches to nutrition care of patients with cystic fibrosis. Top Clin Nutr. 2:10, 1989.
33. Lloyd-Still JD. Cystic fibrosis. In: Lebenthal E, ed. Textbook of gastroenterology and nutrition in infancy, 2nd ed. New York: Raven Press, 1989; 831.
34. Roulet M. Protein-energy malnutrition in cystic fibrosis patients. Acta Pediatr (Suppl 1) 395:43–48, 1994.
35. Hopkins RL. Nutritional management of children with cystic fibrosis. In: Suskind RM, Lewintwer-Suskind L, eds. Textbook of pediatric nutrition. New York: Raven Press, 1993; 375–82.
36. Homnick DN, Spillers CR, Cox SR, Cox JH, Yelton LA, et al. Single- and multiple-dose response relationships of ß-carotene in cystic fibrosis patients. J Pediatr 127:491–94, 1995.
37. Sokol PJ, Reardon MC, Accurso FJ, et al. Fat-soluble vitamin status during the first year of life in infants with cystic fibrosis identified by screening of newborns. Am J Clin Nutr 50:1064–71, 1989.
38. Peters SA, Kelly FJ. Vitamin E supplementation in cystic fibrosis. J Pediatr Gastroenterol Nutr 22(4):341–45, 1996.
39. Mischler EH, Chesney PJ, Chesney RW, et al. Demineralization in CF detected by direct photonabsorptiometry. Am J Dis Child 133:632–35, 1979.
40. Green CJ, Doersuk CF, Stern RC. Symptomatic hypomagnesemia in CF. J Pediatr 107:425–28, 1985.
41. Hamilton RM, Billespie CR, Cook HW. Relationships between levels of essential fatty acids and zinc in plasma in cystic fibrosis patients. Lipids 16:374–76, 1981.
42. Ater JL, Herbst JJ, Landaw SA, et al. Relative anemia and iron deficiency in cystic fibrosis. Pediatrics 71:810–14, 1983.
43. Pencharz PB, Durie PR. Nutritional management of cystic fibrosis. Ann Rev Nutr 13:111–36, 1993.

Suggested Additional Reading

Shalon LB, Adelon JW. Cystic fibrosis: Gastrointestinal complications and gene therapy. Pediatr Clin North Am 43:1, 1996.

Lacaille F, Schmiltz J. Cystic fibrosis. Semin Pediatr Gastroenterol Nutr 4(2):1–15, 1993.

Ramsey BW, Farell PM, Pencharz P, Consensus Committee. Nutrition assessment and management in cystic fibrosis: a consensus report. Am J Clin Nutr 1992; 55, 108–15.

Parent Education Materials

Aspen Reference Group, Caregiver education guide for children with developmental disabilities. Rockville, Md.: Aspen, 1994. (1) Promoting weight gain, (2) Tube feedings.

Cunningham JC, Taussig LM. Cystic fibrosis learning kit. Bethesda, Md.: Cystic Fibrosis Foundation, 1994.

Klein MD, Delaney TA. Feeding and nutrition for the child with special needs: Handouts for parents. Medvescek, CR, ed. Tucson: Therapy Skill Builders, 1994. (1) Cystic fibrosis, (2) Feeding your child with a G-tube.

Luder E. Living with cystic fibrosis: Family guide to nutrition. Raritan, N. J.: McNeilab, 1993.

McNeil's guide to cystic fibrosis for parents and children. McNeil Pharmaceuticals.

Ohio Neonatal Nutritionists. Neonatal nutrition handouts: Cystic fibrosis. Nancy Nevin-Folino, Children's Medical Center, Dayton, Ohio 45404.

Nutrition Care for High-Risk Newborns (Rev. Ed.)
S. Groh-Wargo, M. Thompson, J. Cox, editors

14

BRONCHOPULMONARY DYSPLASIA

Janice Hovasi Cox, MS, RD

Bronchopulmonary dysplasia (BPD) is a chronic lung condition that develops in neonates following hyaline membrane disease, meconium aspiration pneumonia, neonatal pneumonia, congestive heart failure, hypoplastic lungs, pulmonary air leaks, Wilson-Mikity syndrome, or other lung problem that requires treatment with intermittent positive pressure ventilation and supplemental oxygen.[1] Nutritional care during the acute phase of BPD is described elsewhere.[2] This chapter reviews the nutritional problems often encountered in infants and young children during the convalescent stage of BPD after hospital discharge and provides suggestions for treatment.

Nutrition Assessment

Nutrition screening of infants and children with BPD includes an assessment of growth based on age corrected for premature birth (see appendix O, "corrected age"), a review of dietary intake, and feeding history (see appendixes A and B). Growth and nutrition are affected by a variety of factors that may be present for the infant or child with BPD, such as continued need for assisted ventilation, supplemental oxygen, diuretic or anti-inflammatory medications, increased respiratory effort and rate, fatigability, and other diagnoses or conditions associated with premature birth. Feeding problems are common and may require a more in-depth assessment to best meet the patient's needs (see appendixes D and E).

Growth

As with any other infant or young child, weight, length or height, and head circumference are measured routinely and plotted on the National Center for Health Statistics (NCHS) growth charts using age corrected for premature birth (see appendix F). Many reports have documented low percentile rankings for length and weight in infants and children with BPD.[3–11] Factors that are thought to contribute to this growth delay include elevated resting metabolic energy expenditure, increased work of breathing, chronic respiratory tract infections, poor nutritional intake, altered nutrient absorption, gastroesophageal reflux, and relative tissue hypoxia. Many infants who develop BPD are born extremely premature and at extremely low birth weight. These factors may also account for growth delay.

Weight, length, and head growth may lag during the acute state of disease. Head growth usually begins to catch up or grow at an accelerated rate between 32 and 38 weeks' gestation.[12] Length begins to grow at a *normal* rate from 38 to 48 weeks' gestational age, although often not at a catch-up rate as might be expected of prematurely born infants without BPD.[4, 5, 12, 13] Infants and young children in the convalescent stage of BPD usually grow at a normal *rate* throughout the early years. Head circumference usually plots at normal percentile ranks, while length and weight plot at or below normal percentile ranks for corrected age. Catch-up growth may not take place until school age[9, 11] (see figure 14-1). Weight for length or height often plots at or slightly below normal percentile ranks, although occasionally weight for length greater than the 95th percentile is seen with linear growth lag and chronic steroid use. Referral to a registered dietitian should be considered if (1) weight or length for corrected age is at or below the 5th percentile, (2) weight for length or weight for height is at or below the 5th percentile, (3) weight for length or weight for height is above the 95th percentile, or (4) if feeding history indicates feeding problems or inadequate nutritional intake.

Feeding History

Infants and toddlers with BPD often receive breast milk supplements or formulas of higher than usual caloric density to meet their increased nutrient needs. Electrolytes such as potassium chloride or sodium chloride may be added to their feedings. If growth is delayed, a detailed 24-hour diet history or three-day dietary intake record may be needed to determine nutritional adequacy.

Feeding problems may occur, especially if there is continued presence of airway appliances such as nasal cannula, supplemental oxygen, mechanical ventilation, or tracheostomy. The sense of smell is often diminished, which may also decrease taste acuity. Continued respiratory compromise may decrease endurance or ability to efficiently suck and swallow an adequate amount of milk. Repeated noxious experiences in or near the mouth, including airway obstruction, may create oral defensiveness or feeding aversion. Decreased exposure to normal feeding patterns and pleasant oral stimulation may delay normal feeding progression and dietary intake.

Gastroesophageal reflux (GER) is often seen in infants and toddlers with BPD. Frequent episodes of reflux or vomiting can be irritating to the esophagus and can increase the risk for aspiration and respiratory compromise.[14–16] Feeding problems may be best identified by questions asked regarding:

- Distress, fussiness, or arching during feedings
- Frequent difficulty breathing during feedings
- Tiring easily with feedings or frequent difficulty finishing a feeding
- Extended duration of feedings
- Frequency of coughing during feedings
- Delayed progression of feeding skills
- Aversion or refusal of feedings
- Recurrent vomiting (reflux or rumination) (see appendixes A and B).

Referral to a feeding therapist may be indicated for further evaluation and treatment if feeding problems interfere with the infant's/toddler's ability to consume adequate feedings (see table 4-4 and appendixes D and E).

Nutrition Treatment

Nutrients

Infants and young children in the convalescent stage of BPD may require specialized nutrition treatment plans to achieve greatest potential for catch-up growth, lung tissue growth, and oral-motor development. A summary of their nutrient needs is given in table 14-1. Infants with BPD and growth failure have increased resting energy

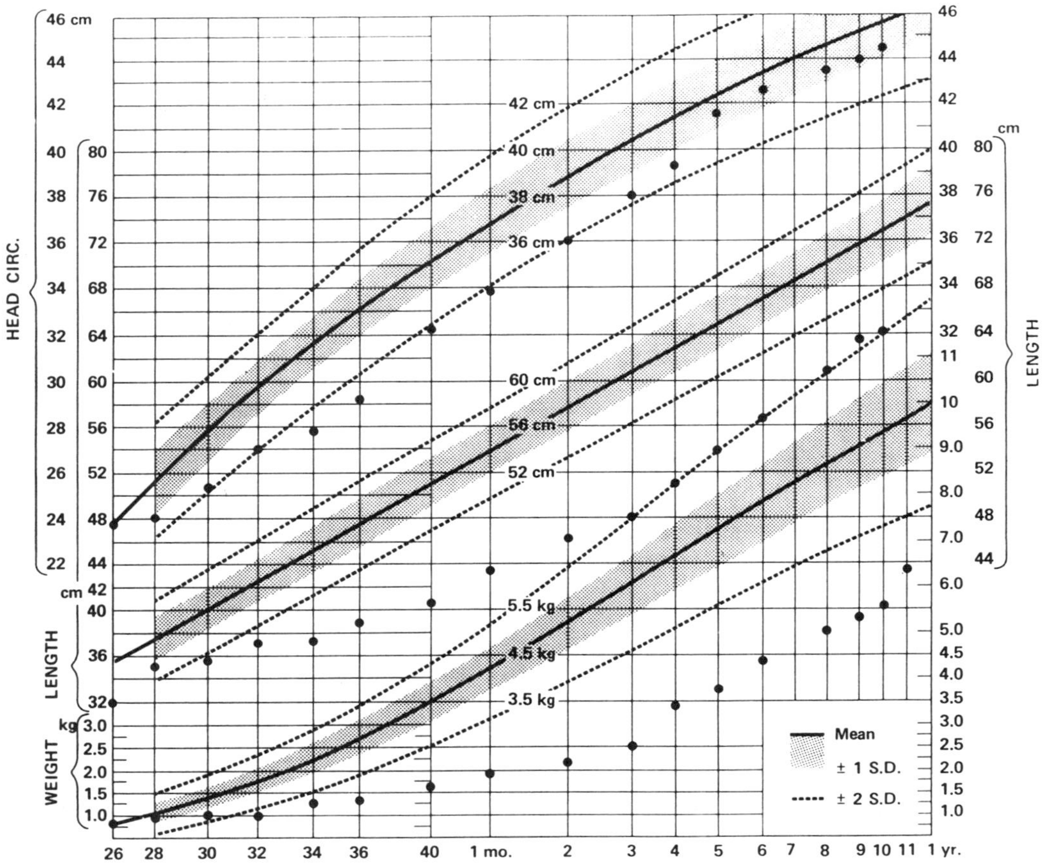

Figure 14-1. Growth chart of an infant with BPD. (From Cox JH[2] and J Pediatr 89:815, 1976. Used with permission.)

expenditure.[10, 17] Although increasing dietary fat may decrease carbon dioxide production, dietary fats may be less well absorbed, leading to lower energy intake and lower weight gain.[18, 19] Protein, mineral, and electrolyte needs may be increased if steroid or diuretic medications are used.[20, 21] (see appendix J).

Fluid tolerance may be limited due to cor pulmonale and left cardiac ventricular hypertrophy, or oral intake may be impaired by continued respiratory compromise or oral skill delay. Decreased fluid tolerance, combined with increased nutrient needs, requires careful planning to ensure adequate nutrition. High-calorie formulas, which may be needed during infancy, are given in table 14-2 with nutrient analyses. Pediatric enteral feeding products such as Pediasure and Kindercal may also be used orally to provide an energy-dense liquid feeding for toddlers.

Feeding

Table 14-3 lists feeding problems common in infants and young children with respiratory compromise, along with their causes and prevention or treatment strategies. Spoon-feedings may be tolerated more easily than liquids given by nipple. Smooth, pureed foods form a cohesive bolus that may be more quickly and easily swallowed, allowing better coordination of swallowing and breathing. Solid foods may be started as early as 3 to 4 months corrected age if needed to enhance development of oral skills. Foods such as cereal, fruit-flavored yogurt, pudding, white or sweet potato, ice cream, sherbet, and similar foods may be given to enhance intake of energy, protein, vitamins, and minerals. Waiting beyond 6 to 8 months corrected age to initiate spoon feedings may further delay oral skill development.[22] Although thickening liquids may be controversial from a nutritional standpoint, this technique may be required to enhance development of normal swallowing skills.[23]

Table 14-1. Nutrient Needs of Convalescent Infants and Toddlers with BPD

Nutrient	Amount	Comments
Fluid	95–150 ml/kg/day (chronic phase) 135–180 ml/kg/day or ↑ (convalescent phase)	Limited during periods of illness when pulmonary edema and reduced cardiac output may be present; more liberal during convalescence; may require diuretics; oral intake may be limited due to fatigue or high respiratory rate; tube feedings may be indicated if oral fluid intake is inadequate
Energy	130–160 kcal/kg/day (infants) 120–150 kcal/kg/day (toddlers)	Increased resting energy expenditure, increased work of breathing, incomplete absorption of fats, and catch-up growth may all contribute to increased needs
Protein	2.5–4.0 gr/kg/day (infants) RDA for ideal weight for length or height, age corrected for prematurity and/or height age (toddlers)	8–12% of total energy intake; higher end of range needed during catch-up growth or chronic corticosteroid use
Electrolytes	1.5–3.5 mEq Na/kg/day 3.5-6.0 mEq K/kg/day	Depending upon cardiac output and effect of diuretics; potassium excretion ↑ with corticosteroids, chlorothiazide and furosemide; sodium needs may be greater if sodium losses exceed fluid losses with diuretic use
Minerals	72–150 mg calcium/kg/day (infants) 1.0–1.5 mg zinc/kg/day (infants) RDA for age, corrected for prematurity and/or height age (toddlers)	Calcium, phosphorus, magnesium, and/or zinc excretion may be enhanced with corticosteroid, diuretic use
Vitamins	RDA for age, corrected for prematurity and/or height age (infants, toddlers)	Ensure normal vitamin D intake, as calcium anc phosphorus metabolism may be altered by corticosteroid or diuretic use, infants may have decreased exposure to sunlight

References: 25–29

Conservative management of GER usually includes small and frequent feedings, prone positioning with head elevated 45°. Thickened feedings may be recommended, but this is controversial. Liquids thickened with cereal may provide a disproportionately large intake of carbohydrate and iron. Alternatively, liquids can be given in close proximity to spoon-feedings of a balanced variety of solid foods in the older infant or toddler. More aggressive management, including medical or surgical options, may need to be explored if GER is associated with chronic upper airway infections, feeding aversion, esophageal irritation, or failure to thrive.[24] (See chapter 6 for additional information on GER and vomiting.)

If oral feedings cannot fulfill fluid or nutrient needs by maximizing nutrient density of feeding, supplemental tube-feedings may be needed. Depending upon the volume of oral feedings tolerated, tube-feedings may be given intermittently after each feeding to enhance satiety, or they may be given continuously during the night to meet daily nutritional needs but interfere minimally with oral feedings during the day. If tube-feeding is needed for a prolonged period (usually longer than two months), a gastrostomy tube may be needed. Prolonged use of nasogastric feeding tubes may cause irritation or erosion of the nares and may interfere with oral skill development.

Hunger and satiety cues may not be as clear when tube-feedings are used. The registered dietitian can help parents detect subtle feeding cues and provide guidance regarding the volume of feeding needed to support optimal growth and development. Increases in feeding volumes are required frequently during infancy (every week or two) and young childhood (every month or two) to meet changing needs during rapid growth. As feeding skills progress, the dietitian can provide guidance for selecting foods and tapering tube-feedings or modifying tube-feeding schedules to enhance hunger-induced motivation for eating while preventing nutritional compromise.

Table 14-2. High-Calorie Formula Recipes and Nutrient Analyses

High-Calorie Formula Recipes and Nutrient Analyses

Ohio Neonatal Nutritionists

Nutrient analysis (based on 100 ml)		Formulas			
		1	2	3	4
ENERGY	cal	99	99	99	103
VOLUME	ml	100	100	100	100
PROTEIN	g	2.38	2.46	2.45	2.68
FAT	g	4.87	5.34	5.42	5.63
CARBOHYDRATE	g	11.8	10.5	10.6	10.8
Calcium	mg	93	147	152	160
Phosphorus	mg	47	83	76	83
Magnesium	mg	3.9	9.2	10.4	11.4
Iron	mg	0.20	1.01	1.47	0.33
Zinc	mg	0.79	1.14	1.30	1.38
Manganese	mcg	10.3	8.7	10.2	13.1
Copper	mcg	127	175	212	222
Iodine	mcg	6.3	10.0	5.6	7.1
Sodium	mg	33.2	35.7	38.4	40.6
Potassium	mg	88.2	118.0	114.3	127.8
Chloride	mg	73.0	73.3	74.3	79.1
Vitamin A	IU	952	501	583	617
Vitamin D	IU	262	108	128	135
Vitamin E	IU	3.6	3.5	3.5	3.9
Vitamin K	mcg	10.3	10.1	10.6	11.6
Thiamine (B_1)	mcg	198	179	213	219
Riboflavin (B_2)	mcg	278	401	515	534
Vitamin B_6	mcg	198	161	208	215
Vitamin B_{12}	mcg	0.24	0.41	0.47	0.49
Niacin	mcg	3173	3161	4137	4307
Folic acid	mcg	27.8	26.6	31.5	33.3
Pantothenic acid	mcg	952	1224	1578	1636
Biotin	mcg	1.6	21.9	30.2	30.3
Vitamin C	mg	27.8	23.9	30.8	31.6
Choline	mg	6.0	12.6	9.5	11.5
Inositol	mg	3.7	5.1	7.5	5.5
Linoleic Acid	mg	793	962	726	565
Taurine	mg	4.7	6.6	6.2	5.4

Ohio Neonatal Nutritionists. Appendix N. High-calorie formula recipes and nutrient analysis. In: Groh-Wargo S, Thompson M, Cox JH, eds. Nutritional care for high-risk newborns. rev. ed. Chicago: Precept Press, 1994; 419–20. Used with permission.

Table 18.3. Feeding Problems Common to Infants with Prolonged Respiratory Problems

Problem	Probable cause	Prevention/intervention strategies
Increased oral defensiveness as evidenced by aversive behaviors	Prolonged and frequently noxious simulation of the oral and nasal areas, such as endotracheal intubation and suctioning, placement of nasogastric or orogastric tube for feedings	During acute phases of treatment:
		Prevent, as possible, the need to change and reposition tubes
		Provide, as tolerated, pleasurable facial and oral stimulation, such as firm facial stroking with bathing and after tube changes, and nonnutritive sucking during awake periods, especially with tube feedings
		During recovery phases of treatment:
		Provide extra-oral stimulation with slow, firm stroking of lips, chin and cheeks prior to oral feeding
		If prolonged tube feeding is anticipated (x months vs. x weeks), gastrostomy tube should be considered to provide feeding volumes and avoid frequent replacement of nasogastric tubes
	Shortness of breath (dyspnea) and increased rate of breathing (tachypnea)	Keep environmental stimulation to a *minimum* (for a fragile infant with respiratory problems, this is a must)
		Monitor infant for signs of readiness (e.g., quiet, alert state) and/or fatigue (glazed expression and floppy muscle tone)
		Increase oxygen flow during feeding. If infant is not on oxygen, suggest using oxygen during feeding
		Allow more quiet, minimal interaction, time-out periods as the infant becomes disorganized and fatigued
Frequent vomiting of feedings	Increased oral/nasal/bronchial secretions	Coordinate feeding with pulmonary treatments, i.e., feed infant after a brief rest period following respiratory treatment and suctioning to clear bronchial secretions
	Increased intake of air with feedings due to inefficient oral-motor coordination	Burp the infant frequently. Consider holding infant in a supported sitting position in care-giver's lap and gently rub infant's back in an upward direction toward infant's left shoulder
	Prolonged use of NG or OG tube resulting in persistent insufficiency of gastroesophageal sphincter	Position infant in reflux position (prone with head elevated 45°) after feeding
		Initiate a team discussion about the long-term medical, physical, and behavioral needs of the infant. Consideration of gastrostomy tube placement, while a medical decision, is often initiated by an experienced care-giver who feeds the infant frequently

(continued on next page)

Table 14-3. Feeding Problems Common to Infants with Prolonged Respiratory Problems (continued)

Problem	Probable cause	Prevention/intervention strategies
Rumination	Lack of attachment to primary caretaker	Establish a primary care team as early as possible, but by at least 3–4 mo corrected age. Include the family in all planning as they desire and as possible
	Inappropriate environment and/or lack of developmentally appropriate environment/activities	Provide age-appropriate developmental intervention through primary care team
		At typical feeding times, promote normal social and developmental behaviors, such as allowing infant to explore food with fingers, as the infant's condition allows
	Decreased communication with care-givers resulting in feelings of lack of control	Provide age-appropriate social and language behaviors and choices, using "signs" and/or augmentative communication as needed
		Feed "on demand"
Impaired ability to tolerate spoon feeding	Delayed exposure to spoon-feeding	Offer strained foods by spoon at 4–6 mo corrected age, as infant's condition allows. Hold infant or place in infant seat for support and provide appropriate social interaction with oral feedings. Allow infant to explore food with fingers and the spoon
	Poor appetite due to fatigue, prolonged illness, and/or psychosocial deprivation	Do not attempt feeding immediately after stressful care procedures (i.e., suctioning and bagging, blood draw); allow for physiological and psychosocial recovery. Do not overstimulate before, during or after feeding; maintain calm, quiet, social atmosphere
		Begin spoon/solid feedings slowly and maintain calm, quiet atmosphere, accepting and praising infant's success. Keep "mealtime" calm, positive, interactive, happy. *Do not force feed*
		Provide consistent exposure to others eating and drinking

Chamberlain JL. Assessment and treatment of feeding problems/dysfunction. In: Groh-Wargo S, Thompson M, Cox JH, eds. Nutritional care for high-risk newborns. rev. ed. Chicago: Precept Press, 1994; 224–25. Used with permission.

References

1. Northway WH. Bronchopulmonary dysplasia: Twenty-five years later. Pediatrics 89:969, 1992.
2. Cox JH. Bronchopulmonary dysplasia. In: Groh-Wargo S, Thompson M, Cox JH, eds. Nutritional care for high-risk newborns. rev. ed. Chicago: Precept Press, 1994; 245–61.
3. Bozinski MEA, Albert JM, Ushanalini V, et al. Bronchopulmonary dysplasia and postnatal growth in extremely premature black infants. Early Human Develop 21:83, 1990.
4. Davidson S, Schrayer A, Wielunsky E, et al. Energy intake, growth, and development in ventilated very-low-birth-weight infants with and without bronchopulmonary dysplasia. Am J Dis child 144:553, 1990.
5. Meisels SJ, Plunkett JW, Roloff DW, et al. Growth and development of preterm infants with respiratory distress syndrome and bronchopulmonary dysplasia. Pediatrics 77:345, 1986.
6. Yu VYH, Orgill AA, Lim SB, et al. Growth and development of very low birthweight infants recovering from bronchopulmonary dysplasia. Arch Dis Child 58:791, 1983.
7. Vohr BR, Bell EF, Oh W. Infants with bronchopulmonary dysplasia: Growth pattern and neurologic and developmental outcome. Am J Dis Child 136:443, 1982.
8. Robertson CMT, Etches PC, Goldson E et al. Eight-year school performance, neurodevelopmental, and growth outcome of neonates with bronchopulmonary dysplasia: A comparative study. Pediatrics 89:365, 1992.
9. Blayney M, Kerem E, Whyte H, et al. Bronchopulmonary dysplasia: Improvement in lung function between 7 and 10 years of age. J Pediatrics 118:201, 1991.
10. Kurzner SI, Garg M, Bautista DB, et al. Growth failure in infants with bronchopulmonary dysplasia: Nutrition and elevated resting metabolic expenditure. Pediatrics 81:379–84, 1988.
11. Vrlenich LA, Bozynski MEA, Shyr Y, et al. The effect of bronchopulmonary dysplasia on growth at school age. Pediatrics 95:855–59, 1995.
12. Manser JI. Growth in the high-risk infant. Clin Perinatol 11:19–40, 1984.
13. Altigani M, Murphy JF, Newcombe RG, et al. Catch-up growth in preterm infants. Acta Pædiatr Scand (suppl) 357:3, 1989.
14. Hyman PE. Gastroesophageal reflux: One reason why baby won't eat. J Pediatr 125:103, 1994.
15. Gluffre RM, Rubin S, Mitchell I. Anti-reflux surgery in bronchopulmonary dysplasia. Am J Dis Child 141:648, 1987.
16. St. Cyr JA, Ferrara TB, Thompson T et al. Treatment of pulmonary manifestations of gastroesophageal reflux in children two years of age or less. Am J Surg 157:400, 1989.
17. Yeh TF, McClean DA, Ajayi OA, et al. Metabolic rate and energy balance in infants with bronchopulmonary dysplasia. J Pediatr 114:448–51, 1989.
18. Pereira GR, Baumgart S, Bennett MJ, et al. Use of high-fat formula for premature infants with bronchopulmonary dysplasia: metabolic, pulmonary, and nutritional studies. J Pediatr 124:605–11, 1994.
19. Boehm G, Bierbach U, Moro G, et al. Limited fat digestion in infants with bronchopulmonary dysplasia. J Pediatr Gastroenterol Nutr 22:161–66, 1996.
20. Adams E. Nutrition for the young child with bronchopulmonary dysplasia. Nutr Focus 6(3):1–6, 1991.
21. Van Foudoever JB, Wattimena JDL, Carnielli VP, et al. Effect of dexamethasone on protein metabolism in infants with bronchopulmonary dysplasia. J Pediatr 124:112–18, 1994.
22. Coyner AB, Zelle RS. Habilitative approaches to facilitate more adaptive oral patterns related to eating and expressive language. In: Developmentally disabled infants and toddlers: Assessment and intervention. Philadelphia: Davis, 1983; 443.
23. Koops BL, Abman SH, Accurso FJ. Outpatient management and follow-up of bronchopulmonary dysplasia. Clin Perinatol 11:101, 1984.
24. Novak DA. Gastroesophageal reflux in the preterm infant. Clin Perinatol 23:305–20, 1996.
25. Lund CL. Collier SB. Nutrition and bronchopulmonary dysplasia. In: Lund CH, ed. Bronchopulmonary dysplasia strategies for total patient care. Petaluma, Calif.: Neonatal Network, 1990; 75.
26. Oh W. Nutritional management of infants with bronchopulmonary dysplasia. In: Bronchopulmonary dysplasia and related chronic respiratory disorders: Report of the 90th Conference on Pediatric Research. Columbus, Ohio: Ross Laboratories, 1986; 96.
27. Farrell PM, Taussig LM, et al. Bronchopulmonary dysplasia and related chronic respiratory disorders. Columbus, Ohio: Ross Laboratories, 1986.
28. National Research Council Food and Nutrition Board. Recommended dietary allowances. 10th ed. Washington D.C.: National Academy of Sciences, 1989.
29. Lucas A, Bishop NJ, King FJ, et al. Randomized trial of nutrition for preterm infants after discharge. Arch Dis Child 67:324–27, 1992.

Parent Education Materials

Klein MD, Delaney TA. Feeding and nutrition for the child with special needs: Handouts for parents. Medvescek, CR, ed. Tucson: Therapy Skill Builders, 1994; Nutrition and feeding for the child with bronchopulmonary dysplasia.

Aspen Reference Group, Caregiver education guide for children with developmental disabilities. Rockville, Md.: Aspen, 1994; (1) Enhancing oral-motor skills, (2) Nutrition for your gastrostomy-fed child, (3) Guidelines for the progression of food textures, (4) Oral treatment techniques, (5) Feeding treatment techniques.

Ohio Neonatal Nutritionists. Neonatal nutrition handouts: Feeding your baby with bronchopulmonary dysplasia. Nancy Nevin-Folino, Children's Medical Center, Dayton, Ohio 45404.

Nutrition Manual for At-Risk Infants and Toddlers
Janice Hovasi Cox, editor

15

PEDIATRIC HUMAN IMMUNODEFICIENCY VIRUS INFECTION

Lori Yelton, MS, RD, and Janice Hovasi Cox, MS, RD

The term *human immunodeficiency virus* or *HIV* infection encompasses all stages of the disease, from asymptomatic to severely symptomatic. The Center for Disease Control (CDC) has classified categories of HIV infection in pediatric patients based on (1) immune suppression and evidence of infection and (2) CD4 helper cell counts or percentages as these relate to diagnosis and prognosis.[1, 2] Infants with moderate to severe signs and symptoms of immune suppression and specific infections are reported to have acquired immunodeficiency syndrome (AIDS).[1, 3]

Reports of the lethal effect of HIV infection in infants and children first appeared in 1982.[4] During the decade and a half since, HIV has become a major child health care problem and has been the most rapidly growing cause of death among children in the United States.[5, 6] Vertical transmission of HIV from mother to child accounts for nearly 90% of pediatric cases in the United States, with an estimated transmission rate of 8–30% in mothers who become infected during pregnancy or lactation.[1, 7–10] Rates of transmission vary, depending upon when the mother's primary infection occurs and when the mother receives medical treatment. The incidence of perinatally acquired HIV infection has declined with improved screening and treatment of HIV-positive women during pregnancy.[11, 12] Intrauterine transmission accounts for 30–50% and intrapartum transmission accounts for 50–70% of cases vertically transmitted.[8, 10] Postnatal transmission of HIV through breast-feeding is greater if the mother acquires the virus and experiences primary infection postnatally.[13]

Definitive diagnosis of HIV in the young infant using antibody tests may be difficult, inasmuch as current tests do not distinguish between maternal and infant antibodies; infants may not completely lose maternal antibodies until 18 months of age.[1, 9] More recently, highly sensitive tests for viral presence have become available. These tests allow the vast majority of infants with HIV to be identified within the first few weeks after their primary infection.[1, 14] Infants born with HIV infection demonstrate a shorter period of clinical latency, averaging 3 years, compared to

The authors wish to thank Kelly York, RD, Department of Nutrition and Dietetics, Medical Center of the University of California, San Francisco, for her critical review of this chapter and her thoughtful suggestions.

7.8 to 11.0 years typically seen in adults.[15] Initial reports held that 50% of the children with AIDS were diagnosed during the first year of life, and 82% were diagnosed by 3 years of age.[9] The mortality from perinatal HIV disease was highest during the first year.[16] More recently, longitudinal studies demonstrate that only 20–30% of perinatally infected infants develop profound immune deficiency and AIDS-defining illness before 1 year of age. Most infants experience a slower progression of disease and survive at least five years.[1] Survival rates of infants and children with AIDS will continue to change as medical treatment improves, but survival rates will also continue to depend on the HIV phenotype, time of infection, time of diagnosis, access to medical care, compliance with medical regimens, as well as the AIDS-defining condition.[17, 18]

As in the adult population, the signs, symptoms, and complications of human immunodeficiency virus-1 infection in infants and children range from asymptomatic to critical illness. Presenting symptoms in infants born with HIV usually occur within four to six months. Although these may be varied or nonspecific, most have nutritional implications, such as failure to thrive, weight loss, feeding difficulties due to neurological changes, chronic or recurrent diarrhea, hypoalbuminemia and persistent oral thrush.[1, 6, 18, 19] Later manifestations may include recurrent bacterial, fungal, and viral infections; chronic interstitial pneumonitis and dyspnea; encephalopathy or developmental delay; and neurological abnormalities, cardiomyopathy, gastrointestinal infections, and malabsorption.[1, 3, 6, 9, 18, 19] These also have nutritional implications.

Although nutrition is affected by the presence of HIV at perhaps every stage of the infection, the converse is also true. Nutrition may affect the course of HIV infection. In fact, there are numerous similarities in immunologic dysfunction between children with chronic protein-energy malnutrition (PEM) and those with AIDS.[6, 20] It is evident that even mild PEM is associated with impaired cell-mediated immunity, with reduced numbers of circulating T lymphocytes, decreased numbers and functioning of CD4 helper cells, impaired secretory immunity, altered phagocytic function, and decreased killer cell activity.[6] Various nutrients, including energy, protein, iron, zinc, selenium, copper, and vitamins A, C, E, pyridoxine, and folate support optimum functioning of the immune system.[21] Various amino acids and nucleotides support cell proliferation and immune system function. Deficiencies of these nutrients may impair immune function, reducing resistance to infection. Chronic infections may preclude intake of adequate nutrition due to anorexia, fever, malaise, and/or diarrhea, further compromising nutritional status and decreasing immunocompetence. Thus, a self-perpetuating cycle is created, ultimately ending in death.

Nutrition may be further compromised by side effects of chronic treatment with antibiotic, antifungal, antiviral, antiparasitic, and immunomodulator medications. Anorexia, nausea, vomiting, diarrhea, fever, and gastrointestinal distress are common side effects. (See appendix J for specific drug/nutrient interactions).

Nutrition Assessment

Because nutrition is intricately involved with HIV, a thorough nutrition assessment should be regularly included in the evaluation of all HIV infants or children, both symptomatic and asymptomatic.[22] Infants born to HIV-positive mothers should be assessed and monitored regularly until HIV status is proven to be negative. Screening tools such as those given in appendixes A, B, and D may be helpful in identifying infants and children who need further assessment or treatment by a registered dietitian and experienced feeding therapist.

Growth Assessment

Although birth weight is not likely to be affected by intrauterine exposure to HIV, poor growth and wasting may occur at any stage of the disease. When infants born to HIV-positive mothers are compared, infants who become HIV positive exhibit lower weight gains, with a preferential decline in lean body mass when compared to infants who experience seroreversion.[23]

Growth status appears to decrease with disease progression. When weight and length status of infants and children (1) diagnosed with AIDS, (2) HIV infected, and (3) exposed to HIV but seronegative were compared in a recent study, 24%, 16.7%, and 9.5%, respectively were below 90% of expected weight-for-height. Linear growth fell below the 10th percentile for 64%, 33%, and 23%, respectively. Severe nutritional depletion characterized both by underweight and low height status was evident in 16%, 3%, and 1%, respectively.[24] Although growth status in this study was found to be normal in 36% of patients with AIDS and 64% of patients with HIV infection, other studies report that up to 90% of children who have moderate to severe suppression of immune function may exhibit growth delay.[6, 25] Because wasting generally precedes opportunistic infections, monitoring of growth and timely nutrition intervention are paramount to increased survival and quality of life.[23]

Poverty or limited economic resources, chronic use of recreational drugs, chronic illness, or depression in mothers with AIDS may make it difficult or impossible for them to care for their infant or child adequately. Diminished growth status may occur due to neglectful care regardless of whether the infant or child is infected with HIV.

Weight, length, and head circumference are monitored regularly and plotted on standard growth charts for sex, age, and gender (see appendix F). Mid-arm circumference and skin fold measurements are useful in identifying changes in muscle and adipose tissues.[26] Frequent measurements provide a more accurate picture of growth status. Changes in nutritional status can then be quickly identified, permitting intervention and prevention of further immunologic compromise caused by nutritional deficiencies.

Clinical Assessment

Anorexia, nausea/vomiting, difficulty swallowing, prolonged feeding times, and delayed progression of feeding skills may be identified using standard nutrition screening tools (see appendixes A, B, and D). When these problems are associated with a deceased intake of breast milk, formula, or food, a registered dietitian should be consulted to provide suggestions for optimizing nutritional intake.

Diarrhea may be a significant factor in compromised nutritional status. Stool frequency, odor, and appearance may help to identify the presence, type, and severity of malabsorption (see chapter 6, table 6-4).

Dietary Intake

Dietary intake may be assessed using a 24-hour recall. If the parent has difficulty providing this information, written records of food intake may be helpful in providing more specific dietary intake information. Evaluation of energy, protein, iron, zinc, and vitamins A, C, E, pyridoxine, and folate intake may helpful in establishing a nutrition therapy plan. Unproven therapies for AIDS may include large doses of vitamins or minerals or other substances that may produce toxic side effects or deficiencies of other nutrients.[18]

Laboratory Assessment

The most common hematological abnormality in children with HIV infection is anemia.[5, 27] Hemoglobin levels may range from 10.5 g/dl to 12 g/dl. Most often, anemia is due to iron deficiency. A recent study concluded that iron deficiency caused by intestinal malabsorption is a significant contributing factor to the presence of anemia.[27] Although oral administration of iron corrects anemia caused by iron deficiency without malabsorption, parenteral administration of iron may be needed to correct hemoglobin levels if anemia is associated with malabsorption.[27] Parenteral iron administration requires that appropriate precautions be taken to reduce risk of anaphylaxis. Red blood cell mean corpuscular volume (MCV) may be elevated during zidovudine (ZDV or AZT) therapy and may mask iron deficiency anemia.[5] Serum iron level measurement may be needed to accurately assess iron status.

Serum albumin allows evaluation of visceral protein stores but may be altered by hydration or infection. If PEM is suspected, serum prealbumin and retinol-binding proteins can be monitored regularly to assess short-term progress of nutrition rehabilitation.

Nutrition Treatment

Nutrition intervention depends upon the stage of disease and the presence of complicating diagnoses or conditions. It is designed to increase quality of health, limit episodes of illness, and reduce medical costs by:

- Providing adequate nutrition to maximize growth potential and support ideal weight for length or height status
- Providing adequate nutrition to prevent further compromise of immunological function and/or developmental progress
- Maintaining optimal nutrition status in spite of medications or other treatments that may alter nutrient needs

- Maintaining optimal nutrition status in spite of feeding problems or delayed development of feeding skills
- Providing support and guidance for the selection of foods and nutrient supplements to maximize oral nutrition or facilitate progression of feeding skills
- Providing parents with adequate information to meet their infant's/child's nutrition needs and limit or prevent nutrition problems.

Recommended treatments for the various nutrition problems associated with HIV and AIDS are listed in table 15-1.

Nutrient Needs

Individual energy and protein needs vary with the age and medical status of the infant or child. Metabolic needs may be increased with fever, stress, infection, and increased respiratory rate.[3] Appendix L provides several methods for estimating normal energy needs for infants and children. Energy needs may be increased by 25–50% above the Recommended Dietary Allowances (RDA) for infants and children with suboptimal growth or increased metabolic needs due to infection.[3,28] If weight status or lean body mass is lower than expected for age and length or height, most sources recommend using ideal weight for length or height to determine energy and protein needs.[28–30] If basal or resting energy expenditure is used to calculate total energy needs, normal activity factors for infants and children range from 1.7 to 2.0, and factors for illness or infection range from 1.2 to 1.8.[31,32] (See figure 15-1 for estimating energy and protein needs.)

Estimating Energy and Protein Needs

1. Smaha ME, Morris V, Gallagher L, et al.[25]

RDA* kcal and protein for age + 25%
or
ideal body weight for length or height × RDA kcal and protein for age

2. Bentler M, Stanish M[26]

Minimum: weight (kg) at 50th percentile for actual height × kcal/kg based on age
Maximum: weight (kg) for age at 50th percentile × kcal/kg based on age

3. Mawson AR, Warrier RP, Kuvibidila S, Suskind RM[6]

kcal and protein at least 1.5 and up to 3 times the RDA for age and weight
or
1000 kcal above requirements per day to gain 1 kg/wk
and at least 2.0 to 3.0 gm protein/kg/day
to reach positive nitrogen balance and prevent weight loss

4. Peterson K, Washington JS, Rathbun J[27†]

$$\text{Catch-up growth requirement (kcal/kg/day and protein gm/kg/day)} = \frac{\text{kcal and protein required for weight age (kcal/kg/day and protein/kg/day)} \times \text{ideal weight for age (kg)}}{\text{actual weight (kg)}}$$

(a) Plot height and weight on NCHS growth charts (appendix F)
(b) Weight age = age at which present weight plots at 50th percentile
(c) Kcal/kg/day and protein/kg/day = recommendations for weight age (appendix L)
(d) Ideal weight for age = 50th percentile weight for age

---

*Recommended Dietary Allowances.[31] See appendix L

†Adapted with permission from Peterson K, Washington JS, Rathbun J. Team management of failure to thrive. J Am Dietet Assoc 84:810. © 1984, American Dietetic Association.

Figure 15-1. Estimating energy and protein needs of infants and children with AIDS. Recommendations for estimating needs using any of these equations provides a starting point. Adjustments to intake are determined by frequent follow-up, measurement of growth progress, and assessment of changes in clinical condition.

Table 15-1. Probable Causes and Intervention Strategies for Nutrition-Related Problems Encountered in Infants and Children with HIV Infection/AIDS

Problem	Possible cause	Nutrition intervention
Anorexia or poor oral intake	Drug therapy, pain, depression, lack of adequate psychosocial stimulation or adequate food; impoverished environment; depressed or chronically ill parent (if mother also has AIDS)	Small, frequent meals and snacks High-calorie infant formula or nutritionally complete supplements High-calorie, nutrient-dense foods Multivitamin/mineral supplements Supplemental tube feedings if oral feedings inadequate Pleasant, relaxed atmosphere; reduce number of distractions during feeding times Favorite foods until child is feeling better Refer parent or caregiver to social worker for resources of nutrition (i.e., WIC, Infant Support Systems) Refer to mental health or social service agency to support family in providing adequate psychosocial environment and stimulation
Nausea/vomiting	Drug therapy; infections that affect gastrointestinal tract	Small, frequent meals and snacks; drink fluids between meals rather than with meals Bland, soft diet or liquid diet Avoid foods with strong odors Serve foods (especially high-protein foods such as meat) cold to eliminate problems with strong odors If vomiting persists, clear liquids with calories and electrolytes, advancing diet as soon as possible, usually within 6–24 hr If nausea/vomiting occurs more often at specific times of day (sometimes related to medication dosing), avoid offering meals or snacks at these times Avoid favorite foods during periods of nausea and vomiting to prevent development of taste aversions to these foods Avoid very sweet or fatty foods Dry, salty foods such as crackers or pretzels may diminish nausea Maintain upright position for 30 to 60 min after meals; (prone position with head of bed elevated at least 45° angle for naps)
Taste and smell changes	Drug therapy, nutrient deficiency or other factors related to the disease	Encourage fresh fruit or use favorite seasoning such as cinnamon, vanilla, or mint to offset unpleasant taste in mouth
Oral/esophageal disorders	Oral or esophageal lesions from thrush (candidiasis), herpes simplex, or hairy leukoplakia	For infants, avoid food with lumps, foods that require chewing, and stringy foods Avoid table foods that are more likely to become stuck: dry foods and foods that require chewing or are difficult for the young child to chew, including nuts, seeds, skins, hulls, bread, raw fruits and vegetables, and meats Swallowing may take longer—allow enough time between mouthfuls; frequent sips of liquid may help "wash down" more solid foods Avoid sticky carbohydrate foods, which may exacerbate fungal infections Stimulate saliva with sour foods/beverages (although citrus or pineapple may cause mouth pain) Use soft, nutrient-dense foods such as eggs, cream soups, ice cream, puddings, ground meats, baked fish, soft cheeses, canned or strained fruits, noodles or rice

Table 15-1. Probable Causes and Intervention Strategies for Nutrition-Related Problems in Infants and Children with HIV Infection/AIDS (continued)

Problem	Possible cause	Nutrition intervention
Oral/esophageal disorders (continued)	Oral or esophageal lesions from thrush (candidiasis), herpes simplex, or hairy leukoplakia	Liquid or pureed diet may be better tolerated. Use a straw for liquids when developmentally ready Dip or soak hard, dry, crisp or rough-textured foods in liquids before eating; some thicker strained foods may require thinning with a little liquid Use cool or room-temperature nutrition supplements to help ease pain; avoid extremes of temperature If swallowing dysfunction is present, may require assessment by experienced feeding therapist, thickened liquids; avoid slippery foods such as gelatin or noodles
Dyspnea	Pneumonia may cause shortness of breath or labored breathing, which may interfere with suck/swallow sequence or eating	Small, frequent meals and snacks Encourage high-calorie, nutrient-dense liquids If patient requires O_2 per cannula or mask, full liquids per straw or tube-feed if nutrient needs cannot be met orally
Lethargy/dementia	Often seen at end-stages of AIDS/HIV disease	Liquid oral supplements or tube feed as deemed necessary If end-stage, maintain comfort
Diarrhea	Drug therapy Contaminated foods, tube feeding or formula Large doses of vitamins, especially ascorbic acid Malabsorption; often seen from bacterial overgrowth, deconjungation of bile acids, and fat malabsorption Hypoalbuminemia Emotional stress Gastrointestinal infections HIV effect on bowel epithelium cells may lead to diarrhea Malabsorption (confirm with a fecal fat test or D-xylose test for carbohydrate malabsorption)	Confirm if drug therapy has side effect Avoid long-term food restrictions, which may cause poor intake Provide frequent, small meals with liquids between meals Replace fluids and electrolytes with oral rehydration solutions, soups, fruit juices, gelatin, and high-potassium foods such as fruits and vegetables; watch for signs of dehydration Serve liquids at room temperature Avoid lactose if there is history of lactose intolerance. Try lactose enzyme supplements; yogurt may be well tolerated even with lactose intolerance and may help reestablish normal gastrointestinal flora Avoid foods high in *insoluble* fiber (bran, seeds, husks) Encourage foods high in *soluble* fiber (oatmeal, cooked dried beans, rice, apples, potatoes, other fruits, vegetables, and grains) If necessary, use elemental infant or pediatric formulas listed in appendix C (given orally, or by tube, continuous drip if necessary). Consider parenteral nutrition if enteral intake is inadequate or poorly tolerated Correct serum albumin parenterally (0.5 – 1 g albumin/kg body weight given over 1–2 days *along with adequate energy and protein intake*) Multivitamin/mineral supplement if nutritional deficiency is suspected See table 15-2 for food safety considerations

References: Bentler M, Stanish M,[29] Raiten DJ,[18] Task Force on Nutrition Support in AIDS[41]

Table 15-2. Calorie and Protein Boosters for Young Children

Basic Principles
Offer small, frequent meals (6 to 8 times a day)
Make every bite or sip count
Limit foods and beverages that are low in calories
Offer a variety of foods—include a variety of colors, textures, and flavors
Carry food with you at all times to be enjoyed while waiting in line, at appointments, traveling

Beverages
Use whole or extra-rich milk instead of nonfat or low-fat milk
Make "super milk" by mixing 1 cup of powdered milk into a quart of whole milk—use as beverage and in preparing other foods
Add instant breakfast drink mix, malt mix, chocolate powder or syrup to milk
Try milkshakes, ice cream sodas, root beer floats, fruit smoothies, eggnog (*no* raw eggs)
Offer soda, juice, nectars, Koolaid, Gatorade, or milk instead of water
Avoid calorie-free beverages such as diet soda or flavored drinks sweetened with artificial sweeteners
Try high-calorie supplements such as Pediasure, Kindercal, Ensure Plus, Sustacal

Foods
Use milk instead of water to prepare cooked cereals, cream soups, hot chocolate
Add powdered milk to sauces, gravies, soups, casseroles, meat loaf, puddings, scrambled eggs, mashed potatoes, pancakes, muffin batters
Use half-and-half or cream on cereal, over fruit, in custards, egg dishes, milkshakes
Top shakes, desserts, fruits, and hot chocolate with whipped cream
Add butter or margarine to vegetables, potatoes, pasta, rice, toast, rolls, muffins, pancakes, hot cereals
Use mayonnaise on sandwiches, in salad dressings, dips, and meat, fish, or vegetable salads
Serve gravy or cream sauce with meats, vegetables, rice, noodles, biscuits, potatoes
Try sour cream on potatoes, in gravies, sauces, dips, or mixed with sugar over fruit
Add cheese to sandwiches, burgers, toast, eggs, potatoes, noodles, vegetables, soups, salads, chili; order extra cheese on pizza, tacos, burgers
Add chopped, hard-cooked eggs to salads, casseroles, sandwich fillings; add an extra egg to pancake batter
Use beaten raw egg to dip chicken, fish, etc. before breading or add to ground meat before cooking
Add *finely chopped or ground* nuts or peanut butter to ice cream, yogurt, puddings, breads, muffins, cookies, pies, cakes, salads
Include refried beans in Mexican meals
Use sugar, syrup, jelly, or jam on toast, sandwiches, crackers; add to hot and cold cereals and yogurt
Use fruits canned in heavy syrup
Add extra butter or margarine and fresh-grated cheese to macaroni and cheese, scalloped potatoes, and other packaged mixes
Consider frying foods instead of baking or broiling
Take advantage of high-calorie fast foods

Used with permission. Department of Nutrition and Dietetics. Hints for adding calories to the diet. San Francisco: Medical Center at University of California, San Francisco, 1996.[37] (Capitalized diet items are manufacturers' registered trademarks.)

Because many nutritional deficiencies of various vitamins and minerals have been reported,[6] most sources recommend vitamin and mineral supplementation in amounts one to two times the RDA for age.[6, 28] Unproven nutritional therapies for AIDS have been proposed, including megadoses of selenium and zinc and vitamins A, C, E, B_{12}, and beta carotene. Toxicity symptoms of fatigue, anorexia, nausea/vomiting, and diarrhea may occur with megadoses of zinc or vitamins A, C, or E. Zinc supplementation is controversial, as excess zinc may impair immunity. Also, copper deficiency may occur with large doses of zinc. No toxicity symptoms have been reported with large doses of vitamin B_{12}, beta carotene, or selenium.[33]

Dietary Recommendations

Breast-feeding. Because HIV status is often not certain in the newborn and because HIV can be transmitted through breast milk, it is not recommended that mothers with HIV infection breast-feed their infants.[34] Standard infant formula is recommended throughout the first year. Other foods may be started at the usual time unless developmental skills are delayed due to chronic illness or neurological compromise.

Table 15-3. Food Safety Considerations for Children with HIV Infection

Avoid raw protein foods, such as uncooked eggs, rare meat, and sushi. Do not allow these foods to come in contact with other foods; hands, cutting boards, counters, knives, or other utensils should be thoroughly washed after contact with uncooked foods
Thoroughly cook poultry and meat (internal temperature 165°F)
Thoroughly cook eggs; do not use cracked eggs
Avoid soft cheese, hot dogs, or cold cuts from delicatessen counters to reduce risk of listeriosis infection
Thaw frozen meats in the refrigerator or microwave oven, not at room temperature
Wash fruits and vegetables thoroughly
Use only pasteurized milk
Keep hot foods hot (cooked to 165 to 212°F and held at 140 to 165°F)
Keep cold foods cold (refrigerator should be 35 to 40°F; freezer should be 0°F)
Do not allow foods to stand at temperatures between 45°F and 140°F for more than 2 hr
Refrigerate perishable foods immediately upon return from the store. Store foods that have been opened in airtight containers or a moisture/vaporproof wrap. Don't crowd or overpack foods in the refrigerator
Avoid moldy or spoiled foods
Do not use foods after the recommended expiration date on the label
Always wash hands before handling food. Young children may need adult supervision during handwashing
Avoid drinking lake, river, or stream water. Even accidental swallowing while swimming carries risk of cryptosporidiosis and giardiasis

Note: HIV is not spread by food or water. Disposable utensils, dishes, and trays are *not* needed for meals served in the institutional setting. Use of regular dishes improves temperature control of foods and makes meals more attractive. Routine sanitation standards for food preparation, storage, serving, dishwashing, and cleaning should be maintained.

References: Raiten DJ[18] and Centers for Disease Control and Prevention[40]

Formula and food. Nutrient-dense foods are recommended, with additional calories or protein when suboptimal intake or growth, chronic infection, or nutrition deterioration occurs. (Infant formulas and nutritional supplements are listed in appendix C.) Calorie-dense formulas such as those used for infants or young children with bronchopulmonary dysplasia or congenital heart disease may also be used (see tables 12-4 and 14-2). Lists of high-calorie and high-protein foods are given in table 15-2 and are available for parent education from several sources.[35,36]

Lactose intolerance. If lactose intolerance is present, milk-based infant formula, milk, and other dairy foods may need to be temporarily eliminated or restricted in the diet. Because these foods are generally excellent sources of protein, minerals, and many vitamins, it is best to not eliminate them unless absolutely necessary. Lactase, an enzyme that breaks down lactose into its component monosaccharides, may be added to milk or other dairy products to decrease lactose content. Not all lactose-free "imitation" milk products contain the nutrients normally found in infant formula or milk, including adequate amounts of protein, minerals, and B-complex vitamins. Pellagra, beriberi, iron deficiency anemia, and zinc and essential fatty acid deficiency have been identified in an infant fed an "imitation" milk product that provides less the 2% of the RDA for B-complex vitamins, zinc, iron, and essential fatty acids.[38] If milk and dairy products must be eliminated or severely restricted, a registered dietitian can provide suggestions for maintaining optimal nutrition. (Lactose-free formulas and supplements that provide complete nutrition are listed in appendix C.)

Protein. If protein intolerance or malabsorption is present, infant and pediatric formulas are available that contain hydrolyzed protein, as listed in appendix C. Because hydrolyzed protein formulas may also contain glucose polymers in place of sweeter tasting carbohydrates, they may not be well accepted. Flavors may be added using unsweetened powdered drink mixes or flavor packets provided by various companies that make feeding supplements. Hydrolyzed protein formulas may be accepted if they are mixed in gradually increasing proportions with a more accepted formula.

Fat. If fat malabsorption is present, infant or pediatric formulas are available that contain medium-chain triglycerides. Low-fat diets are not routinely recommended because fat is an excellent source of energy. Although malabsorbed fat may contribute to loose, frothy, or foul-smelling stools, reducing fat intake further reduces net fat and energy absorption and may cause essential fatty acid deficiency and further decline in growth.[39]

Food safety. Achlorhydria and compromised immune function make food-borne illness a particular concern in infants and children with AIDS. (Recommendations for food safety are given in table 15-3[18, 40]). Hands should be thoroughly washed with antimicrobial soap after toileting, handling of soil or raw foods (especially poultry, meat, or eggs), and before handling or eating food. Young children may need adult supervision during handwashing.

Enteral/parenteral nutrition. When disease advancement occurs and oral intake cannot meet estimated needs in spite of supplements and/or concentrated feedings, a more aggressive route of nutrition may be necessary. When well absorbed, nasogastric tube feedings often improve growth in HIV-infected children.[41, 42] If oral, pharyngeal, or esophageal lesions are present, or if the estimated need for tube-feeding exceeds one to two months, gastrostomy tube placement may be indicated.[42, 43] Standard infant and pediatric formulas may be used, as listed in appendix C. If diarrhea is present, using a formula with fiber or adding small amounts of rice cereal or banana may help to thicken or reduce the number of stools. Semielemental formulas may be given to enhance absorption.

When tube-feedings are needed to provide adequate nutrition, oral feeding should be encouraged as much as possible to maintain feeding skills.[44] Tube-feedings are often given during the night, with oral feedings offered during the day. When most or all of the child's nutrient needs are met at night, daytime meals and snacks can be more pleasurable because there is less pressure to consume large amounts of food or certain kinds of foods that are nutrient dense.

Although enteral feedings are preferred because they help maintain bowel integrity and immune status, infants and children unable to tolerate oral or enteral feedings may require parenteral nutrition to support significant increases in body weight and improve quality of life.[45] Special care is needed to avoid sepsis or other catheter-related complications, just as with other immunocompromised individuals.[44] Parenteral nutrition can be administered in the home setting with adequate parent training and supervision.

Parents must be active partners in making decisions about all aspects of their infant's or child's health care. They may understandably refuse what may be perceived as "invasive" nutritional therapies, such as surgical placement of tubes or catheters, especially if the infant or child is nearing the end stages of disease. Information must be presented to parents in a way that meets the individual medical, physical, and psychosocial needs of the child and the family. Learning styles, abilities, and functional levels of literacy and understanding must be accommodated to allow parents to make informed decisions.

References

1. Chadwick EG, Yogev R. Pediatric AIDS. Pediatr Clin North Am 42:969–92, 1995.
2. Centers for Disease Control and Prevention. 1994 Revised classification system for human immunodeficiency virus infection in children less than 13 years of age. MMWR 43:No. RR-12, 1994.
3. Gallagher LM, Evans S, Smaha ME. Pediatric acquired immunodeficiency syndrome. In: Queen PM, Lang CE, eds. Handbook of pediatric nutrition. Gaithersburg Md.: Aspen, 1993; 384–99.
4. Oleske J, Minnelor A, Cooper R, et al. Immune deficiency syndrome in children. JAMA 249:2345–49, 1993.
5. Burroughs MH, Edelson PJ. Medical care of the HIV-infected child. Pediatr Clin North Am 38:45–67, 1991.
6. Mawson AR, Warrier RP, Kuvibidila S, et al. Pediatric AIDS and nutrition. In: Suskind RM, Suskind-Lewinter L, eds. Textbook of pediatric nutrition, 2d ed. New York: Raven Press, 1993; 447–55.
7. Gabiano C, Tovo PA, deMartino M, et al. Mother-to-child transmission of human immunodeficiency virus type 1: Risk of infection and correlates of transmission. Pediatrics 90:369–74, 1992.
8. Krivine A, Firtion G, Cao L, et al. HIV replication during the first weeks of life. Lancet 339:1187–89, 1992.
9. Falloon J, Eddy J, Weiner J, Pizzo PA. Medical progress: Human immunodeficiency virus infection in children. J Pediatr 114:1–30, 1989.
10. Connor EM, Sperling RS, Gelber R, et al. Reduction of maternal-infant transmission of human immunodeficiency virus type 1 with zidovudine treatment. N Engl J Med 331:1173–80, 1994.
11. Mauskopf J, Paul J, White A, et al. The economic impact of treatment of HIV-positive women and their newborns with zidovudine: Implications for HIV screening. XI International Conference on AIDS. Vancouver, B.C., Canada, 1996. abstract 6047.

12. Lindegren ML, Byers B, Fleming P, et al. A decline in the incidence of perinatally acquired (PA) AIDS in the United States. XI International Conference on AIDS. Vancouver, B.C., Canada, 1996. abstract 2593.
13. Dunn DT, Newel ML, Ades AE, et al. Risk of human immunodeficiency virus type 1 transmission through breastfeeding. Lancet 340:585–88, 1992.
14. Owens DK, Holodniy M, McDonald TW, et al. A meta-analytic evaluation of the polymerase chain reaction for the diagnosis of HIV infection in infants. JAMA 275:1342–48, 1996.
15. Berkleman RL, Heywoard WL, Stehr-Grees JK, Curran JW. Epidemiology of human immunodeficiency virus infection and acquired immunodeficiency syndrome. Am J Med 86:761–70, 1989.
16. Scott G, Hutto C, Makuch R, et al. Survival in children with perinatally acquired human immunodeficiency virus type I infection. N Engl J Med 321:179–91,1989.
17. Munoz-Fernandez MA, Navarro J, Obregon E, et al. Longitudinal study of infants with vertically acquired HIV-1 infection: Immunological and virological markers of disease progression. XI International Conference on AIDS. Vancouver, B.C., Canada, 1996. abstract 3438.
18. Raiten DJ. Nutrition and HIV infection: A review and evaluation of the extant knowledge of the relationship between nutrition and HIV infection. Nutr Clin Prac 6:1-S, 1991.
19. Dworkin B, Wormser GP, Rosenthal WS, et al. Gastrointestinal manifestations of acquired immunodeficiency syndrome, a review of 22 cases. Am J Gastroenterol. 80:774–78, 1985.
20. Ortiz R Bentancourt M. Cell proliferation in bone marrow cells of severely malnourished animals. J Nutr 114:472–76, 1984.
21. Cunningham-Rundles S. Effects of nutritional status on immunological function. Am J Clin Nutr 35:1202–10, 1983.
22. Position of the American Dietetic Association and the Canadian Dietetic Association: Nutrition intervention in the care of persons with human immunodeficiency virus infection. J Am Diet Assoc 94:1042–45, 1994.
23. Miller TL, Evans SJ, Orav EJ, et al. Growth and body composition in children infected with the human immunodeficiency virus-1. Am J Clin Nutr 57:588–92, 1993.
24. Gaston J, Nesheim S, Sawyer M. Prevalence of malnutrition in children infected with HIV. XI International Conference on AIDS. Vancouver, B.C., Canada, 1996. abstract 4249.
25. Sato HK, Grumach AS, Jacob CMA, et al. Pediatric AIDS in a Brazilian population: 10 years of follow-up. XI International Conference on AIDS. Vancouver, B.C., Canada, 1996. abstract 2320.
26. Frisancho AR. Anthropometric standards for the assessment of growth and nutritional status. Ann Arbor: University Press, 1990.
27. Castaldo A, Tarallo L, Palomba E, et al. Iron deficiency and intestinal malabsorption in HIV disease. J Pediatr Gastroenterol Nutr 22: 359–63, 1996.
28. Smaha ME, Morris V, Gallagher L, et al. Section XVII. AIDS and HIV+. In: Wooldridge NH, Spinozzi N, Isaacs JS, et al., eds. Quality assurance criteria for pediatric nutrition conditions: A model. Chicago: American Dietetic Association, 1993.
29. Bentler M, Stanish M. Nutrition support of the pediatric patient with AIDS. J Am Diet Assoc 87:488–91, 1987.
30. Peterson K. Failure to thrive. In: Queen PM, Lang CE, eds. Handbook of pediatric nutrition. Gaithersburg, Md.: Aspen, 1993; 376.
31. National Research Council, Food and Nutrition Board. Recommended dietary allowances, 10th ed. Washington DC:National Academy of Sciences, 1989.
32. Thorn K. The Harris-Benedict equation: a simple plan for nutrition intervention in HIV/AIDS. J Care Mgt 1:10–18, 1995.
33. Dwyer JT, Bye RL, Holt PL, et al. Unproven nutrition therapies for AIDS: What is the evidence? Nutr Today 23:25–3, 1988.
34. Black RF. Transmission of HIV-1 in the breastfeeding process. J Am Diet Assoc 96;267–74, 1996.
35. Aspen Reference Group. Caregiver education guide for children with developmental disabilities. Rockville, Md.: Aspen, 1996.
36. Klein MD, Delaney TA. Feeding and nutrition for the child with special needs: Handouts for parents. Medvescek CR, ed. Tucson: Therapy Skill Builders, 1994.
37. Medical Center at University of California San Francisco Department of Nutrition and Dietetics. Hints for adding calories to the diet. San Francisco, 1996.
38. Personal experience. Case presentation, pediatric grand rounds, Children's Hospital at Bronson, Kalamazoo, Mich. Feb. 1995.
39. Pettei MJ, Daftary S, Levine JJ. Essential fatty acid deficiency associated with the use of a medium-chain-triglyceride formula in pediatric hepatobiliary disease. Am J Clin Nutr 53:1217, 1991.
40. Centers for Disease Control and Prevention. USPHS/UDSA Guidelines for the prevention of opportunistic infections in persons infected with human immunodeficiency virus: A summary. MMWR 44(no. RR-8):31, 1995.
41. Task Force on Nutrition Support in AIDS. Guidelines for nutrition support in AIDS. Nutrition 5:39–46, 1989.
42. Henderson RA, Saavendra JM, Perman JA, et al. Effect of tube feeding on growth of children with symptomatic human immunodeficiency virus infection. J Pediatr Gastroenterol Nutr 18:429–34, 1994.
43. Miller TL, Awnetwant EL, Evans S, et at. Gastrostomy tube supplements for HIV-infected children. Pediatrics 96:696–702, 1995.

44. Giacomet V, Ruga E, Rampon O, et al. Central venous catheter in HIV infected children receiving total parenteral nutrition for severe failure to thrive. XI International Conference on AIDS. Vancouver, B.C., Canada, 1996. abstract 4242.
45. Nicholas SW, Leung J, Fennoy I. Guidelines for nutritional support of HIV-infected children. J Pediatr 119:S59–S62, 1991.

Suggested Reading

Task Force on Nutrition Support in AIDS. Guidelines for nutrition support in AIDS. Nutrition 5(1); Jan/Feb 1989; 39–46.

Suskind RM, Suskind-Lewinter L. Pediatric AIDS and nutrition. In: Textbook of pediatric nutrition. 2d. ed. New York: Raven Press, 1993.

Gallagher LM, Evans S, Smaha ME. Pediatric acquired immunodeficiency syndrome. In: Queen PM, Lang CE, eds. Handbook of pediatric nutrition. Gaithersburg, Md.: Aspen, 1993; 384–99.

Position of the American Dietetic Association and the Canadian Dietetic Association: Nutrition intervention in the care of persons with immunodeficiency virus infection. J Am Diet Assoc 94(9):1042–45, 1994.

Gordan AN. CE AHP 8658. Nutritional aspects of the AIDS patient. Syllabus used with a videotape for hospital satellite network. Hospital Satellite Network, 1988.

Parent Education Materials

Klein MD, Delaney TA. Feeding and nutrition for the child with special needs. Handout for parents: Nutrition and feeding for the child with HIV. Medvescek CR, ed. Tucson: Therapy Skill Builders, 1994.

Aspen Reference Group. Caregiver education guide for children with developmental disabilities: Nutrition for children with HIV. Rockville, Md.: Aspen, 1996.

Centers for Disease Control and Prevention (CDC) National AIDS Clearinghouse, P.O. Box 6003, Rockville, Md. 20849-6003; 1-800-458-5231. (1) Because you love them: a parents' planning guide. Child Welfare League of America, Nov. 1994 (D251); (2) Eating defensively: Foods safety advice for persons with AIDS. FDA. (D533) (also available in videotape V466).

Appendix A

Early Intervention Nutrition Screening Form

and

Referral Criteria

Massachusetts Department of Public Health

EARLY INTERVENTION NUTRITION SCREENING FORM

To be completed by screener. Refer to protocols for instructions on completing each question. To determine if further assessment is needed, see Nutrition Referral Criteria.

DEMOGRAPHICS

1. Screening Date: 1. ☐☐/☐☐/☐☐
2. Child's ID No.: 2. ☐☐☐☐☐☐☐☐
3. Child's Sex: **(M)** Male **(F)** Female 3. ☐
4. Date of Birth: 4. ☐☐/☐☐/☐☐
5. Birth Weight: 5. ☐☐.☐ kgs or ☐☐ lbs. ☐☐ oz.
6. Birth Length: 6. ☐☐.☐ cm. or ☐☐ in ☐/ 8th

reported by caregiver ☐ or found in medical record ☐

7. Gestational age: 7. ☐☐

ANTHROPOMETRICS

8. Date of measurements: 8. ☐☐/☐☐/☐☐
9. Weight: 9. ☐☐.☐ kg. or ☐☐ lb. ☐☐ oz.
10. Length/height: 10. ☐☐.☐ cm. or ☐☐ in ☐/ 8th
11. How was the child measured? 1=standing, 2=lying down 11. ☐

PERCENTILES

12. Weight/AGE 12. ☐☐ to ☐☐ centile
13. Height/AGE 13. ☐☐ to ☐☐ centile
14. Weight/Height 14. ☐☐ to ☐☐ centile

LAB WORK

15. Date of Hemoglobin or Hematocrit: 15. ☐☐/☐☐/☐☐
16. HEMOGLOBIN ☐☐.☐ gms/100ml or 17. HEMATOCRIT ☐☐.☐ percent
18. Date of FEP or Lead (PB): 18. ☐☐/☐☐/☐☐
19. FEP ☐☐.☐ ug/dl or 20. LEAD(PB) ☐☐.☐ ug/dl
21. Does this child have any of the following diagnoses or chronic medical conditions? Yes ☐ No ☐

(**Check all that apply**)

___ Down Syndrome	___Failure to Thrive	___Cardiac
___ Cerebral Palsy	___Fetal Alcohol Syndrome	___Kidney
___ Spina Bifida	___Cystic Fibrosis	___Seizure Disorders
___ Anemia	___Neuromuscular	___Poor Growth
___ Respiratory	___Liver	___Gastrointestinal

Other(specify)____

Ask parent/caregiver the following questions. All questions can be answered with a 'Yes" or 'No' response. Check the appropriate box next to each question. A **YES** response indicates a possible nutritional risk, a **NO** response indicates no nutritional risk in that particular area.

		YES	NO
22. Does your child have any food allergies?	22.	☐	☐
23. Does your child take any medications on a regular basis? (excluding vitamins, iron, flouride or other minerals) (a) If yes, which one(s)?__________	23.	☐	☐
24. Does your child experience any of the following? (**Circle all that apply**): 1. diarrhea 2. constipation 3. vomiting/reflux	24.	☐	☐
25. Does your child use a feeding tube or other special feeding equipment?	25.	☐	☐
26. Do any of the following apply to your child at his/her present age? (**Circle all that apply**) 1. 7 mo. of age or older and has not started using cup yet 2. 9 mo. of age or older and does not finger feed yet 3. 12 mo. of age or older and drinks liquids primarily from the bottle 4. 19 mo. of age or older and does not use a spoon yet	26.	☐	☐
27. Does your child experience any of the following? (**Circle all that apply**) 1. difficulty with sucking 2. difficulty with swallowing 3. difficulty with chewing 4. gagging	27.	☐	☐
28. If your child uses the bottle, does he/she take the bottle to bed?	28.	☐	☐
29. Do you add solid foods to the bottle?	29.	☐	☐
30. If your child is under 12 months, and drinks formula, is he/she drinking less than 24 ounces per day?	30.	☐	☐
31. If your child is over 12 months old, does he/she reject any of the following foods: (**Circle all that apply**) 1. milk 2. meats 3. vegetables 4. fruits	31.	☐	☐
32. Does your child do anything that upsets you at mealtimes such as refusing to eat, excessive throwing of food or utensils, or other? (explain)__________	32.	☐	☐
33. Do you ever find that you are almost out of food at the end of the month?	33.	☐	☐
34. Do you have any questions or concerns about your child's nutrition and feeding? If yes, specify__________	34.	☐	☐
35. If you are currently breastfeeding, do you have any questions or concerns? If yes, specify__________	35.	☐	☐

Bayerl CT and Ries JD. Early start: Nutrition services in early intervention in Massachusetts. Zero to three 12:29-31, 1992. Used with permission. Developed for Early Intervention Nutrition Services, Bureau of Parent, Child, and Adolescent Health, Massachusetts Department of Public Health, Office of Nutrition, 150 Tremont Street, Boston MA 02111 (617) 624-5070.

Early Intervention Nutrition Referral Criteria

Check the "Yes" column next to any nutritional risk that applies to the infant or child.

If **ONE or more of the following** apply, refer infant or child to a nutritionist/or registered dietitian for further assessment. If you need assistance locating a qualified nutritionist, contact the Office of Nutrition at the Massachusetts Department of Public Health. (617) 624-5070

YES

______ Weight for age is **below the 10th percentile**
______ Length/height for age is **below the 10th percentile**
______ Weight for length/height is **below the 10th percentile**
______ Weight for length/height is **above the 95th percentile**

______ Hemoglobin: 11 gms/dl or LESS
______ Hematocrit: 34% or LESS
______ FEP: 35 μg/dl or GREATER
______ Lead (Pb): 10 μg/dl or GREATER

Infant or child has any of the following diagnoses or chronic medical conditions:

Down Syndrome	Cardiac	Failure to Thrive
Cerebral Palsy	Seizure Disorder	Cystic Fibrosis
Fetal Alcohol Syndrome	Gastrointenstinal	Anemia
Spina Bifida	Respiratory	Liver
Neuromuscular	Poor Growth	Kidney

If **TWO or more of the following apply**, refer infant or child to a nutritionist/R.D. for further assessment.

YES

______ History of food allergies.

_____ Medications taken on a regular basis.

______ Chronic problems with diarrhea, constipation, and/or vomiting/reflux.

______ Any of the following feeding skill delays:

1. 7 months of age or older and has not started using cup yet
2. 9 months of age or older and does not finger feed yet
3. 12 months of age or older and drinks liquids primarily from the bottle
4. 19 months of age or older and does not use a spoon yet

______ Difficulty with sucking, swallowing, chewing, or gagging.

______ Bottle to bed (night or nap time).

______ Formula intake is less than 24 ounces in 24 hours (for infants 0-12 months of age).

______ Meals regularly lack one or more of the basic foods (meat, milk, fruits, or vegetables).

______ Mealtime behavior frustrating to parent.

______ Lack of food in household to meet child's or family's needs.

______ Nutrition or eating habits of child are a concern to parent.

______ Breastfeeding questions or concerns of mother.

Bayerl CT and Ries JD. Early start: Nutrition services in early intervention in Massachusetts. Zero to three 12:29-31, 1992. Used with permission. Developed for Early Intervention Nutrition Services, Bureau of Parent, Child, and Adolescent Health, Massachusetts Department of Public Health, Office of Nutrition, 150 Tremont Street, Boston MA 02111 (617) 624-5070.

Appendix B

Nutrition Screening Form
and
Referral Criteria

Janice Hovasi Cox, MS, RD

NUTRITION SCREENING FORM

Infant/Child's Name ______________________________ DOB __________ Chart # __________

Weight _____ ; _____ %ile Length/Height _____ ; _____ %ile

Head Circumference _____ ; _____ %ile Weight for Length/Height _____ %ile

1. Does your baby/child have any chronic illness or medical condition? Yes No If yes, please list ____________________
____

2. Does your baby or child drink: (Indicate by checkmark all that apply and estimate amount per 24 hours.)

[ ] Breastmilk	____________	[ ] Whole Cow's Milk	____________
[ ] Similac, Enfamil, Gerber, Good Start	____________	[ ] Low Fat Milk (2%)	____________
[ ] Isomil, Prosobee, Gerber Soy	____________	[ ] Skim Milk (1/2%, 1%)	____________
[ ] Alimentum, Nutramigen, Pregestimil	____________	[ ] Goat's Milk	____________
[ ] Pediasure, Kindercal	____________	[ ] Other ____________	

NOTE: If the amount listed above is <24 oz for an infant, <16 oz for a toddler, or > 32 oz for either to check volume you may ask: How many cans of formula do you use/<u>week</u>? Powdered ___ (1 can makes 96 oz); Liquid Concentrate ___ (1 can makes 26 oz)

Is your baby/child enrolled on the WIC Program? YES NO Do you ever buy formula? YES NO If so, how much? _____

3. If your baby/child is on formula, how is it prepared? Are other supplements added?

[ ] Follow directions on can	[ ] Cereal	[ ] Sodium
[ ] Add more water than directions call for	[ ] Moducal/Polycose	[ ] Potassium
[ ] Add less water than directions call for	[ ] Microlipid/Oil	[ ] Other ____________

4. If your baby/child is on formula, is the formula iron fortified? YES NO If no, why not? ____________________
____

5. Does your baby/child take vitamin or mineral supplements? Vitamins-ADC Multivitamin Iron Fluoride Other ________

6. Does your baby/child take a bottle to bed? YES NO If yes, what is in the bottle? ____________________

7. How does your baby/child eat? (Circle all that apply.)

   Breast Bottle Cup Spoon Fingers Fork Infant Feeder Feeding Tube

8. Does your baby/child regularly eat: (Circle all that apply.)

   Strained/pureed/baby foods: cereal juice fruit vegetable meat dinners egg yolk

   Table foods: cereal bread pasta
   juice fruit vegetable
   meat poultry fish beans peanut butter cheese

NUTRITION SCREENING FORM (continued)

9. How often does your baby/child eat? every _____ hours; _____ times a day; _____ meals; _____ snacks

10. How do you know your baby/child is hungry? (Circle all that apply.)

Awakens Sucks on hands or fingers Fussy Cries Screams Says word/words that mean food Points

11. How do you know your baby/child is full? (Circle all that apply.)

Stops eating Falls asleep Spits out food or nipple Turns away from food or feeder Plays with food or is easily distracted

12. What describes your baby's/child's usual feeding behavior?

[ ] Seems to enjoy eating, takes feedings easily, good appetite

[ ] Happy at beginning of feeding, then often gets fussy or distressed during feedings

[ ] Frequently has trouble breathing while eating

[ ] Often does not wake for feeding, tires easily with feedings, or often has difficulty finishing feedings

[ ] Eats slowly, usually takes more than 30 minutes (infant)/45 minutes (toddler) to eat (excluding time for diaper changes, play, etc.)

[ ] Usually has difficulty sucking, swallowing, or chewing

[ ] Frequently gags, coughs, or chokes during feedings

[ ] Refuses to eat, is difficult to feed, fussy throughout most of feeding, arches backward, or doesn't seem to enjoy eating

[ ] Picky eater, seems to eat very little, not interested in food or eating, or has poor appetite

13. Does your baby/child spit up or vomit?

Amount: _______________ Frequency: occasionally every day during or after every feeding

14. Usual stool frequency: _______________ Description: yellow/green white/grey brown seedy soft/mushy liquid hard

Usual urine frequency: _______________

15. Does your baby/child take any medicines (other than vitamin or mineral supplements)? Yes No

If yes, please list ____

16. Do you have any questions or concerns about your baby's/child's nutrition? ______________________

____

Interviewer's Signature ________________________________ Date ______________

CRITERIA FOR REFERRAL TO REGISTERED DIETITIAN

Anthropometric 'red flags'	Clinical 'red flags'	Feeding/diet 'red flags'
Weight for age or weight for length at or below 5th percentile Weight for age or weight for length at or above 95th percentile Weight loss or significant decline in percentile ranking, particularly if weight precedes length in decline	*Vomiting*—chronic vomiting, particularly if accompanied by other signs and symptoms such as: diarrhea or dehydration; growth faltering, pain or obvious discomfort or frequent respiratory tract infections; diarrhea, atopic dermatitis or wheezing; forceful vomiting, or vomitus which contains bile (green) or blood (red or "coffee ground" appearance)	Low iron formula, Similac Special Care, Enfamil Premature Formula, goat's milk, or a product other than an infant formula for infants Adding more or less water than can directions call for; supplements added to formula
Poor rate of weight gain for age (corrected age in infants and toddlers up to 24 mo): <20 g/day (<5 oz/wk) — term – 3 mo <15 g/day (<3½ oz/wk) — 3 – 6 mo <10 g/day (<2 oz/wk) — 6 – 9 mo <7 g/day (<1½ oz/wk) — 9 – 12 mo <1 kg (2 lb)/6 mo — 1 – 2 yr <0.7 kg (1½ lb)/6 mo — 2 – 5 yr	*Diarrhea*—frequent/chronic loose, watery, large, bulky or unusually foul smelling stools, particularly if accompanied by other signs and symptoms such as vomiting or dehydration, gas and bloating, skin breakdown in diaper area; grey, white or pale colored stools. Note: Stools of breast-fed babies may be quite frequent (often occur with every feeding) during the first few weeks of life *Constipation*—hard, dry, infrequent stools which are difficult to pass.	Cow's milk as the main source of nutrition during the first year *instead of formula or breast milk*; low-fat milk *(especially skim milk)* <2 yr of age <24 oz formula/day for infants; <16 oz milk/day for toddlers and no other significant source of dairy products in diet; >32 oz cow's milk/day for toddlers (over 1 yr of age) Use of infant feeders, tube feedings or parenteral nutrition (TPN or "hyperal")
Disproportional head growth See chapter 5 for complete discussion of normal and "at risk" growth patterns	*Chronic illness* or medical conditions such as: AIDS/HIV+, multiple allergy/food intolerance, bronchopulmonary dysplasia, cyanotic cardiac anomalies, cerebral palsy, cystic fibrosis, Down syndrome, failure to thrive, fetal alcohol syndrome or other intrauterine drug exposure, gastrointestinal disease, kidney or liver disease, seizure disorder, spina bifida	Infants >6 mo corrected age not yet starting spoon feedings or toddlers >12 mo of age not yet taking finger foods; daily food intake regularly excludes one or more basic food groups >12 mo of age Feeding duration >30 min for infants or >45 min for toddlers (excluding breaks for diapering, playing, etc.); <5 feedings/day for infants; <4 feedings/day for toddlers
	Chronic use of medications such as antibiotics, anticholinergics, anticonvulsants, antidiuretics, laxatives or others that may affect nutritional status See chapter 6 for complete discussion of clinical signs and symptoms	Parents have difficulty interpreting or responding appropriately to feeding cues Fussy or distressed during feeding; has trouble breathing during feeding; difficult to wake for feedings, tires easily or has difficulty finishing feedings; frequently gags, coughs or chokes during feedings; refuses to eat, is difficult to feed, or arches backwards when feeding; mealtimes are frustrating to parent or infant/child Parents have nutrition questions or concerns not addressed in standard nutrition education materials

Appendix C

Formula Composition and Indication Chart

Compiled by the Dietary Department, Children's Hospital, Columbus, Ohio
Edited by Peggy Rasche, MS, RD, LD,
and Melody Thompson, MS, RD, LD

and

Recipes for Varying Caloric Density of Standard Formulas

Product (manufacturer) (Caloric density)	g/100 ml CHO	Protein	Fat	mg/100 ml (mEq/100 ml) Na	K	Fe	Osmolality (mOsm/kg of H_2O) Macronutrient sources Nutrients per 100 ml Comments/indication
				HUMAN, COW AND GOAT MILK			
Human milk (mature) (20 kcal/oz) (0.67 kcal/ml)	7.2	1.0	3.9	18 (0.8)	53 (1.3)	0.3	**(300)** CHO—lactose PRO—human milk FAT—human milk Iron, vitamin D and fluoride supplementation should be considered
Cow milk, whole[+] (20 kcal/oz) (0.67 kcal/ml)	4.9	3.5	3.5	51 (2.2)	159 (3.9)	trace	**(290)** CHO—lactose PRO—cow milk (casein predominant) FAT—butterfat Not recommended for infants less than 1 yr of age
Cow milk, 2%[+] (15 kcal/oz) (0.5 kcal/ml)	4.9	3.5	2.0	51 (2.2)	159 (4.0)	trace	**(300)** CHO—lactose PRO—cow milk (casein predominant) FAT—butterfat Not recommended for infants or toddlers less than 2 yr of age
Cow milk, skim[+] (10 kcal/oz) (0.33 kcal/ml)	4.9	3.5	trace	53 (2.3)	169 (4.3)	trace	**(300)** CHO—lactose PRO—cow milk (casein predominant) Not recommended for infants and children less than 2 yr of age
Goat milk[+] (20 kcal/oz)	4.4	3.7	3.9	51 (2.3)	208 (5.3)	trace	**(267)** CHO—lactose PRO—goat milk FAT—butterfat Not recommended for infants less than 1 yr of age. Tuberculosis and brucellosis may be passed through unpasteurized goat milk. Most commercial products are now fortified with folic acid and vitamin D. Check labels

[+]Included for comparison purposes. These products are *not* recommended for use as infant formulas.

Product (manufacturer) (Caloric density)	g/100 ml CHO	Protein	Fat	mg/100 ml (mEq/100 ml) Na	K	Fe	Osmolality (mOsm/kg of H_2O) Macronutrient sources Nutrients per 100 ml Comments/indication
				STANDARD INFANT FORMULAS			
Enfamil (Mead Johnson) (20 kcal/oz) (0.67 kcal/ml)	7.0	1.5	3.8	18 (0.8)	73 (1.9)	1.3 [0.3 w/o Fe]	**(300)** CHO—lactose PRO—whey, nonfat cow milk protein (whey: casein ratio 60:40) FAT—palm olein; soy, coconut, and sunflower oils
Enfamil (Mead Johnson) (24 kcal/oz) (0.8 kcal/ml)	8.3	1.8	4.5	22 (1.0)	87 (2.2)	1.5 [0.4 w/o Fe]	**(360)** CHO—lactose PRO—whey, nonfat cow milk protein (whey: casein ratio 60:40) FAT—palm olein; soy, coconut, and sunflower oils
Gerber Baby Formula (Gerber) (20 kcal/oz) (0.67 kcal/ml)	7.3	1.5	3.7	22 (1.0)	73 (1.9)	1.2 [0.1 w/o Fe]	**(320)** CHO—lactose PRO—nonfat milk (whey: casein ratio is 18:82) FAT—palm olein; soy, coconut, and sunflower oils
Good Start (Carnation) (20 kcal/oz) (0.67 kcal/ml)	7.3	1.6	3.4	16 (0.7)	65 (1.7)	1.0	**(260)** CHO—lactose (70%), maltodextrin (30%) PRO—*partially* hydrolyzed demineralized whey *Not* indicated for known allergy to cow milk protein
Lactofree (Mead Johnson) (20 kcal/oz) (0.67 kcal/ml)	7.0	1.5	3.7	20 (0.9)	74 (1.9)	1.2	**(200)** CHO—corn syrup solids PRO—nonfat milk (whey: casein ratio is 18:82) FAT—oleo, coconut, safflower, and soybean oils Contains no lactose, but is not recommended for galactosemia
Similac (Ross Laboratories) (20 kcal/oz) (0.67 kcal/ml)	7.2	1.5	3.6	19 (0.8)	73 (1.9)	1.2 [0.2 w/o Fe]	**(300)** CHO—lactose PRO—nonfat milk (whey: casein ratio is 18:82) FAT—soy oil, coconut oil (also corn oil in powder)
Similac (Ross Laboratories) (24 kcal/oz) (0.8 kcal/ml)	8.5	2.2	4.3	27 (1.2)	107 (2.7)	1.5 [0.2 w/o Fe]	**(380)** CHO—lactose PRO—nonfat milk (whey: casein ratio is 18:82) FAT—soy oil, coconut oil
Similac (Ross Laboratories) (27 kcal/oz) (0.9 kcal/ml)	9.6	2.5	4.8	313 (1.3)	120 (3.1)	0.2	**(430)** CHO—lactose PRO—nonfat milk (whey: casein ratio is 18:82) FAT—soy oil, coconut oil

Product (manufacturer) (Caloric density)	g/100 ml			mg/100 ml (mEq/100 ml)			Osmolality (mOsm/kg of H_2O) Macronutrient sources Nutrients per 100 ml Comments/indication
	CHO	Protein	Fat	Na	K	Fe	
FOLLOW-UP AND TODDLER FORMULAS							
Carnation Follow-up (Carnation) (20 kcal/oz) (0.67 kcal/ml)	8.9	2.6	2.6	26 (1.1)	91 (2.3)	1.3	**(300)** CHO—lactose, corn syrup solids PRO—nonfat milk FAT—palm, soy, coconut, and high-oleic safflower oils For infants 6–12 mo of age who are eating solid foods
Carnation Follow-up Soy (Carnation) (20 kcal/oz) (0.67 kcal/ml)	6.8	2.1	3.7	28 (1.2)	78 (2.0)	1.3	**(300)** CHO—maltodextrin (potato) PRO—soy protein isolate FAT—soy oil For infants 6–12 mo of age who are eating solid foods. Calcium 90 mg, phosphorus 60 mg
Enfamil Next Step (Mead Johnson) (20 kcal/oz) (0.67 kcal/ml)	7.4	1.8	3.4	28 (1.2)	87 (2.2)	1.2	**(270)** CHO—corn syrup solids, lactose PRO—nonfat milk FAT—palm olein; soy, coconut and high-oleic sunflower oils For toddlers 1–3 yr of age
Enfamil Next Step Soy (Mead Johnson) (20 kcal/oz) (0.67 kcal/ml)	8.0	2.2	2.9	31	101	1.2	**(260)** CHO—corn syrup solids, sucrose PRO—soy protein isolate FAT—palm olein; soy, coconut and high-oleic sunflower oils For toddlers 1–3 yr of age. L-carnitine added
Similac NeoCare—See formulas designed for growing low-birth-weight infants							
Similac Toddler's Best (Ross Laboratories) (20 kcal/oz) (0.67 kcal/ml)	7.3	2.3	3.1	27 (1.2)	125 (3.2)	1.2	**(350)** CHO—sucrose, lactose PRO—nonfat milk FAT—high-oleic safflower oil, coconut and soy oils For toddlers 1–3 yr of age. Available in vanilla, chocolate, and berry flavors

Product (manufacturer) (Caloric density)	g/100 ml CHO	Protein	Fat	mg/100 ml (mEq/100 ml) Na	K	Fe	Osmolality (mOsm/kg of H_2O) Macronutrient sources Nutrients per 100 ml Comments/indication
SOY FORMULAS (MILK-FREE AND LACTOSE-FREE)							
Alsoy (Carnation) (20 kcal/oz) (0.67 kcal/ml)	6.8	2.1	3.7	28 (1.2)	78 (2.0)	1.3	**(300)** CHO—maltodextrin (potato) PRO—soy protein isolate FAT—soy oil Calcium 68 mg, phosphorus 42 mg
Carnation Follow-up Soy—See follow-up and toddler formulas							
Enfamil Next Step Soy—See follow-up and toddler formulas							
Gerber Soy (Gerber) (20 kcal/oz) (0.67 kcal/ml)	6.8	2.0	3.6	32 (1.4)	78 (2.0)	1.2	**(230)** CHO—corn syrup solids, sucrose PRO—soy protein isolate, L-methionine, taurine FAT—palm olein; soy, coconut, sunflower oils L-carnitine added
Isomil (Ross Laboratories) (20 kcal/oz) (0.67 kcal/ml)	6.8	1.8	3.7	30 (1.3)	73 (1.9)	1.2	**(240)** CHO—corn syrup solids, sucrose PRO—soy protein isolate, L-methionine, taurine FAT—soy oil, coconut oil L-carnitine added
Isomil-DF (Ross Laboratories) (20 kcal/oz) (0.67 kcal/ml)	6.8	1.8	3.7	30 (1.3)	73 (1.9)	1.2	**(240)** CHO—corn syrup solids PRO—soy protein isolate, L-methionine, taurine FAT—soy oil, coconut oil L-carnitine added
Isomil-SF (Ross Laboratories) (20 kcal/oz) (0.67 kcal/ml)	6.8	1.8	3.7	30 (1.3)	73 (1.9)	1.2	**(180)** CHO—corn syrup solids PRO—soy protein isolate, L-methionine, taurine FAT—soy oil, coconut oil L-carnitine added. Sucrose free. Lactose free
Prosobee (Mead Johnson) (20 kcal/oz) (0.67 kcal/ml)	6.8	2.0	3.6	24 (1.1)	82 (2.1)	1.3	**(200)** CHO—corn syrup solids PRO—soy protein isolate, L-methionine, taurine FAT—palm olein; soy, coconut, and high-oleic sunflower oils L-carnitine added

Product (manufacturer) (Caloric density)	g/100 ml CHO	 Protein	 Fat	mg/100 ml (mEq/100 ml) Na	 K	 Fe	Osmolality (mOsm/kg of H_2O) Macronutrient sources Nutrients per 100 ml Comments/indication
HUMAN MILK AND HUMAN MILK FORTIFIERS USED FOR GROWING LOW-BIRTH-WEIGHT INFANTS							
Preterm human milk (20 kcal/oz) (0.67 kcal/ml)	6.6	1.4	3.9	25 (1.1)	57 (1.5)	0.1	**(290)** CHO—lactose PRO—human milk FAT—human milk Calcium 25 mg, phosphorus 13 mg, vitamin D 2 IU. Data compiled for 14th day of lactation from 20 studies
Preterm human milk + Enfamil Human Milk Fortifier (Mead Johnson) 100 ml milk + 4 pkts HMF (24 kcal/oz) (0.8 kcal/ml)	9.3	2.1	4.0	32 (1.4)	73 (1.9)	0.1	**(380)** CHO—lactose; corn syrup solids, lactose PRO—human milk; whey protein concentrate and casein FAT—human milk Calcium 115 mg, phosphorus 60 mg, vitamin D 210 IU
Preterm human milk + Similac Natural Care (Ross Laboratories) 50 ml milk + 50 ml SNC (22 kcal/oz) (0.73 kcal/ml)	7.6	1.8	4.2	30 (1.3)	81 (2.1)	0.2	**(300)** CHO—lactose; corn syrup solids, lactose PRO—human milk; cow milk, demineralized whey FAT—human milk; medium-chain triglycerides, corn and coconut oils Calcium 98 mg, phosphorus 49 mg, vitamin D 62 IU
Enfamil Human Milk Fortifier—4 packets (Mead Johnson) (14 kcal)	2.7	0.7	0.1	7 (0.3)	16 (0.4)	0.0	— CHO—corn syrup solids, lactose PRO—whey protein concentrate and casein FAT—negligible < 0.1 g Calcium 90 mg, phosphorus 45 mg, vitamin D 210 IU; designed to be mixed 4 packets in 100 ml human milk
Similac Natural Care (Ross Laboratories) (24 kcal/oz) (0.8 kcal/ml)	8.5	2.2	4.4	35 (1.5)	105 (2.7)	0.3	**(300)** CHO—lactose, corn syrup solids PRO—cow milk, demineralized whey; whey; casein ratio 60:40 FAT—medium-chain triglycerides, corn and coconut oils Calcium 170 mg, phosphorus 85 mg, vitamin D 120 IU; designed to be mixed in a 1:1 ratio with human milk or given at alternate feedings to low-birth-weight infants receiving human milk

Product (manufacturer) (Caloric density)	g/100 ml			mg/100 ml (mEq/100 ml)			Osmolality (mOsm/kg of H_2O) Macronutrient sources Nutrients per 100 ml Comments/indication
	CHO	Protein	Fat	Na	K	Fe	
FORMULAS DESIGNED FOR GROWING LOW-BIRTH-WEIGHT INFANTS							
Enfamil Premature Formula (Mead Johnson) (20 kcal/oz) (0.67 kcal/ml)	7.4	2.0	3.4	26 (1.1)	70 (1.8)	1.3 [0.2 w/o Fe]	**(244)** CHO—corn syrup solids, lactose PRO—cow milk, whey protein concentrate; whey: casein ratio 60:40 FAT—medium-chain triglycerides, soy and coconut oils Calcium 110 mg, phosphorus 55 mg, vitamin D 180 IU
Enfamil Premature Formula (Mead Johnson) (24 kcal/oz) (0.8 kcal/ml)	8.9	2.4	4.1	31 (1.4)	83 (2.1)	1.5 [0.2 w/o Fe]	**(380)** CHO—corn syrup solids, lactose PRO—cow milk; whey protein concentrate; whey: casein ratio 60:40 FAT—medium-chain triglycerides, soy and coconut oils Calcium 132 mg, phosphorus 66 mg, vitamin D 220 IU
Similac NeoCare (Ross Laboratories) (22 kcal/oz) (0.73 kcal/ml)	7.6	1.9	4.0	24 (1.0)	104 (2.7)	1.3	**(290)** CHO—corn syrup solids, lactose PRO—nonfat milk; whey protein concentrate; whey: casein ratio 50:50 FAT—soy, high-oleic safflower, medium-chain triglycerides and coconut oils Calcium 77 mg, phosphorus 46 mg, vitamin D 59 IU; designed as an enriched formula for use by low-birth-weight infants after hospital discharge
Similac Special Care (Ross Laboratories) (20 kcal/oz) (0.67 kcal/ml)	7.2	1.8	3.6	29 (1.3)	87 (2.2)	1.2 [0.3 w/o Fe]	**(250)** CHO—corn syrup solids, lactose PRO—nonfat milk, whey protein concentrate; whey: casein ratio 60:40 FAT—medium-chain triglycerides, soy and coconut oils Calcium 122 mg, phosphorus 61 mg, vitamin D 100 IU
Similac Special Care (Ross Laboratories) (24 kcal/oz) (0.8 kcal/ml)	8.5	2.2	4.4	35 (1.5)	104 (2.7)	1.5 [0.3 w/o Fe]	**(300)** CHO—corn syrup solids, lactose PRO—nonfat milk, whey protein concentrate; whey: casein ratio 60:40 FAT—medium-chain triglycerides, corn and coconut oils Calcium 145 mg, phosphorus 72 mg, vitamin D 120 IU

Product (manufacturer) (Caloric density)	g/100 ml			mg/100 ml (mEq/100 ml)			Osmolality ($mOsm/kg$ of H_2O) Macronutrient sources Nutrients per 100 ml Comments/indication
	CHO	Protein	Fat	Na	K	Fe	
FORMULAS FOR SPECIAL NUTRITIONAL NEEDS							
Alimentum (Ross Laboratories) (20 kcal/oz) (0.67 kcal/ml)	6.9	1.9	3.7	30 (1.3)	80 (2.0)	1.2	**(370)** CHO—sucrose, corn syrup solids PRO—casein hydrolysate, taurine, L-carnitine FAT—medium-chain triglycerides, safflower oil, soy oil Hypoallergenic formula for infants/toddlers sensitive to intact proteins. Also for fat malabsorption associated with pancreatic insufficiency or cholestasis
Neocate (SHS) (20 kcal/oz) (0.67 kcal/ml)	7.8	2.1	3.0	25 (1.1)	104 (2.7)	1.2	**(280)** CHO—corn syrup solids PRO—L-amino acids; taurine, L-carnitine, L-glutamine FAT—hybrid safflower oil, refined vegetable oils: coconut, soy Elemental infant formula for those with impaired gastrointestinal function or sensitivity to intact protein. Available only as powder. 1⅓ cups powder + 28 oz water yields 1 qt formula
Nutramigen (Mead Johnson) (20 kcal/oz) (0.67 kcal/ml)	9.1	1.9	2.6	32 (1.4)	73 (2.1)	1.3	**(320)** CHO—corn syrup solids, modified cornstarch (lactose and sucrose free) PRO—casein hydrolysate FAT—palm olein, soy, coconut, and high-oleic sunflower oils Hypoallergenic formula for infants/toddlers sensitive to intact proteins
Portagen (Mead Johnson) (20 kcal/oz) (0.67 kcal/ml)	7.7	2.3	3.1	33 (1.4)	83 (2.1)	1.3	**(320)** CHO—corn syrup solids, sucrose PRO—caseinate FAT—medium-high triglycerides 85%, corn oil 15% For infants/toddlers who do not efficiently digest, absorb, or utilize long-chain fatty acids as in chylothorax or chylous ascites
Similac Special Care (Ross Laboratories) (20 kcal/oz) (0.67 kcal/ml)	7.2	1.8	3.6	29 (1.3)	87 (2.2)	1.2 [0.3 w/o Fe]	**(250)** CHO—corn syrup solids, lactose PRO—nonfat milk, whey protein concentrate; whey: casein ratio 60:40 FAT—medium-chain triglycerides, soy and coconut oils Calcium 122 mg, phosphorus 61 mg, vitamin D 100 IU
Pregestimil (Mead Johnson) (20 kcal/oz) (0.67 kcal/ml)	7.0	1.9	3.8	26 (1.2)	73 (1.9)	1.3	**(320)** CHO—corn syrup solids, modified corn starch, dextrose PRO—casein hydrolysate FAT—medium-chain triglycerides, corn, high-oleic safflower and soy oils Hypoallergenic formula for infants/toddlers sensitive to intact proteins; also for fat malabsorption associated with pancreatic insufficiency or cholestasis
Similac PM 60:40 (Ross Laboratories) (20 kcal/oz) (0.67 kcal/ml)	6.9	1.6	3.8	16 (0.7)	58 (1.5)	0.2	**(280)** CHO—lactose PRO—whey protein concentrate, caseinate; whey: casein ratio 60:40 FAT—soy and coconut oils + corn oil in powder For infants predisposed to hyperphosphatemia; low renal solute load

Product (manufacturer) (Caloric density)	g/100 ml CHO	Protein	Fat	mg/100 ml (mEq/100 ml) Na	K	Fe	Osmolality (mOsm/kg of H_2O) Macronutrient sources Nutrients per 100 ml Comments/indication
NUTRITIONALLY COMPLETE PRODUCTS FOR TUBE OR ORAL FEEDING OF CHILDREN AGES 1–10 YEARS							
Kindercal (Mead Johnson) (30 kcal/oz) (1.06 kcal/ml)	13.5	3.4	4.4	37 (1.6)	131 (3.4)	1.1	**(310)** CHO—maltodextrin, sucrose PRO—caseinates, milk protein concentrate FAT—canola, medium-chain triglycerides, corn and high-oleic sunflower oils Contains 0.63 g soy fiber/100 ml; vanilla flavor
Neocate One + (SHS) (30 kcal/oz) (1.06 kcal/ml)	14.6	2.5	3.5	20 (0.9)	93 (2.4)	0.8	**(835)** CHO—maltodextrin, sucrose PRO—L-amino acids FAT—medium chain triglycerides, canola and high-oleic sunflower oils Elemental for those with impaired gastrointestinal tract function or sensitivity to intact protein; orange-pineapple flavor
Pediasure (Ross Laboratories) (30 kcal/oz) (1.06 kcal/ml)	11.0	3.0	5.0	38 (1.7)	131 (3.4)	1.4	**(310)** (with fiber, 345) CHO—corn syrup solids, sucrose PRO—caseinate, whey protein concentrate FAT—high-oleic safflower, soy, and medium-chain triglyceride oils Product available with or without soy fiber 0.5 g/100 ml; vanilla, chocolate, berry flavors
Peptamen Junior (Clintec) (30 kcal/oz) (1.06 kcal/ml)	13.8	3.0	3.8	46 (2.0)	132 (3.4)	1.4	**(260)** CHO—maltodextrin, corn starch PRO—hydrolyzed whey protein FAT—medium-chain triglycerides, soy and canola oils Peptide-based for use with impaired gastrointestinal function or inability to tolerate intact protein or free amino acids; grape, cherry, bubble gum, blue raspberry, chocolate, vanilla flavors
Vivonex Pediatric (Sandoz) (24 kcal/oz) (0.8 kcal/ml)	12.6	2.4	2.4	40 (1.7)	120 (3.1)	1.0	**(360)** CHO—maltodextrin, modified starch PRO—L-amino acids FAT—medium-chain triglycerides and soy oils Elemental for those with impaired gastrointestinal function or sensitivity to intact protein; unflavored; vanilla, cherry-vanilla, raspberry, orange-pineapple, lemon-lime flavor packets available

Product (manufacturer) (Caloric density)	g/100 ml CHO	 Protein	 Fat	mg/100 ml (mEq/100 ml) Na	 K	 Fe	Osmolality (mOsm/kg of H_2O) Macronutrient sources Nutrients per 100 ml Comments/indication
NUTRITION SUPPLEMENT PRODUCTS ADDED TO MILK							
Carnation Instant Breakfast mixed with whole milk as directed (Carnation) (30 kcal/oz) (1.03 kcal/ml)	13.2	5.6	3.1	94 (4.1)	275 (7.0)		(677–715 depending upon flavor) CHO—lactose; lactose, sucrose PRO—milk protein; casein, egg white, whey FAT—butterfat Chocolate, vanilla, strawberry, coffee, chocolate malt flavors
Carnation Instant Breakfast NO SUGAR—mixed with low-fat (2%) milk as directed (Carnation) (22.5 kcal/oz) (0.75 kcal/ml)	8.6	5.6	2.0	109 (4.7)	274 (7.0)		CHO—aspartame, lactose PRO—milk protein; casein, egg white, whey FAT—butterfat Vanilla, chocolate, chocolate malt, strawberry flavors
Delmark Instant Breakfast mixed with whole milk as directed (Delmark) (30 kcal/oz) (1.0 kcal/ml)	13.3	5.4	3.2	79 (3.4)	226 (5.8)		CHO—lactose; lactose, sugar PRO—milk protein; nonfat dry milk FAT—butterfat Vanilla, chocolate, strawberry flavors

Product (manufacturer)	kcal/g	Source	g/tbsp	Comments
				MODULAR COMPONENTS—CARBOHYDRATE
Dextrose (hydrous)	3.4	Corn sugar	9.5	Monosaccharide. Caution: increases osmolality
Fructose	4.0	Fruit sugar	12	Monosaccharide; used for intolerance to corn sugar or other sugars Caution: increases osmolality
Honey	3	Fructose, glucose	20	40% fructose, 35% glucose, 2% sucrose, 23% water; unpasteurized honey *contraindicated* for infant less than 1 yr of age due to risk of botulism
Karo, light (Best Foods)	3	Corn syrup	20	Also contains sugar, vanilla and salt (115 mg Na/100 g)
Moducal Powder (Mead Johnson)	3.8	Glucose polymer (corn product)	8	Low osmolality and minimal sweetness (70 mg Na/100 g powder)
Polycose Liquid	2	Glucose polymer (corn product)	15	Low osmolality and minimal sweetness
Polycose Powder	3.8	Glucose polymer (corn product)	6	Low osmolality and minimal sweetness (115 mg Na/100 g powder)
Rice cereal (dry) (Heintz)	3.8	Rice	2.4	Added to thicken liquid feedings. 1 tbsp dry provides: 0.2 g protein, 0.1 g fat, 1.9 g CHO, 9 calories, 1.1 mg iron
Sucrose	4	Cane or beet	12	Disaccharide. Caution: increases osmolality
Thick-It (Milani Foods)	4.4	Modified cornstarch	4	Instant food thickener for infants/toddlers with dysphagia or swallowing impairment. Maintains desired consistency over time better than added cereal

Product (manufacturer)	kcal/g	Source	g/tbsp (g protein/tbsp)	Other nutrients per tbsp
		MODULAR COMPONENTS—PROTEIN		
Casec (Mead Johnson)	3.7	Calcium caseinate	4.7 (4.1)	75 mg calcium, 38 mg phosphorus, 5.6 mg sodium, 0.5 mg potassium
Instant nonfat dry milk (various brands)	3.5	Cow milk	4.3 (1.5)	52 mg calcium, 47 mg phosphorus, 24 mg sodium, 73 mg potassium, 2.4 g lactose, 15.6 kcal
ProMod (Ross Laboratories)	4.3	Whey, soy	4.0 (3.0)	15.6 mg calcium, 15.6 mg phosphorus, 9.2 mg sodium, 39 mg potassium

Product (manufacturer)	kcal/g	Source	g/tbsp (g fat/tbsp)	Other nutrients per tbsp
		MODULAR COMPONENTS—FAT		
Corn oil	8.6	Corn	14 (14)	Primarily oleic and linoleic unsaturated fatty acids. Linoleic acid 55%
MCT oil (Mead Johnson)	8.3	Fractionated coconut oil	14 (14)	Medium chain triglycerides: C_8 and C_{10} saturated fatty acids; absorbed directly into portal system. Bile salts and lipase not necessary for digestion and absorption. Does not contain essential fatty acids
Microlipid (Mead Johnsonl)	4.5	Safflower oil	15 (7.5)	50% fat in water emulsion; 74% essential fatty acids; maintains emulsion for prolonged periods of time, convenient addition to tube feedings

Product (manufacturer)	kcal/oz	Na	K	Cl	Citrate	Ca	PO_4	Mg	Osmolality mOsm/kg H_2O	Amount/source of carbohydrate g/L
		mEq/L								
					ORAL ELECTROLYTE SOLUTIONS					
Infalyte (Mead Johnson)	3.9	50	25	45	34	—	—	—	200	30 g/L glucose polymers
Pedialyte (Ross Laboratories)	3	45	20	35	30	—	—	—	250	25 g/L dextrose
Rehydralyte (Ross Laboratories)	3	75	20	65	30	—	—	—	305	25 g/L dextrose
Resol (Wyeth-Ayerst)	2.5	50	20	50	34	4	5	4	269	20 g/L dextrose
Ricelyte (Mead Johnson)	3.8	50	25	45	34	—	—	—	200	32 g/L rice syrup solids

RECIPES FOR VARYING CALORIC DENSITY OF STANDARD INFANT FORMULAS (SIMPLIFIED FOR HOME USE)

Preparation of Infant Formula Using One 13-oz Can of Liquid Formula

Desired (and actual) caloric density (kcal/oz)	Water (fluid oz)
20 (20 or 0.67 kcal/cc)	13 (1 can)
24 (24.8 or 0.84 kcal/cc)	8 (1 cup)
27 (27.4 or 0.93 kcal/cc)	6 (3/4 cup)
30 (30.6 or 1.03 kcal/cc)	4 (1/2 cup)

Liquid infant formula concentrate contains 40 kcal/oz (1.35 kcal/cc).

1 fl oz = 29.6 cc

Preparation of Infant Formula Using 1 Cup of Powdered Formula Concentrate*

Desired (and actual) caloric density (kcal/oz)	Water Approximate volumes† (fluid oz)	Final volume of formula† (fluid oz)
20 (20 or 0.67 kcal/cc)‡	29 (3 1/3 cups)	32 oz (1 qt)
24 (24.6 or 0.83 kcal/cc)	22 (2 3/4 cups)	26 oz (3 3/4 cups)
27 (26.7 or 0.9 kcal/cc)	20 (2 1/2 cups)	24 oz (3 cups)
30 (29.0 or 0.98 kcal/cc)	18 (2 1/4 cups)	22 oz (2 3/4 cups)

*One level measuring cup of powdered infant formula contains approximately 640 kcal. One loosely packed scoop contains about 44 kcal and one firmly packed tbsp contains about 40 kcal for most powdered infant formulas.

†One cup of formula powder displaces approximately 1/4 cup of water, so water volumes are approximate. Final volume of formula prepared provides calorie density listed

‡1 fl oz = 29.6 cc

Note: The caloric density of formulas prepared from powder may vary significantly due to different techniques used in measuring powder. For this reason, it is strongly recommended that liquid formula concentrates be used whenever possible to make formula of higher caloric density.

Appendix D

Feeding History Form

Karen Gray, OTR, and Wendy King, PT

FEEDING HISTORY FORM

Infant/Child's Name____________________ DOB________ Age________ (CA______) Chart#__________

Primary caregivers: (Circle all that apply.)
Parent   Babysitter   Foster parent   Other ____________________

Person giving history:
Parent   Babysitter   Foster parent   Other ____________________

Feeding history--caregiver's description of the baby's/child's behaviors:
Feeding and feeding problem(s):

____

____

Sleep/wake cycle: (Circle hours when baby/child is usually awake.)

12^{mid} 1 2 3 4 5 6 7 8 9 10 11 12^{noon} 1 2 3 4 5 6 7 8 9 10 11

When does your baby/child usually eat?

12^{mid} 1 2 3 4 5 6 7 8 9 10 11 12^{noon} 1 2 3 4 5 6 7 8 9 10 11

How do you know your baby/child is hungry? (Circle all that apply.)
Awakens   Sucks on hands or fingers   Fussy   Cries   Screams   Says word/words that mean food   Points

How does your baby/child act when first given the breast/bottle or spoon? (Circle all that apply.)
Excited/happy/eager   Sleepy/not really interested   Fussy/distressed/uncomfortable   Arches/pulls away from nipple/spoon

How does your baby/child act during the feeding? (Circle all that apply.)
Happy/eager   Concentrates on eating   Easily distracted from eating   Tires easily   Fretful/fussy/distressed   Sleepy/tired
Has trouble breathing while eating   Must be burped frequently   Frequently: gags   coughs   chokes

Does your baby/child act differently for breast/bottle feedings and spoon feedings? Yes No If yes, how? ________________

____

In what position is your baby/child during feedings? _____lap/cradled in arms _____infant seat _____laying flat on back

_____high chair _____walker _____regular chair other____________________

What "utensils" are used for feeding your baby/child? _____breast _____bottle (give type:____________________)

_____nipple (give type:____________________) ______spout cup ______open cup _______straw

_____spoon _____fingers _____fork _____infant feeder other____________________

What types of foods are easiest for your infant/child to eat? ____________________

What types of foods are most difficult for your infant/child to eat? ____________________

Does your baby/child prefer foods at a certain temperature? ____________________

How long does it take your baby/child to finish a meal? ______< 30 minutes ______30-45 minutes ______> 45 minutes

How do you know your baby/child is full? (Circle all that apply.)
Stops eating   Falls asleep   Spits out food or nipple   Turns away from food or feeder   Plays with food or is easily distracted

Does your baby/child:
Drool? _____seldom _____frequently _____constantly
Have trouble breathing during feedings? _____seldom _____frequently _____constantly
Cough, gag, or choke during feedings? _____seldom _____frequently _____constantly
Have colds or nasal congestion? _____seldom _____frequently _____constantly
Have problems with respiratory illness, asthma, or pneumonia? Yes No

Signed____________________ Date ________

Appendix E

Feeding Observation Form

Karen Gray, OTR, and Wendy King, PT

FEEDING OBSERVATION FORM

Infant/Child's Name________________ DOB__________ Age________(CA______) Chart#______________

State of Alertness: (Circle all that apply.)

Beginning of feeding:	1	2	3	4	5	6
During feeding:	1	2	3	4	5	6
End of feeding:	1	2	3	4	5	6

State description*:
1 = Deep sleep, no movement, regular breathing
2 = Light sleep, eyes shut, some movement
3 = Dozing, eyes opening and closing
4 = Awake, eyes open, minimal movement
5 = Wide awake, vigorous movement
6 = Crying

Does state of alertness prevent adequate feeding? Yes No

Motor control/body tone/feeding position: (Circle all that apply.)

Flexion:	neck	shoulders	trunk	arms	hips	knees
Extenson:	neck	shoulders	trunk	arms	hips	knees

Are there stress signals during feeding? Yes No If yes, describe ______________________

Describe position: ______________________

____

Oral-motor evaluation: (Circle all that apply.)

Lips: retracted pursed loose cleft normal

Tongue: elevated retracted bunched/humped flat protruded asymmetric normal

Jaw: recessed hangs open clenched asymetric thrusts large excursions clonus tremors normal

Palate: high arched cleft: hard soft normal

Sucking/swallow/breathing evaluation: (Circle all that apply.)

Initiation of sucking:	Normal	Suspect	Abnormal
Strength of sucking:	Normal	Suspect	Abnormal
Suction:	Normal	Suspect	Abnormal
Lip closure around nipple:	Normal	Suspect	Abnormal
Compression of nipple:	Normal	Suspect	Abnormal
Pauses:	Normal	Suspect	Abnormal
Rhythm:	Normal	Suspect	Abnormal
Management of secretions:	Normal	Suspect	Abnormal
Breathing during feeding:	Normal	Suspect	Abnormal
Coordination with breathing:	Normal	Suspect	Abnormal
Coughing/Choking:	Never	Sometimes	Frequently

Is there a difference between nutritive and non-nutritive sucking? Yes No

Spoon feeding evaluation: (Circle all that apply.)

Anticipation of spoon:	Normal	Suspect	Abnormal
Mouth opens for spoon:	Normal	Suspect	Abnormal
Tongue position:	Normal	Suspect	Abnormal
Sucks food off spoon:	Normal	Suspect	Abnormal
Bolus formation:	Normal	Suspect	Abnormal
Swallow:	Normal	Suspect	Abnormal
Gagging/Coughing/Choking:	Normal	Suspect	Abnormal
Chewing:	Normal (for age)	Suspect	Abnormal

Acceptance of textures: Liquid Thickened Liquid Smooth Lumpy Crisp Chewy Mixed

Is acceptance of textures: Normal Suspect Abnormal (for age)

Does baby/child retain food/pouch food in mouth? Yes No

Does food leak or dribble out of mouth? Yes No

Does baby/child vomit frequently or forcefully? Yes No

Is vomitus reswallowed (rumination)? Yes No

Recommendations:

Referrals:

Signed______________________ Date__________

*Morgan AM. Phys Ther 68 (9): 1357, 1988.

Appendix F

National Center for Health Statistics Growth Charts

Girls from Birth to 36 Months
Length for Age

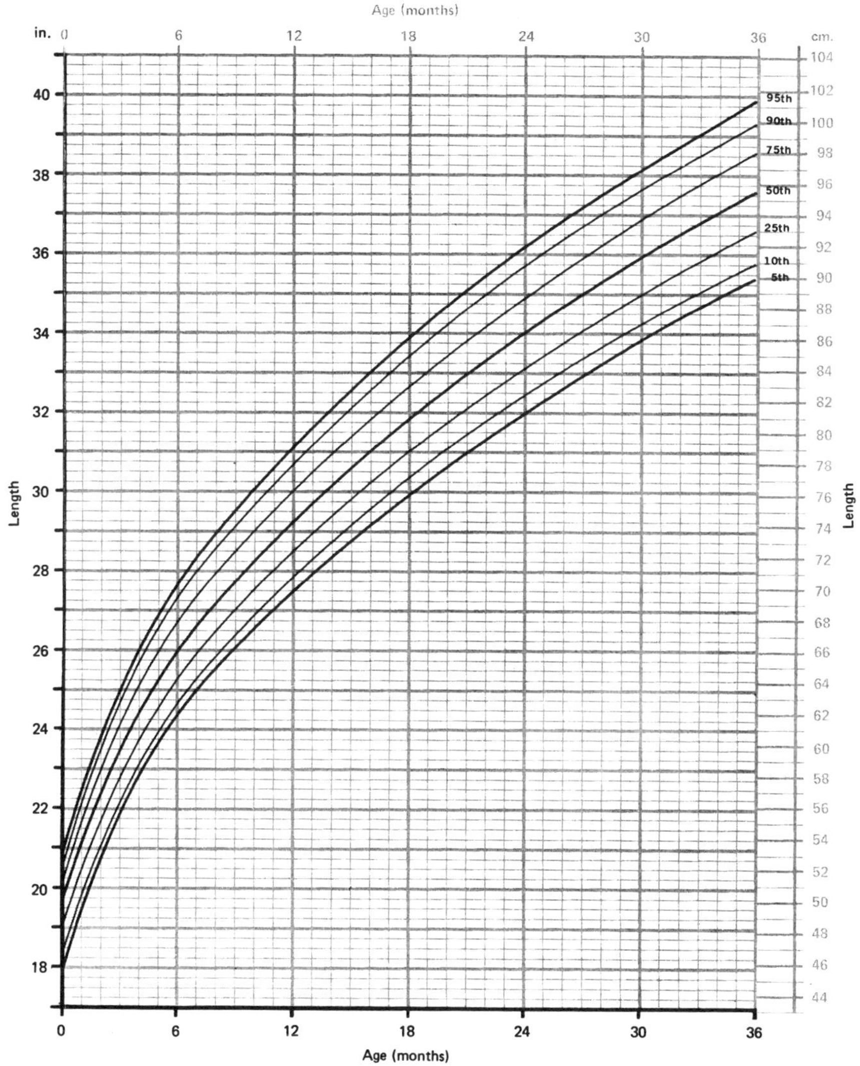

Girls from Birth to 36 Months
Weight for Age

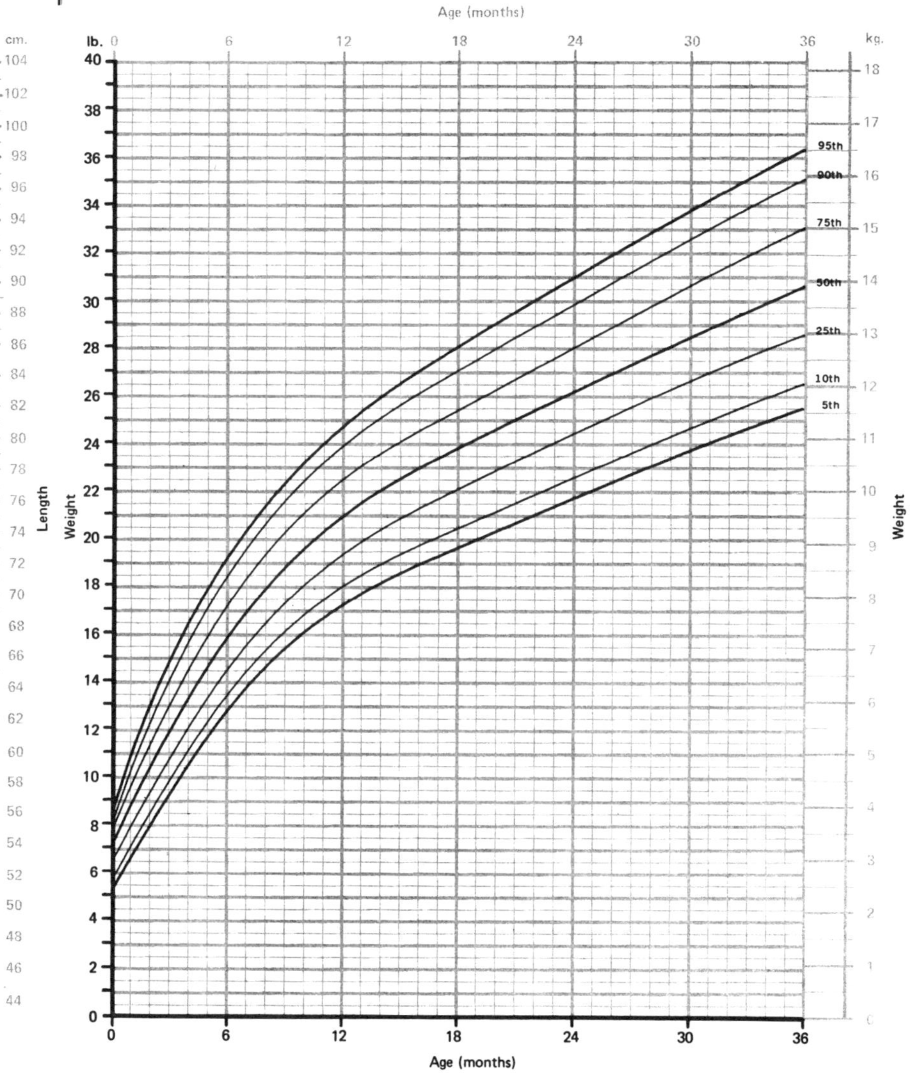

Hamill PVV, Drizd TA, Johnson CL, et al. Physical growth: National Center for Health Statistics percentiles. Amer J Clin Nutr 32:607–29, 1979. Used with permission of Mead Johnson Nutritionals Division, Mead Johnson and Company, Evansville, Indiana.

GIRLS FROM BIRTH TO 36 MONTHS

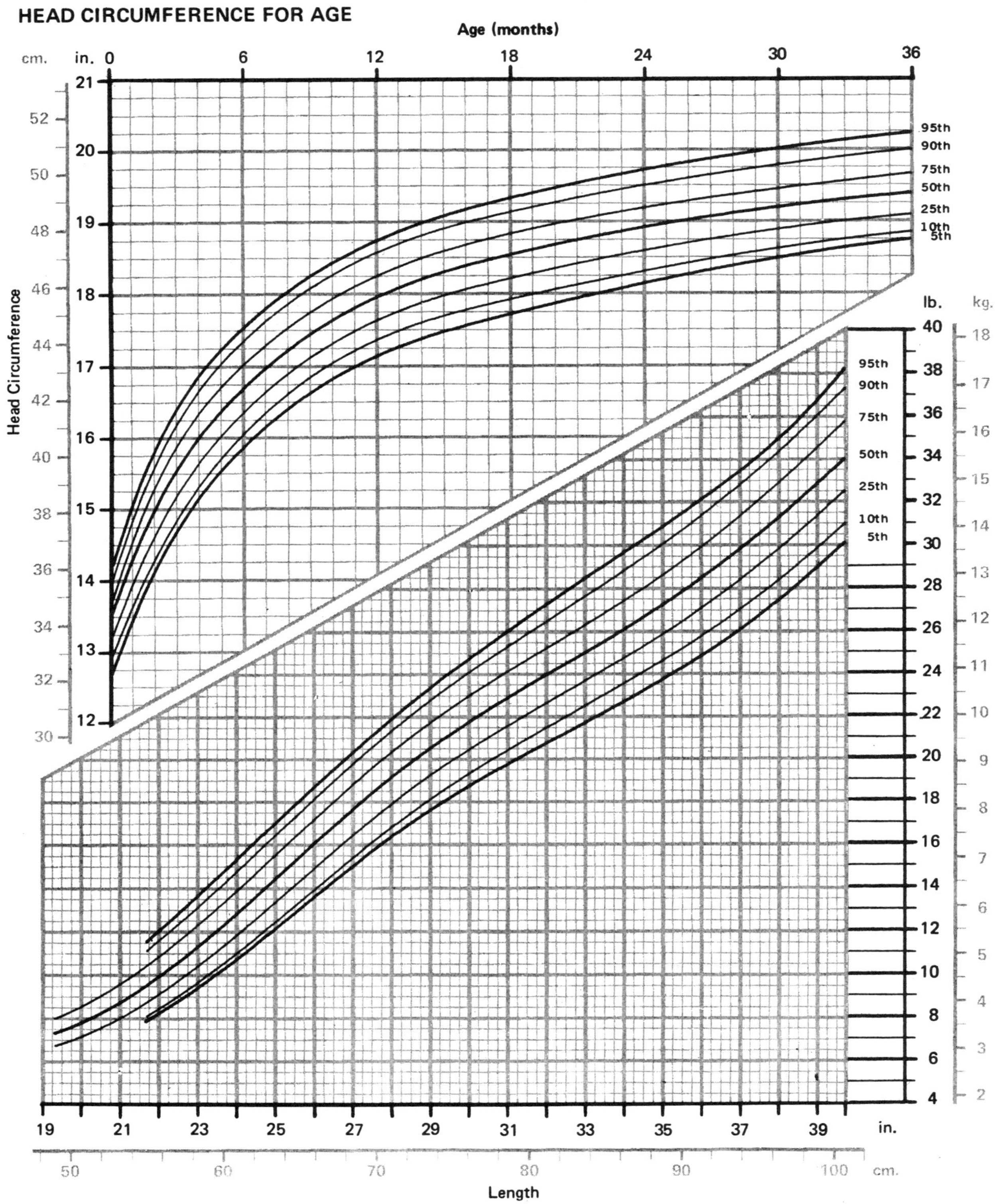

WEIGHT FOR LENGTH

Hamill PVV, Drizd TA, Johnson CL, et al. Physical growth: National Center for Health Statistics percentiles. Amer J Clin Nutr 32:607–29, 1979. Used with permission of Mead Johnson Nutritionals Division, Mead Johnson and Company, Evansville, Indiana.

Boys from Birth to 36 Months Length for Age

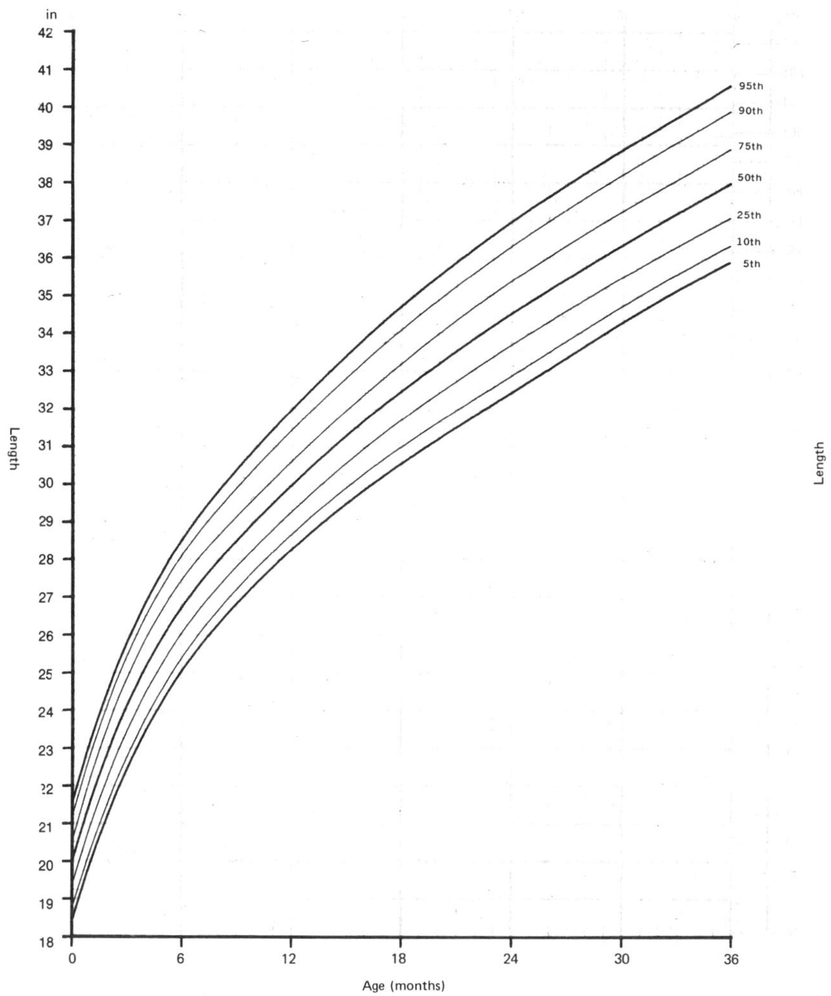

Boys from Birth to 36 Months Weight for Age

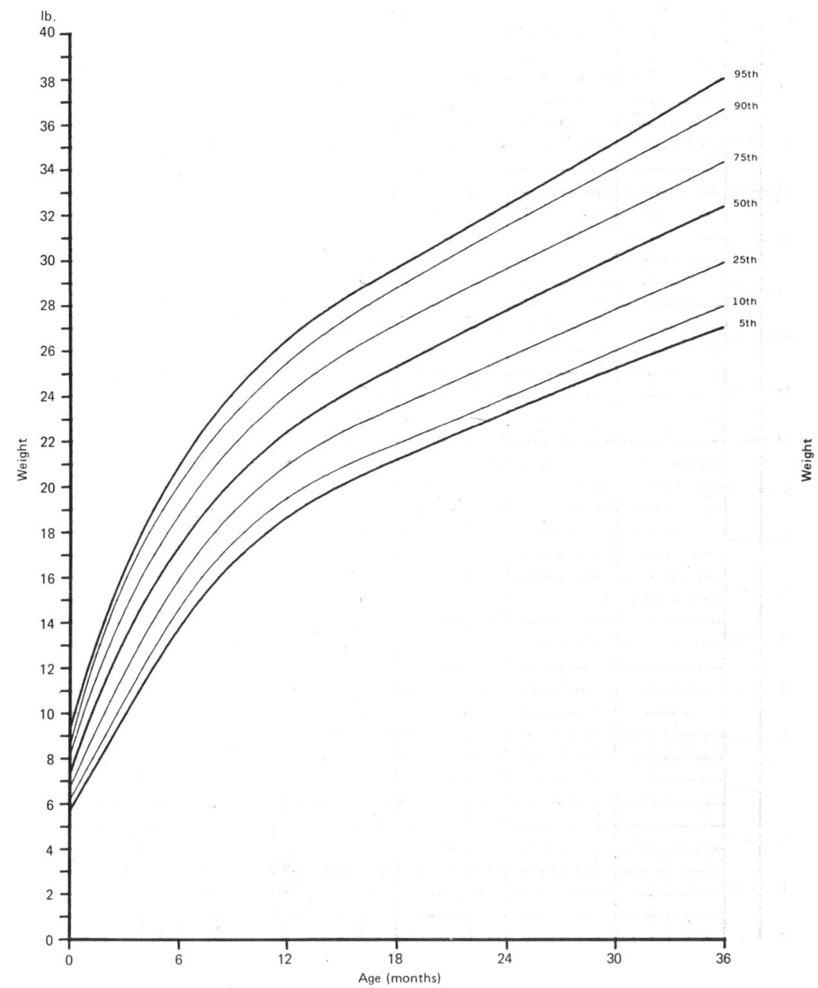

Hamill PVV, Drizd TA, Johnson CL, et al. Physical growth: National Center for Health Statistics percentiles. Amer J Clin Nutr 32:607–29, 1979. Used with permission of Mead Johnson Nutritionals Division, Mead Johnson and Company, Evansville, Indiana.

Boys from Birth to 36 Months
Head Circumference for Age and Weight for Length

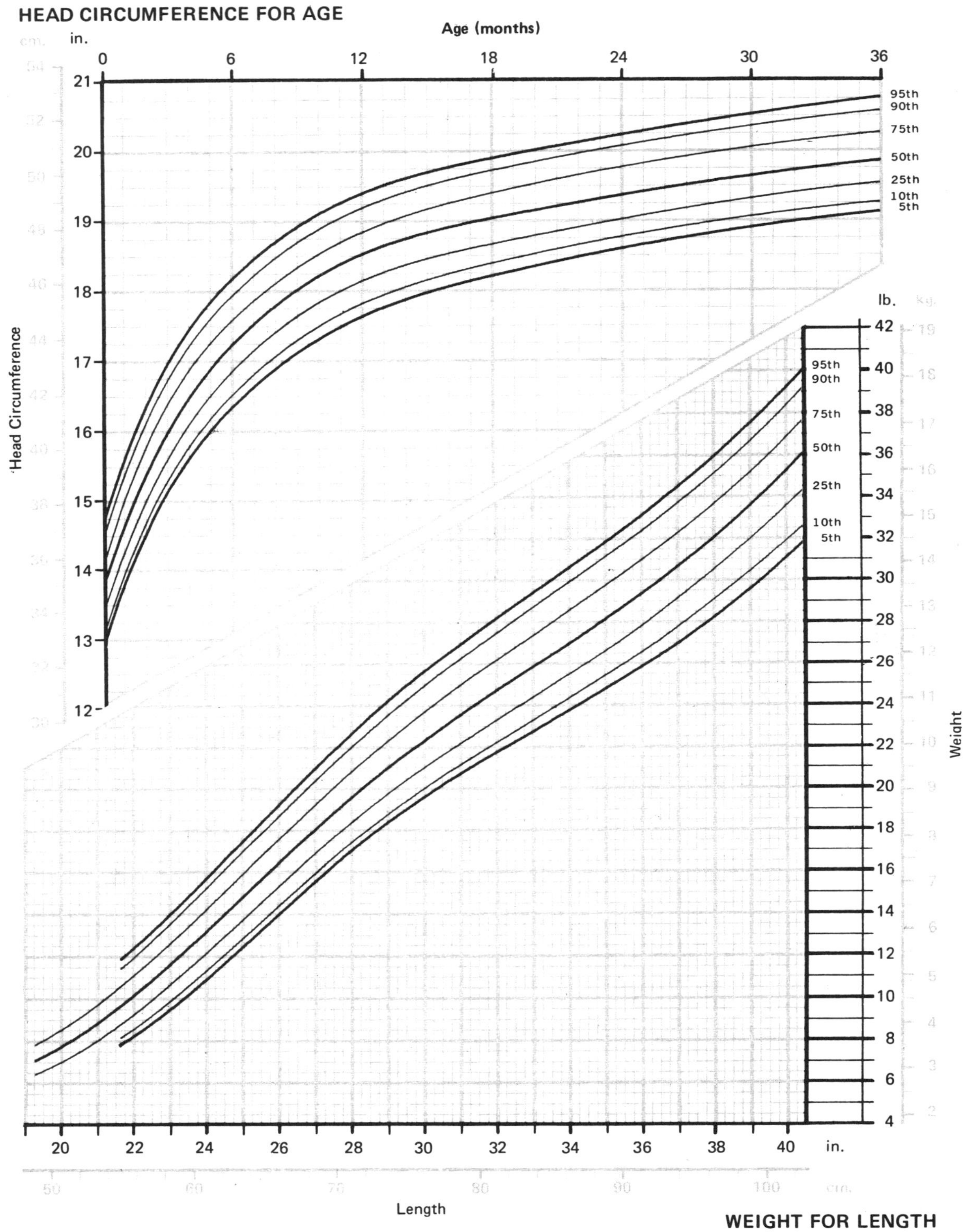

Reprinted by permission of U.S. Department of Health and Human Services, Public Health Service, Health Resources Administration, National Center for Health Statistics, and Center for Disease Control.

Appendix G

Oregon Growth Record for Infants

OREGON GROWTH RECORD FOR INFANTS

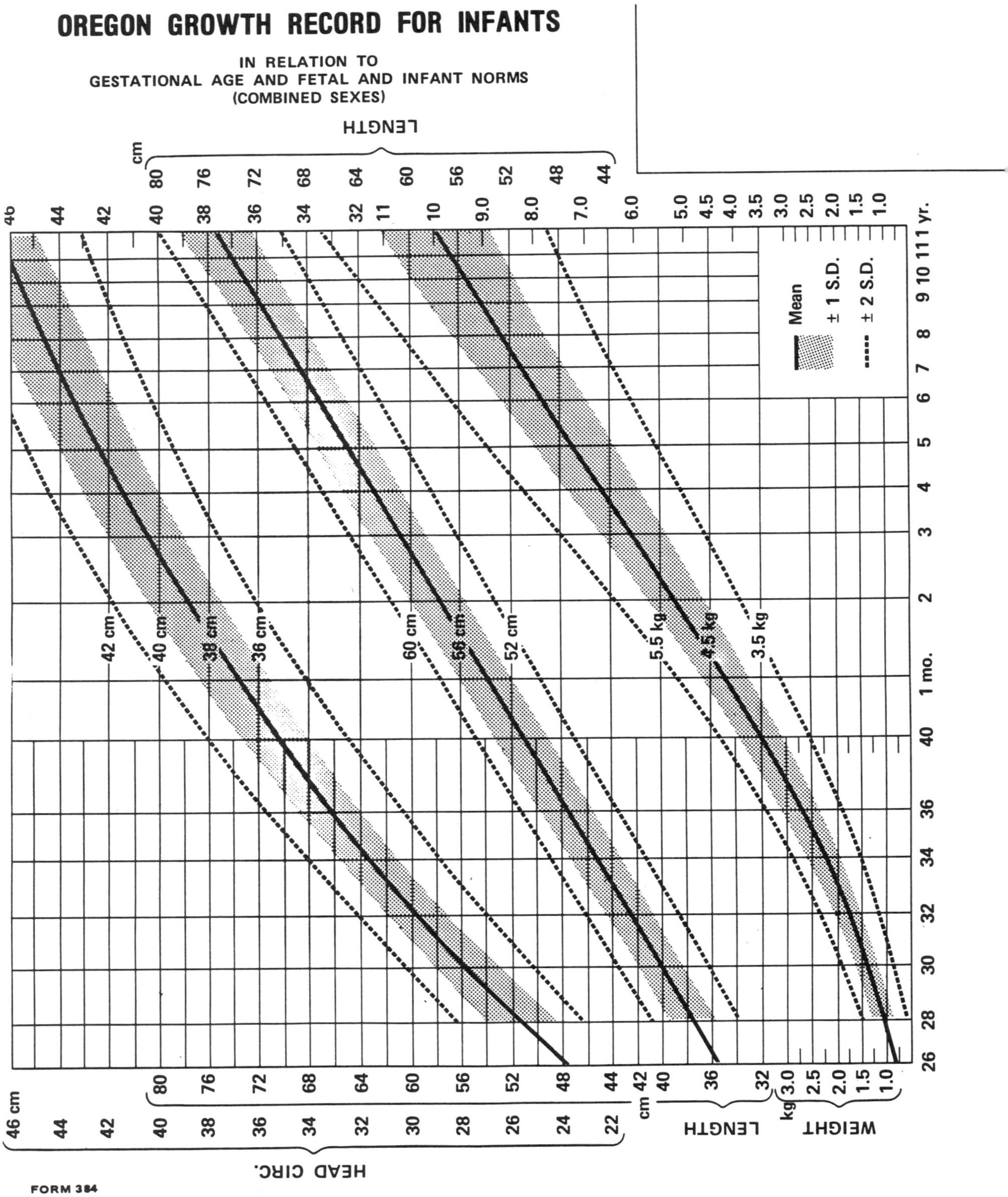

Babson SG and Benda GI. Growth graphs for the clinical assessment of infants of varying gestational age. J Pediatr 89:815, 1976. Reprinted with permission of CV Mosby Co.

Appendix H

Infant Health and Development Program Growth Percentiles

Very Low Birth Weight Premature Boys

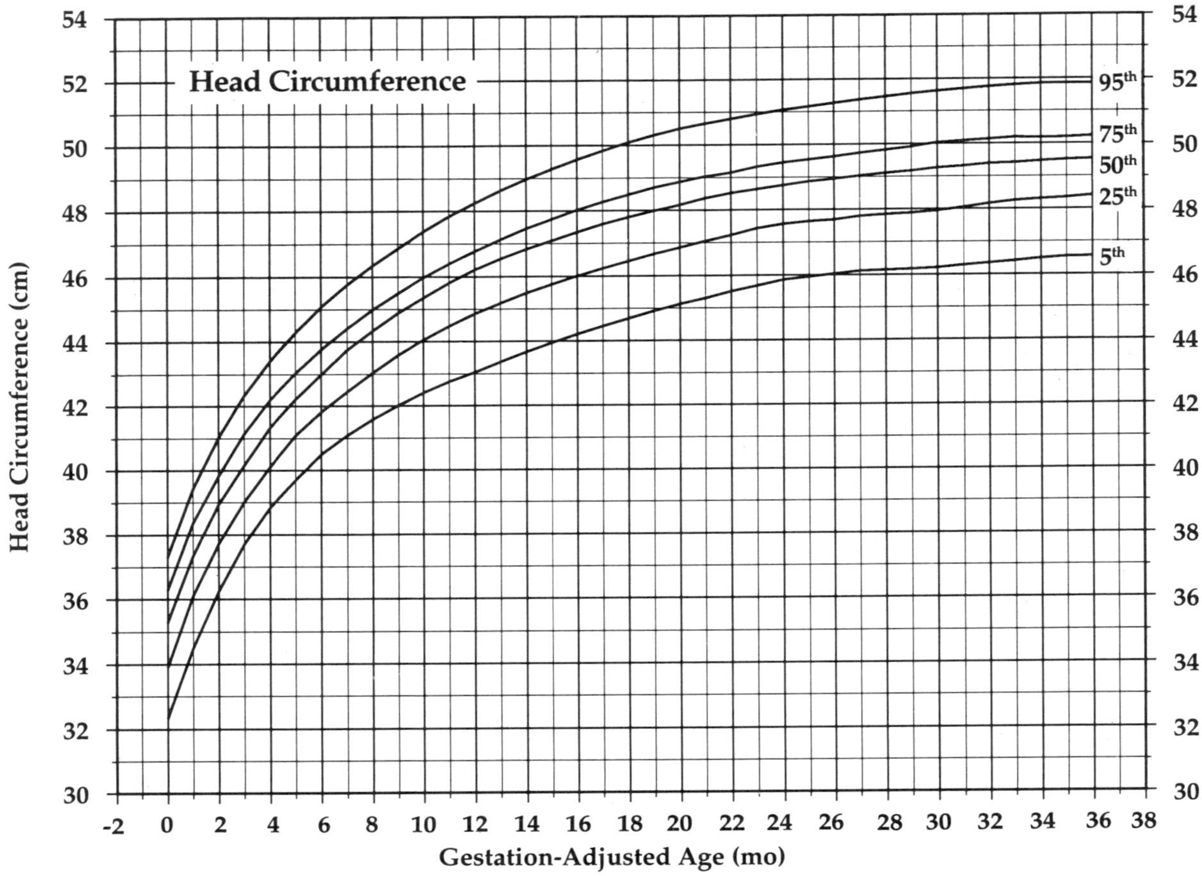

Very Low Birth Weight Premature Boys

Name________________________________

Record #____________________________

ROSS PEDIATRICS

(≤1500 g BW, ≤37 wk GA)

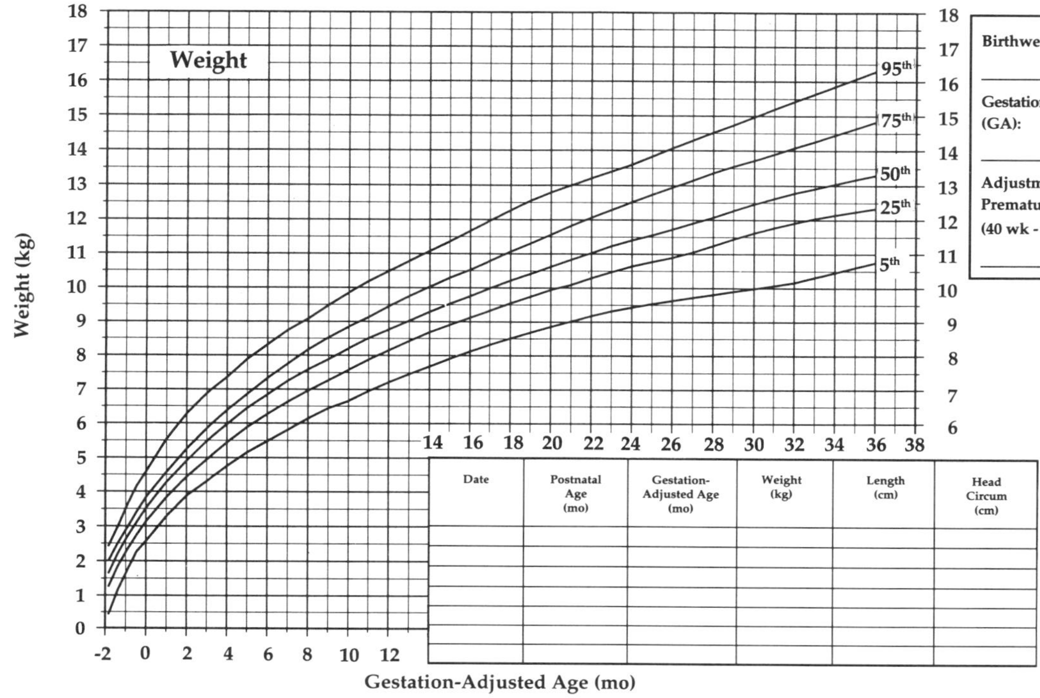

Date	Postnatal Age (mo)	Gestation-Adjusted Age (mo)	Weight (kg)	Length (cm)	Head Circum (cm)

Birthweight (BW): __________ g

Gestational Age (GA): __________ wk

Adjustment for Prematurity (40 wk - GA): __________ wk

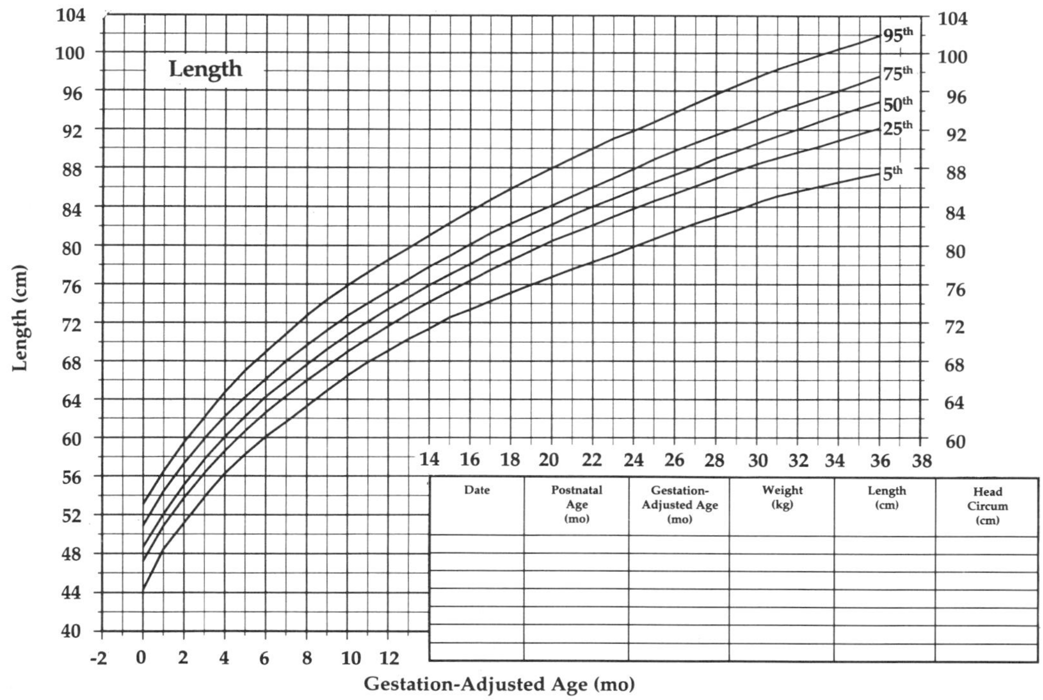

Date	Postnatal Age (mo)	Gestation-Adjusted Age (mo)	Weight (kg)	Length (cm)	Head Circum (cm)

Very Low Birth Weight Premature Girls

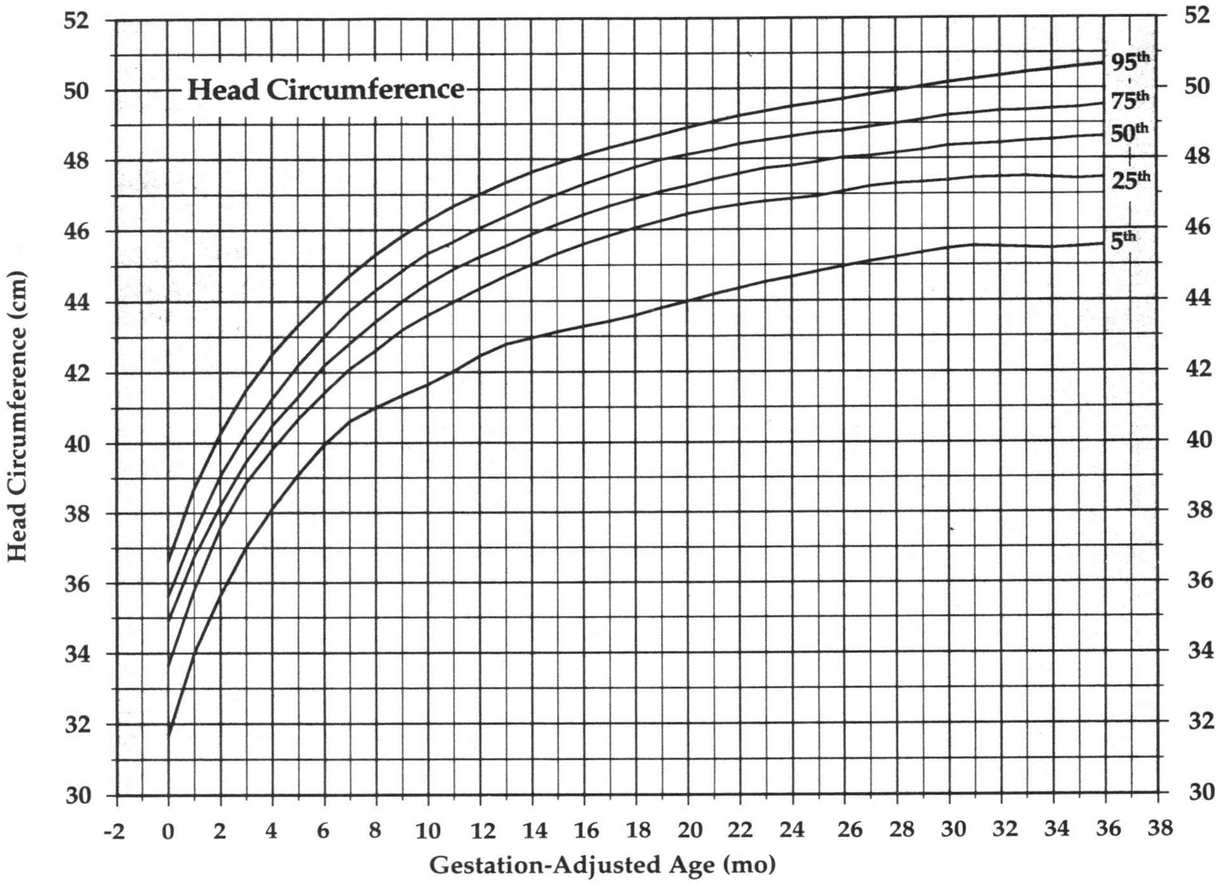

Very Low Birth Weight Premature Girls

Name________________________________

Record #____________________________

(≤1500 g BW, ≤37 wk GA)

ROSS PEDIATRICS

Birthweight (BW): ________g

Gestational Age (GA): ________wk

Adjustment for Prematurity (40 wk - GA): ________wk

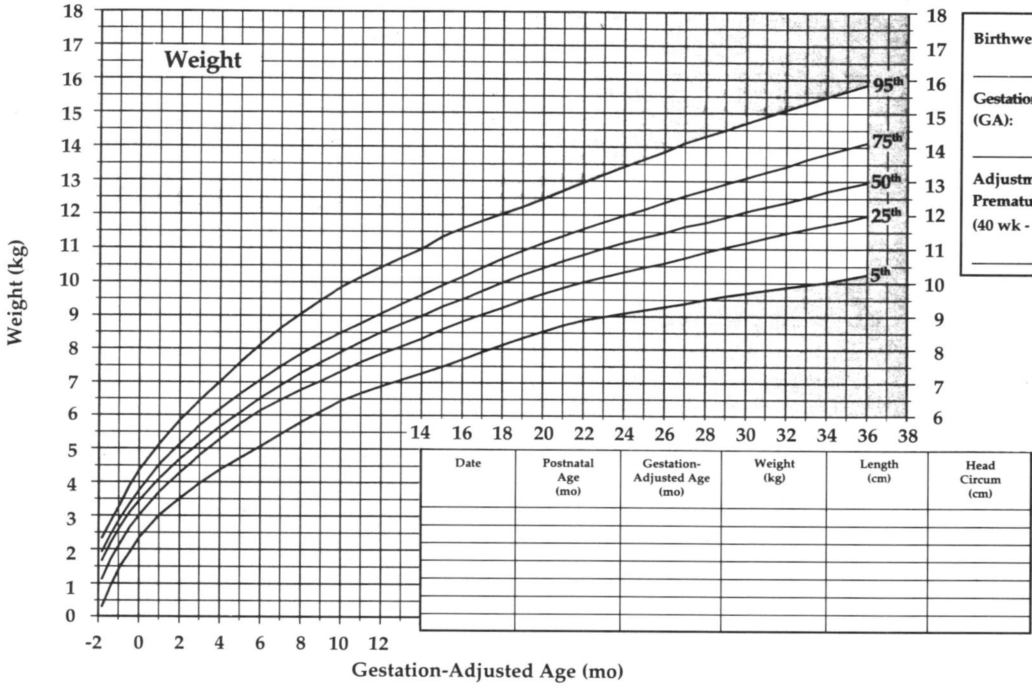

Date	Postnatal Age (mo)	Gestation-Adjusted Age (mo)	Weight (kg)	Length (cm)	Head Circum (cm)

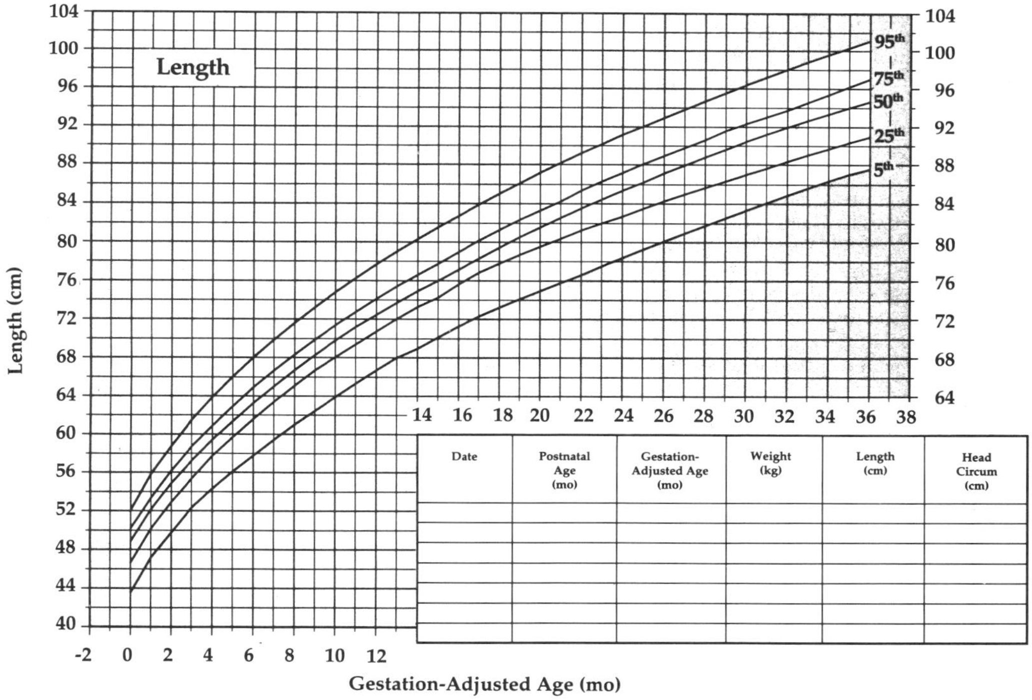

Date	Postnatal Age (mo)	Gestation-Adjusted Age (mo)	Weight (kg)	Length (cm)	Head Circum (cm)

Low Birth Weight Premature Boys

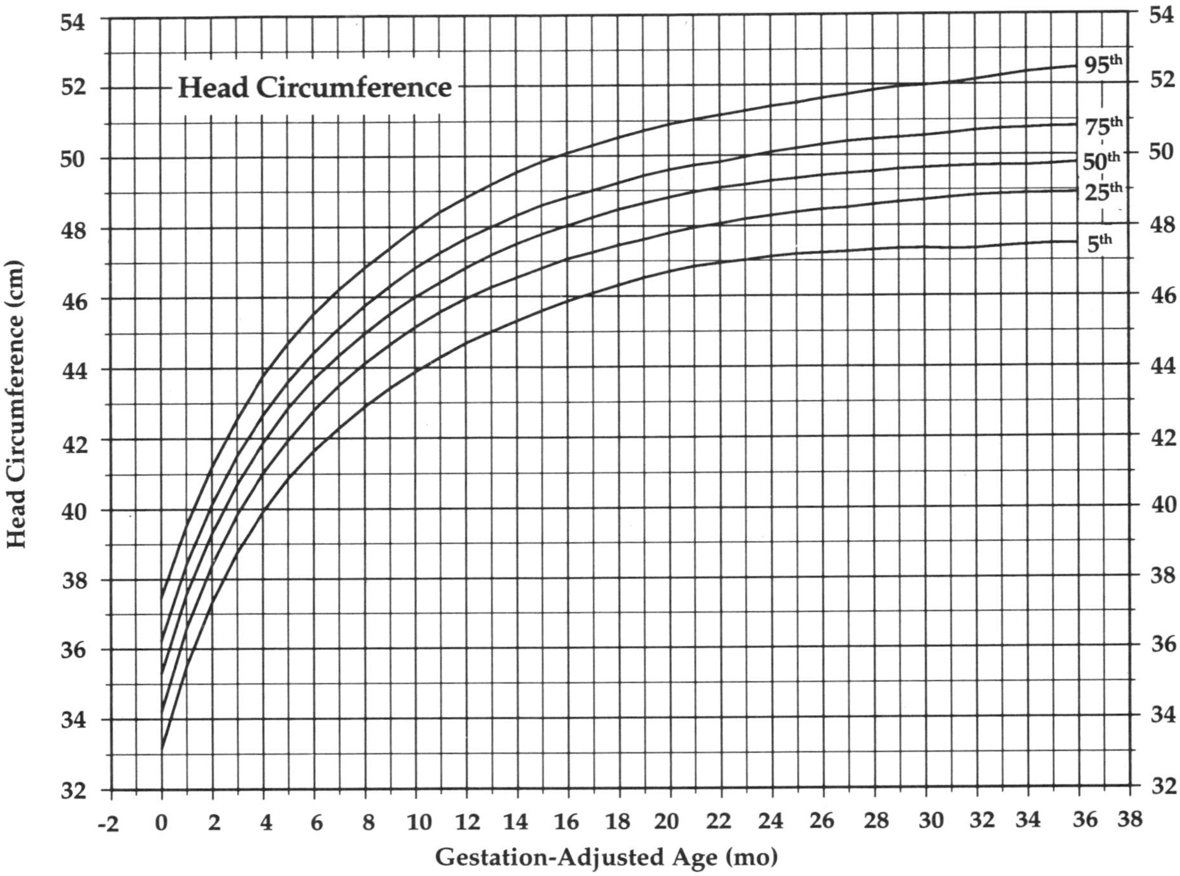

Low Birth Weight Premature Boys

(1501 to 2500 g BW, ≤37 wk GA)

Name______________________________

Record #____________________________

ROSS PEDIATRICS

Birthweight (BW): _________ g

Gestational Age (GA): _________ wk

Adjustment for Prematurity (40 wk - GA): _________ wk

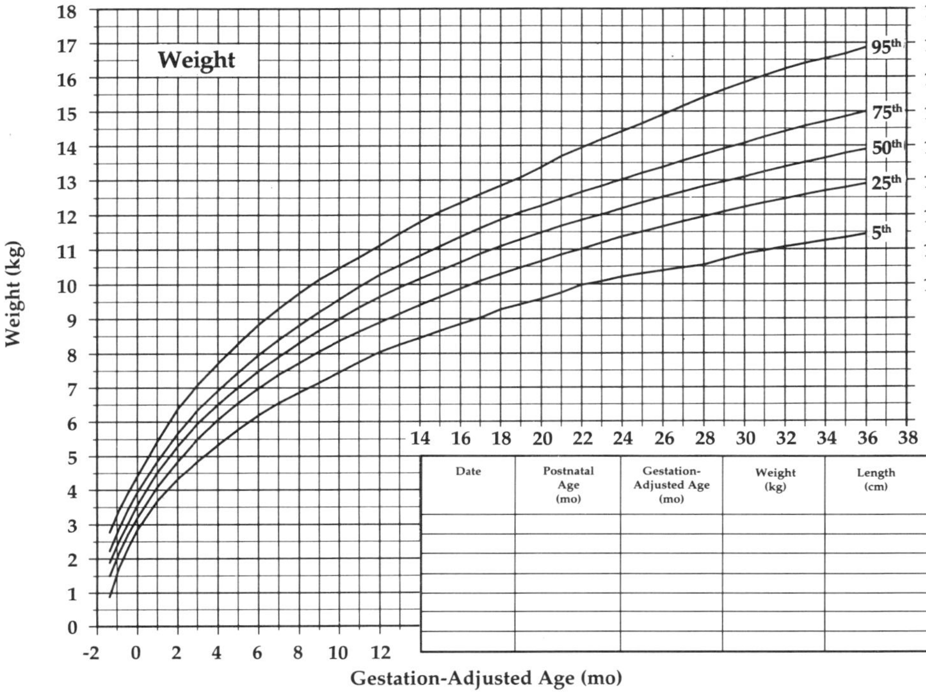

Date	Postnatal Age (mo)	Gestation-Adjusted Age (mo)	Weight (kg)	Length (cm)	Head Circum (cm)

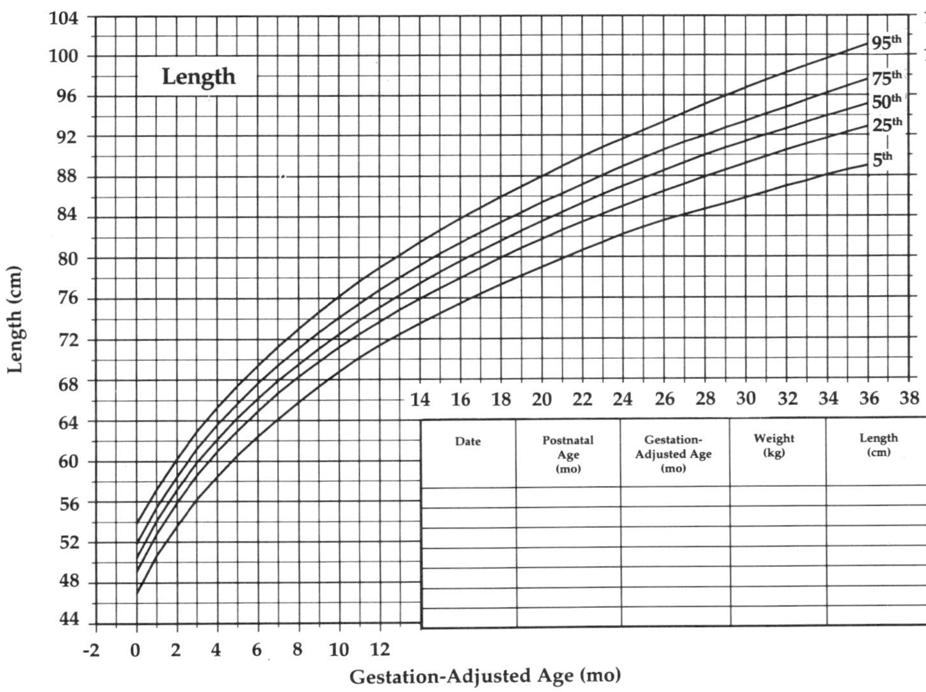

Date	Postnatal Age (mo)	Gestation-Adjusted Age (mo)	Weight (kg)	Length (cm)	Head Circum (cm)

Low Birth Weight Premature Girls

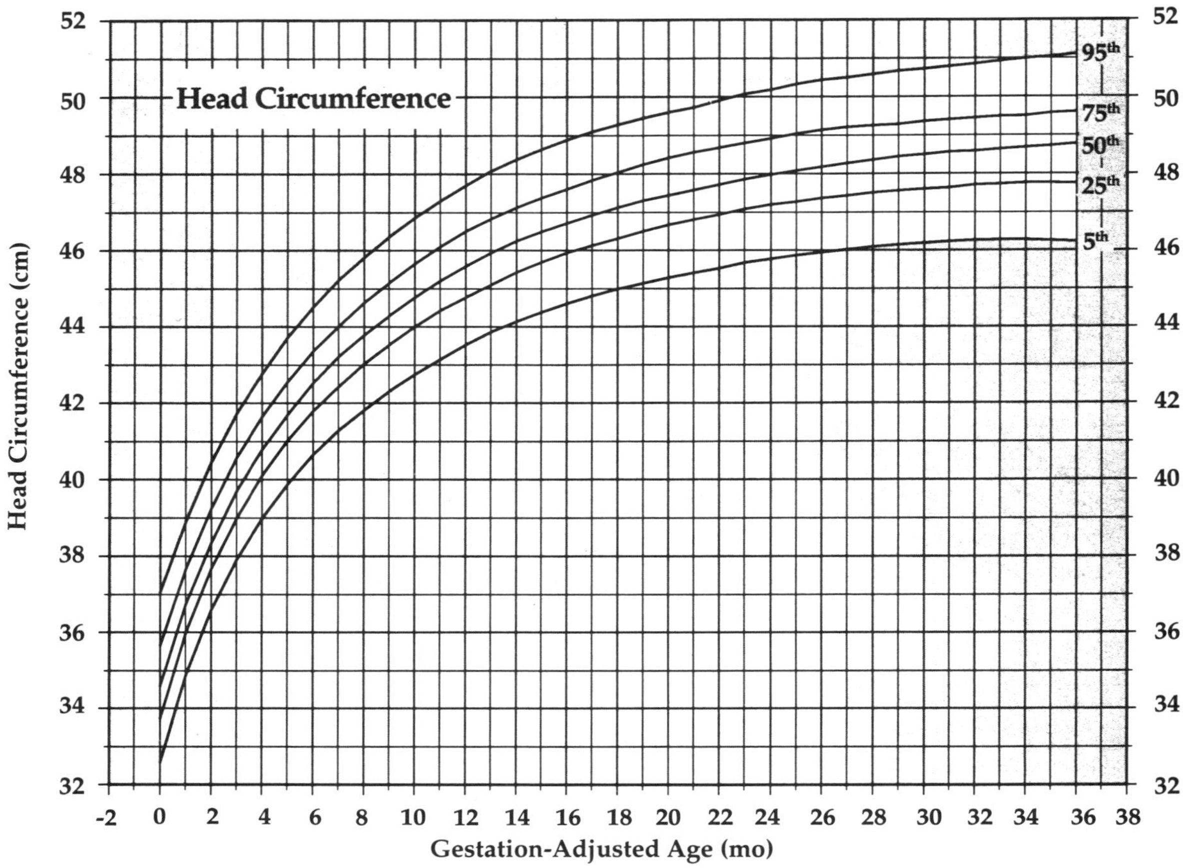

Low Birth Weight Premature Girls

(1501 to 2500 g BW, ≤37 wk GA)

Name________________________________

Record #_____________________________

ROSS PEDIATRICS

Birthweight (BW): ________ g
Gestational Age (GA): ________ wk
Adjustment for Prematurity (40 wk - GA): ________ wk

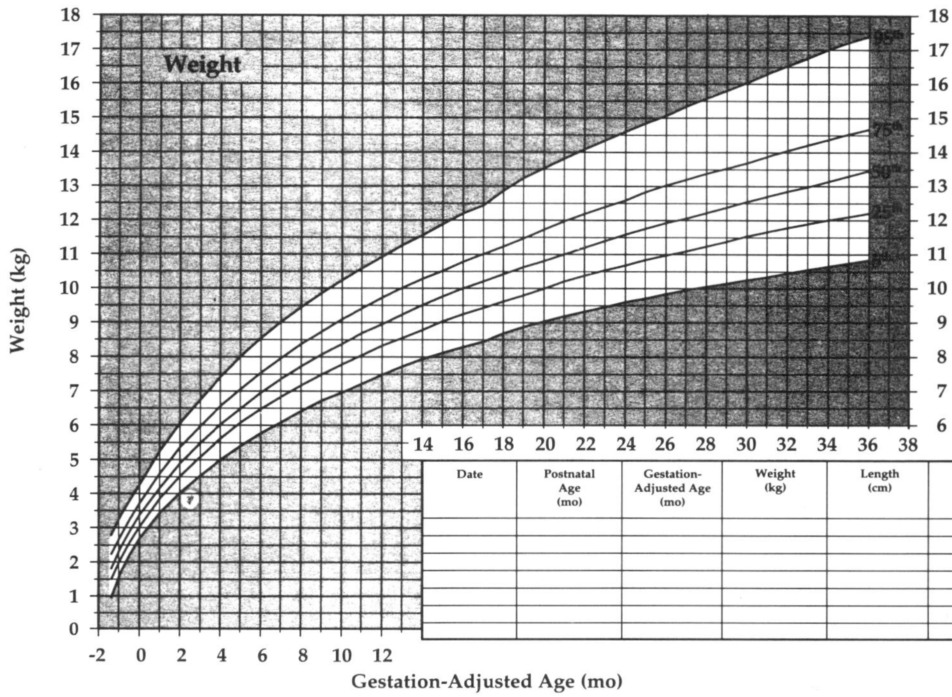

Date	Postnatal Age (mo)	Gestation-Adjusted Age (mo)	Weight (kg)	Length (cm)	Head Circum (cm)

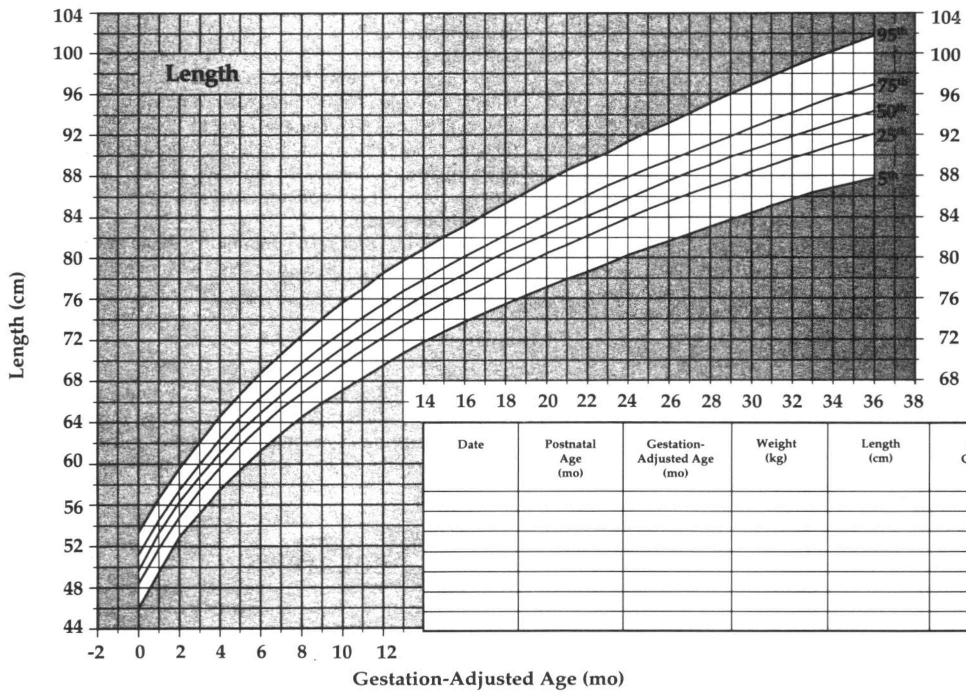

Date	Postnatal Age (mo)	Gestation-Adjusted Age (mo)	Weight (kg)	Length (cm)	Head Circum (cm)

Appendix I

Gairdner-Pearson Growth and Development Record

Boys: Preterm-2 years
Length/Weight/Head Circumference

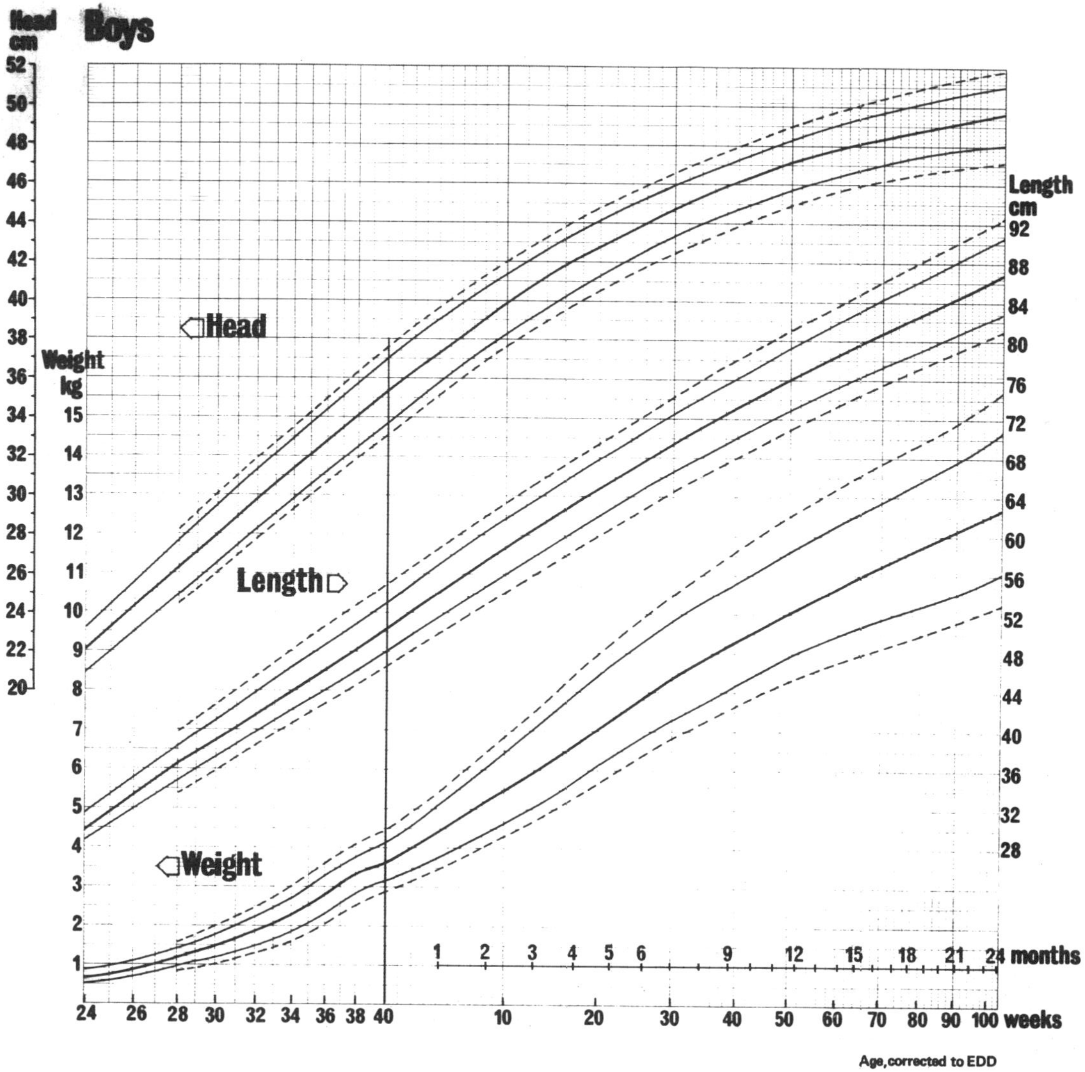

Chart prepared by Gairdner, D. and Peterson, J. First published in Archives of Disease in Childhood 46:783, 1971. Present edition includes data from Lucas, A. et al. Early Hum Develop 13:313, 1986; Yudkin, P.L. et al. Early Hum Develop 15:45, 1987; and Kitchen, W.H. et al. Aust Pædiatr J. 17:72, 1981. Reprinted with permission. Ref. GPB3, © Castlemead Publications, 1988.

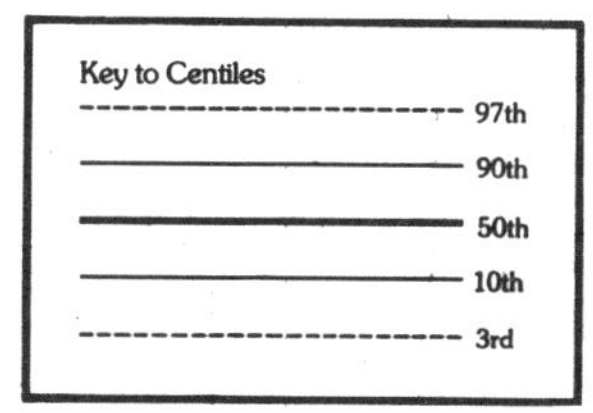

Girls: Preterm-2 years
Length/Weight/Head Circumference

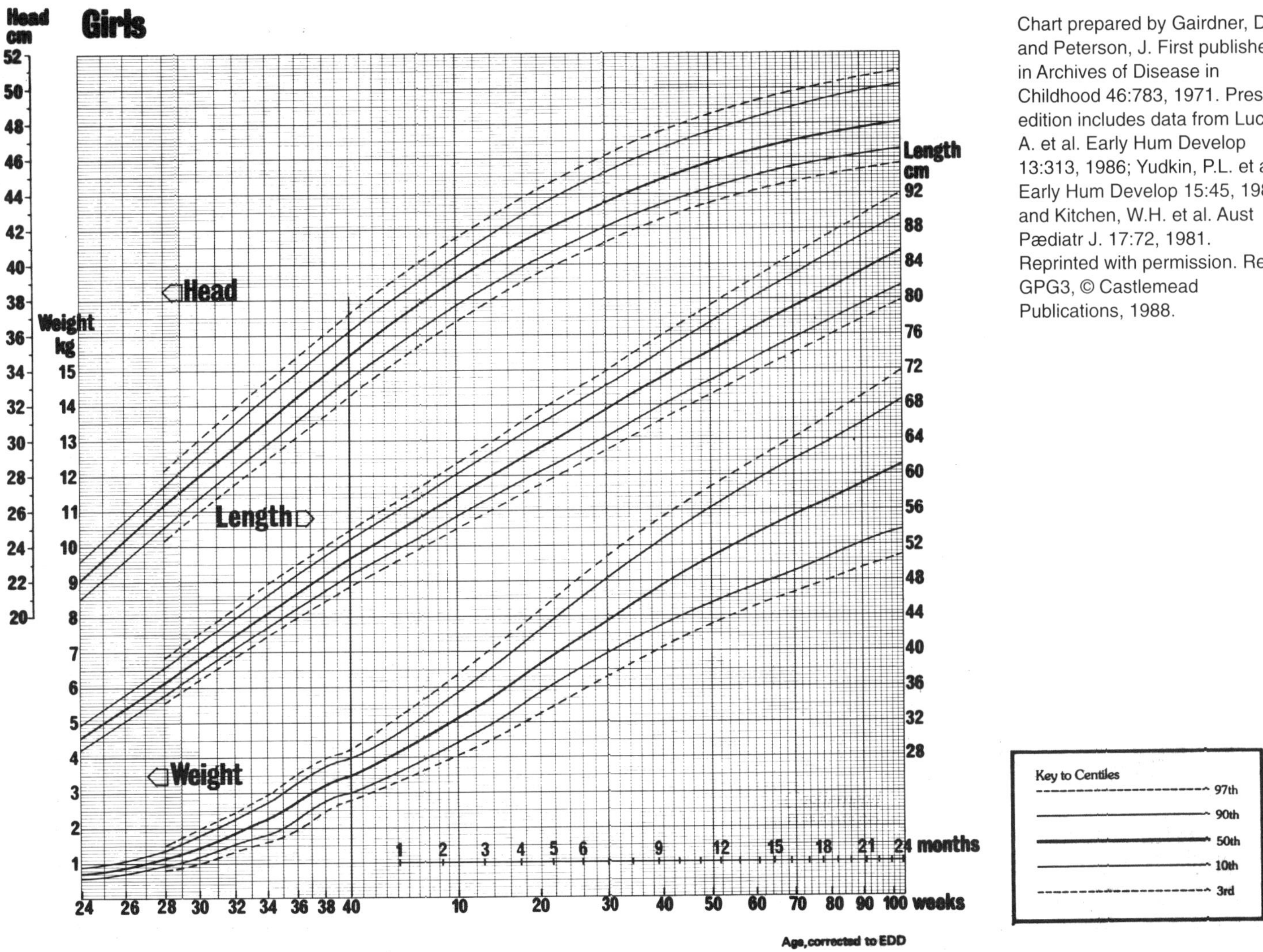

Chart prepared by Gairdner, D. and Peterson, J. First published in Archives of Disease in Childhood 46:783, 1971. Present edition includes data from Lucas, A. et al. Early Hum Develop 13:313, 1986; Yudkin, P.L. et al. Early Hum Develop 15:45, 1987; and Kitchen, W.H. et al. Aust Pædiatr J. 17:72, 1981. Reprinted with permission. Ref. GPG3, © Castlemead Publications, 1988.

Appendix J

Drug/Nutrient Interactions

Dena Goldberg, PhD, RD

Medications	Gastrointestinal side effects	Indirect nutritional side effects	Direct nutritional side effects
Anticonvulsants			
Carbamazepine (Tegretol)	Nausea/vomiting, diarrhea	Dry mouth, anorexia, dizziness, drowsiness	
Clorazepate dipotassium (Tranxene)	Constipation, diarrhea	Dry mouth, drowsiness, confusion	Altered vitamin D metabolism ↓ serum folic acid
Clonazepam (Klonopin)	Nausea/vomiting, constipation, encopresis, diarrhea, gastritis	Drowsiness, anorexia, ↑ appetite, sore gums	Weight gain or loss
Phenytoin (Dilantin)	Nausea/vomiting	Gingival (gum) hyperplasia, ↓ taste acuity, confusion, drowsiness, tube-feedings may ↓ bioavailability of drug	↑ vitamin D metabolism ↓ serum levels of folic acid, vitamin D, calcium, phosphorus, and magnesium
Phenobarbital	Nausea/vomiting, constipation	Dizziness, drowsiness, depression	↑ vitamin D and K metabolism ↓ serum folic acid B_6, B_{12}, C ↓ serum Ca, Mg; may cause ↓ bone density/osteomalacia
Valproic acid (Depakene, Depakote)	Nausea/vomiting, indigestion, diarrhea	Drowsiness, anorexia	↓ serum carnitine
Corticosteroids			
Prednisone/prednisolone Dexamethasone (Decadron)	Gastrointestinal ulceration	↑ appetite with ↑ weight gain, occasional glucose intolerance	Sodium and fluid retention Hypertension; osteoporosis due to ↓ absorption Ca, P and altered metabolism of vitamin D; increased renal excretion of Ca, Zn, K, vitamin C; negative nitrogen balance due to ↑ catabolism and ↑ synthesis; may inhibit growth
Cardiac Medications			
Digoxin, digitoxin, digitalis	Nausea/vomiting, diarrhea	Anorexia, decreased weight	

Medications	Gastrointestinal side effects	Indirect nutritional side effects	Direct nutritional side effects
Diuretics			
Furosemide (Lasix)		Hyperglycemia	↑ excretion and ↓ blood/serum levels of Na, K, Cl, Ca, Mg; chronic use associated with nephrocalcinosis
Hydrochlorothiazide (Diuril, Oretic, Esidrix)		Hyperglycemia	↑ excretion Na, K, Cl, Mg, P, Zn, B_2 and bicarbonate; ↓ Ca excretion
Spironolactone (Aldactone)	Cramps, diarrhea, nausea/vomiting		Hyponatremia, hyperkalemia; ↑ excretion of Na, Cl, Mg, Ca; K sparing
Triameterene (Dyrenium)			Hyponatremia, hyperkalemia
Antibiotics			
Wide variety	Diarrhea; may alter intestinal flora		↓ vitamin K synthesis with altered intestinal flora; other nutrient effects vary
Trimethoprim sulfamethoxazole	Pancreatitis, glossitits, stomatitis	Anorexia, glucose intolerance	Folate deficiency
Antireflux			
Cimetidine (Tagamet)		Drowsiness	↓ B_{12} and iron absorption
Bronchodialator			
Theophylline	Nausea, gastrointestinal tract irritation	Hyperglycemia, anorexia, dizziness, nervousness, insomnia	Feeding intolerance Avoid extremes of protein and carbohydrate intake
Laxatives/stool softners			
Sodium phosphate (Fleet Phospho-Soda)	Abdominal cramps/diarrhea		
Mineral oil			↓ absorption vitamins A, D, E, K
Muscle Relaxants			
Dantrolene (Dantrium)	Nausea/vomiting, diarrhea	Anorexia, drowsiness, dizziness, weakness	
Baclofen (Lioresal)	Nausea/vomiting, constipation	Drowsiness, dizziness, weakness, confusion, headache	

Medications	Gastrointestinal side effects	Indirect nutritional side effects	Direct nutritional side effects
Stimulants			
Dexedrine Methylphenidate (Ritalin)		↓ appetite	↓ intake, poor growth
Chemotherapeutic Agents			
Alkylating agents: cyclophosphamide, ifosfamide, cisplatin, dacarbazine, melphalan	Nausea/vomiting, mucositis, diarrhea		
Plant alkyloids: vincristine, vinblastine, etoposide	Nausea/vomiting, mucositis, constipation		
Antimetabolite: methotrexate, 6-mercaptopurine, cytarabine, 6-thioguanine	Nausea/vomiting, mucositis		
Antivirals			
Zidovudine (ZDV) Azidothymidine—AZT (Retrovir)	Nausea, edema of tongue and lips, mouth ulcers, constipation	Dysgeusia, fatigue	Reduced serum vitamin B_{12}
Acyclovir (Zovirax)	Nausea/vomiting, diarrhea, sore throat	Dysgeusia	
Ganciclovir (Cytovene)	Nausea	Anorexia	
Dextran sulfate		Poor wound healing	
Foscarnet (Foscavir)	Nausea	Renal dysfunction, fatigue, neurologic impairment	Calcium imbalance, hyperphosphatemia
Rifabutin (Mycobutin)	Fatigue	Anorexia, dysguesia	
Sulfadiazine	Nausea/vomiting, diarrhea	Anorexia	Absorption of drug ↓ when given with food

Medications	Gastrointestinal side effects	Indirect nutritional side effects	Direct nutritional side effects
Anti-infective			
Pentamidine (Pentam)	Nausea/vomiting, pancreatitis	Dysguesia, hypoglycemia	Folate deficiency
Antifungals			
Amphotericin B (Fungizone)	Nausea/vomiting, diarrhea	Nephrotoxicity, anorexia	Weight loss, possible decreased potassium and magnesium levels
Ketoconazole (Nizoral)	Nausea/vomiting, abdominal pain		Decreased sodium
Nystatin (Mycostatin)	Nausea/vomiting, diarrhea, gastrointestinal distress	Fever	
Immunomodulators			
Interleukin-2		Fever, anorexia	
Cyclosporine	Nausea/vomiting	Anorexia	
Sodium diethyl dithiocarbamate	Nausea	Fever	
Methionine enkephalin	Nausea, abdominal cramps		

Note: Names of drugs that are capitalized and enclosed in parentheses are manufacturers' registered trademarks.

References:
Physician's desk reference. Montvale, N.J.: Medical Economics Data Co., 1996.
Raiten DJ. Nutrition and HIV infection: A review and evaluation of the extant knowledge of the relationship between nutrition and HIV infection. Nutr Clin Prac 6:1–S, 1991.

Appendix K

Estimating Fluid Requirements

FLUID REQUIREMENTS FOR INFANTS AND CHILDREN

Weight of patient (kg)	Fluid requirement (ml)
1–10	100 per kg
11–20	1000 + 50/kg for each kg > 10 kg
> 20	1500 + 20/kg for each kg > 20 kg
or > 10	1500–2000 per m^2

Fluid needs may be increased in the following clinical conditions:
- fever—↑ 13% for every degree centigrade
- hot weather—↑ 50–100%
- sweating—↑ 5–25 ml/100 kcal/day

Note: Fluid needs closely parallel energy needs.

Example:

A 3-year-old who weighs 15 kg (BSA 0.64 m^2) requires:

1000 ml + (5 × 50 ml) = 1250 ml
(or about 83 ml/kg/day; calorie needs are about 85 kcal/kg/day)

or 1500–2000 ml/m^2 × 0.64 m^2 = 960–1280 ml/day
(which is about 64–85 ml/kg/day)

References: Kerner JA Jr, ed. Manual of pediatric parenteral nutrition. New York: John Wiley and Sons, 1983.
Nelson WE, Behrman RE, Vaughan VC, eds. Nelson's textbook of pediatrics, 12th ed. Philadelphia: Saunders, 1983; 231.

Appendix L

Estimating Energy Needs

ENERGY UTILIZATION OF INFANTS

	Preterm	Kcal/kg/day 0–6 mo	6–12 mo
Basal	55	55	55
Activity	15	17	20
SDA	8	7	7
Stool loss	12	11	13
Subtotal	90	90	95
Growth†	40–85	20–40	5–15
Total	130–175	110–130	100–110

†5 kcal/g weight gain

Reprinted by permission of Pediatrics. Reichman B, Chessex P, Putet G, et al. Partition of energy metabolism and energy cost of growth in the very low-birth-weight infant. Pediatrics 69: 446, 1982.

ESTIMATING CALORIE NEEDS FOR INFANTS AND CHILDREN

Age (yr)	Total energy needs (kcal/kg/day)	Total protein needs (g/kg/day)
0.0–0.5	108	2.2
0.5–1.0	98	1.6
1–3	102	1.2
4–6	90	1.1

Note: Energy needs vary greatly depending on activity levels, stage of growth phase, and with individual constitution. Calculations often include *ideal body weight for length or height* in kilograms, rather than actual weight if infant or child is markedly under or over weight for length or height.

References:
World Health Organization (WHO). Energy and protein requirements, report of a joint FAO/WHO/UNU Expert consultation. Geneva: World Health Organization; 1985, Technical report series 724.

National Research Council Food and Nutrition Board. Recommended Dietary Allowances. 10th ed. Washington DC: National Academy of Sciences, 1989.

ESTIMATING CALORIE NEEDS FOR INFANTS AND CHILDREN (LOWREY)

Age (yr)	BMR (kcal/kg)	SDA + EXC (kcal/kg)	Activity (kcal/kg)	Growth (kcal/kg)	Total (kcal/kg)
0–0.5	55	20	17	20	112
0–5.1	55	17	20	13	105
1–2	40	17	22	11	90
3–4	40	14	21	10	85

BMR = basal metabolic rate, which is similar to REE ± < 10%; it is this component of energy expenditure that is increased during fever or other stress.
SDA = specific dynamic action or energy required for digestion and absorption.
EXC = energy lost through excreta.

Note: Energy needs vary greatly, depending on activity levels, stage of growth phase, and with individual constitution. It is usually recommended that ideal weight for length or height ("expected" weight for length or height or 50th percentile weight for length or height) be used to calculate caloric needs. However, if muscle mass is lower or higher than normal, estimated "lean body weight" may be used.

Reference: Lowrey GH. Growth and development in children, 6th ed. Chicago: Year Book Publishers, 1973.

Appendix M

Nomogram for Estimating Body Surface Area

BODY SURFACE AREAS

Nomogram for estimation of children's body surface area
from height and body mass*

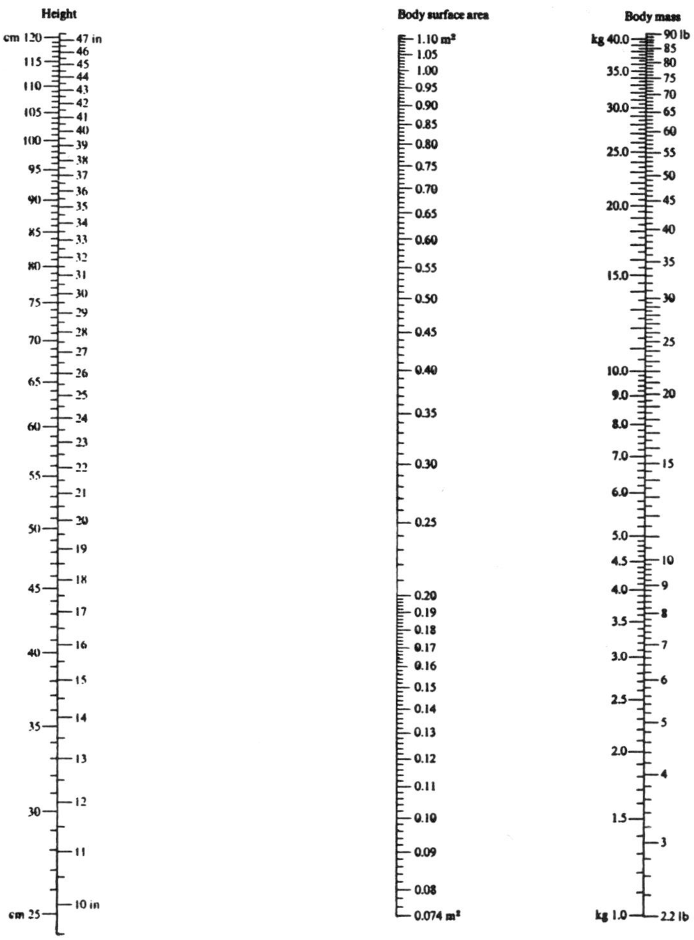

*From the formula of Du Bois and Du Bois. *Arch Intern Med.* 1916;17:863.
$S = M^{0.425} \times H^{0.725} \times 71.84$; $\log S = \log M \times 0.425 + \log H \times 0.725 + 1.8564$
[S: body surface area (in cm^2); *M:* body (mass in kg); *H:* height (in cm)]

Body surface area of children. (From Lentner C, ed. *Geigy Scientific Tables.* 8th ed. Vol. 5 Ciba-Geigy, Basel, 1990:105-106.)

Reprinted with permission from Behrman RE, Kliegman RM, Arvin AM, eds. Nelson textbook of medicine, 15th ed. Philadelphia: Saunders, 1996; 2079.

Appendix N

Method for Determining Mid-Arm Muscle Area

DETERMINING MID-ARM MUSCLE AREA

The upper arm muscle area is often used to estimate skeletal muscle status. When triceps skin fold measurements are greater than the 85th percentile, arm muscle area may be overestimated and estimates should be interpreted with caution.

1. Measure upper mid-arm circumference (UMC) at the mid-point between the acromion process (the body projection cf the scapula that forms the point of the shoulder) and the elbow with the arm relaxed and the elbow extended.

2. Measure the triceps skin fold (TSF) approximately 1 cm proximal to the upper arm midpoint.

3. Upper arm muscle area (cm^2) $= \frac{[\text{UMC in cm} - (3.14 \times \text{TSF in cm})]^2}{12.57}$

Normal triceps skin fold (50th percentile for toddlers, ages 1 to 3 years is 1.0 cm (10 mm); 5th percentile is 0.6 cm (6 mm), and 95th percentile is 1.6 cm (16 mm.)*

Normal arm muscle area for boys and girls ages 1 to 3 years:*

Boys' arm muscle area (cm^2) percentiles

Age	5th	10th	15th	25th	50th	75th	85th	90th	95th
1–1.9	9.7	10.4	10.8	11.6	13.0	14.6	15.4	16.3	17.2
2–2.9	10.1	10.9	11.3	12.4	13.9	15.6	16.4	16.9	18.4
3–3.9	11.2	12.0	12.6	13.5	15.0	16.4	17.4	18.3	19.5

Girls' arm muscle area (cm^2) percentiles

Age	5th	10th	15th	25th	50th	75th	85th	90th	95th
1–1.9	8.9	9.7	10.1	10.8	12.3	13.8	14.6	15.3	16.2
2–2.9	10.1	10.6	10.9	11.8	13.2	14.7	15.6	16.4	17.3
3–3.9	10.8	11.4	11.8	12.6	14.3	15.8	16.7	17.4	18.8

*Frisancho AR. New norms of upper limb fat and muscle areas for assessment of nutritional status. Am J Clin Nutr 34:2540–45, 1981. Used with permission.

Appendix O

Glossary of Terms and Acronyms

Terms Used To Describe Age, Size, or Growth

appropriate for gestational age (AGA)—weight, length, and head circumference measurements that plot ≥ 10th percentile and ≤ 90th percentile at birth

body mass index (BMI)—a weight-to-length or weight-to-height relationship, calculated as follows:

$$\frac{\text{weight (kg)} \times 100}{\text{height (cm)}^2}$$

Used to assess chronic energy deficiency in young children.

Its value in infancy is questionable.

catch-up growth—In research studies, no uniform definition is used, but may be one of the following:

- an *individual* infant who achieves a growth parameter that is above –2 SD from the mean of the same postconceptual age term-born infant
- a *rate* of growth greater than average for postconceptual age, or
- a *group* of infants whose mean weight, length, or head circumference coincides with the mean for the same postconceptual age term-born infants

In clinical practice, the term refers to an individual infant who is growing at a faster rate than expected for postconceptual age, catch-up growth being complete when genetic potential for corrected age is reached.

chronological age—age of infant from birth to present; also called postnatal age

corrected age—age from birth, minus the number of weeks premature; e.g., an infant born at 32 weeks' gestation is born 8 weeks before term; to calculate corrected age for this infant, subtract 8 weeks (or roughly 2 months) from age since birth (at 3 months from birth, this infant has a corrected age of 1 month)

extremely low birth weight (ELBW)—birth weight less than 1000 g or 2 lb 3 oz

gestational age (GA)—the number of completed weeks that have elapsed between the first day of the last normal menstrual period (not the presumed time of conception) and the date of delivery, usually 38-42 weeks; also called postconceptual age (although technically not equal, GA and postconceptual age are often used interchangeably)

height age—age at which a child's height would plot at the 50th percentile

large for gestational age (LGA)—weight, length, and head circumference measurements that plot above the 90th percentile for gestational age at birth

low birth weight (LBW)—birth weight less than 2500 g or 5 lb 8 oz

NCHS—National Center for Health Statistics growth charts (see chapter 5)

ponderal index—a weight-to-length relationship calculated as follows:

$$\frac{\text{weight (g)} \times 100}{\text{length (cm)}^3}$$

Often used in conjunction with gestational age to estimate stunting and wasting that occurred in utero

premature—birth at less than 37 weeks' gestational age

small for gestational age (SGA)—weight, length, and head circumference measurements that plot below the 10th percentile for gestational age at birth

term—birth at 37 to 42 weeks' gestational age; 40 weeks' gestational age is used as term for calculating "corrected age"

very low birth weight (VLBW)—infant with birth weight less than 1500 g or 3 lb 5 oz

Terms Used To Describe Early Intervention Services

community based—services planned, designed, and delivered in the locale in which a family resides

comprehensive—services that cover a broad range of needs including health, education, psychosocial

coordinated care—care that is planned and implemented to consider the comprehensive range of needs and services, forming a cohesive therapeutic program

culturally competent—understanding and skill in working constructively with persons of various values, traditions, beliefs, and customs based on culture

family centered care—care that reflects acknowledgement and respect for the needs, priorities, choices, and strengths of families; care that supports normal living patterns

Terms/Acronyms Used to Describe Feeding or Feeding Behaviors

dysfunctional feeding—feeding behavior involving sucking, swallowing, breathing coordination, chewing, moving of food bolus within the oral/pharyngeal structures, all of which prevent normal nutriture due to neuromuscular dysfunction rather than immature structure or function

ET tube—endotracial tube, a tube placed into the trachea to provide mechanical ventilation; precludes feeding by mouth unless a tracheostomy is in place to bypass the epiglottis

GT—gastrostomy tube, a feeding tube placed through an opening in the abdomen into the stomach

jaw thrust—strong downward extension of jaw, which may appear locked open. The child may have difficulty closing mouth

JT—jejunostomy tube, a feeding tube placed through an opening in the abdomen into the jejunum; a tube may sometimes be placed into the stomach and passed through the pyloric sphincter into the jejunum

lip retraction—tight drawing back of lips so that they form a tight line over mouth and cannot assist in sucking food from spoon or cup

nasal regurgitation—loss of liquid or food through nose during sucking or swallowing

NG—nasogastric tube used for feeding, or, in cases of intestinal blockage, it may be used for suctioning

OG—oral gastric tube used for feeding, or, in cases of intestinal blockage, it may be used for suctioning

rumination—reswallowing stomach contents that are willfully regurgitated

tongue retraction—pulling tongue back into pharyngeal space, an action that may interfere with breathing and make insertion of nipple difficult; makes it difficult for child to handle food in mouth

tongue thrust—strong movement of extension and protraction before or during feeding; tongue appears thick and bunched. It is difficult to insert nipple or spoon, and food may be ejected from mouth

tonic bite reflex—strong closure of jaw when teeth or gums are stimulated. Child may have difficulty opening or closing jaw after reflex cited

Acronyms Used to Indicate a Medical Diagnosis

AIDS—acquired immunodeficiency syndrome
BPD—bronchopulmonary dysplasia
CF—cystic fibrosis
CHD—congenital heart disease
CHF—congestive hearth failure
CP—cerebral palsy
DI—diabetes insipidus
DD—developmental delay
DM—diabetes mellitus
FAS—fetal alcohol syndrome
FTT—failure to thrive
HIV—human immunodeficiency virus
ICH—intracranial hemorrhage, usually graded 1 (mild) to IV (severe)
IODM—infant of a diabetic mother
MMC—myelomeningocele
PEM—protein-energy malnutrition
PDA—patent ductus arteriosus
SBS—short bowel syndrome
TEF—tracheoesophageal fistula

References

American Academy of Pediatrics and American College of Obstetricians and Gynecologists. Guidelines for perinatal care. 3d ed. Chicago: the Academy and the College, 1992.
Klaus MH, Fanaroff AA. Care of the high risk neonate. 3d ed. Philadelphia: Saunders, 1986.
Morris SE. Oral-motor development: normal and abnormal. In: Wilson JM, ed. Oral-motor function and dysfunction in children. Chapel Hill, N.C.: University of North Carolina, Division of Physical Therapy, 1977.
Pipes PL, Trahms CM. Nutrition in infancy and childhood. 5th ed. St. Louis: Mosby, 1993.

INDEX